THE **ESSENTIAL**
FLOWER ESSENCE
BOOK

THANK YOU

Samantha and Dean
Ian Hayward for his creative IT, design and support
Angela Rockel for her impeccable Clean Text and support
All the Flower Essence producers and educators
And all my clients over the years!

MARK WELLS

Mark has been in private practice as a Naturopath & Counsellor for over three decades. He has been extensively involved in teaching Flower Essence Therapy, lecturing, and facilitating courses in Australia and Internationally. His background includes a Bachelor of Biological Sciences from La Trobe University prior to graduating in Naturopathy at the Southern School of Natural Therapies. Mark is a published author of multiple books in the natural therapies area and has conducted formal research at Victoria University into the efficacy of flower essences. Mark has also completed a Master of Social Science (Human Relations/Counselling) at Swinburne University, Melbourne. Over his many years in practice, and in his personal life, Mark has found that the flower essences have emerged as coping and healing tools capable of initiating profound change.

THE **ESSENTIAL** FLOWER ESSENCE BOOK

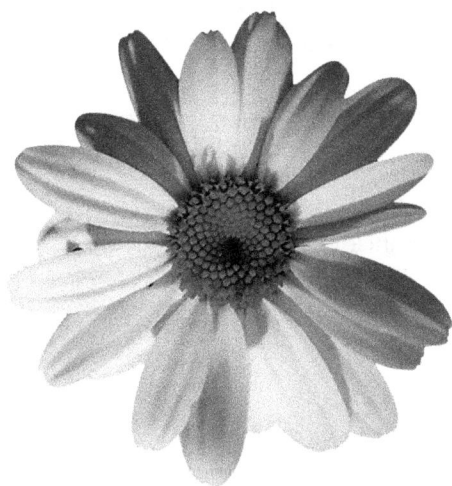

MARK WELLS

HSP Health
PO Box 79
Kew East, 3102
Melbourne, Australia
Text copyright © Mark Wells 2015

Telephone: 0409 985 970
wells@hsphealth.com.au

Second Printing 2019 by Wells Naturopathic Centre (WNC)
Third Printing 2023 by HSP Health

Cover design by Alanna Rance
(Little Nook Creative)

Editing by Clean Text

Interior layout by Ian Hayward

Printed in Australia by IngramSpark Melbourne, Australia
ISBN 978-0-646-93698-7

Contents

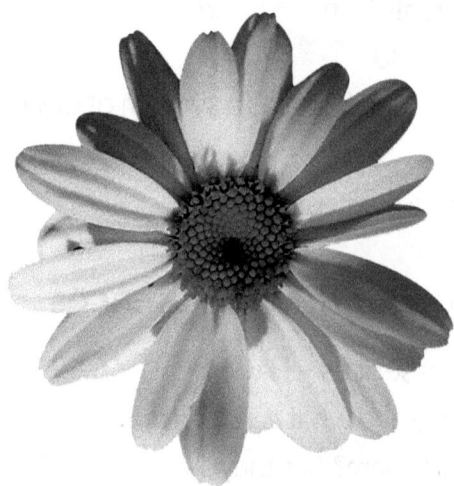

Introduction

From time immemorial, plants, animals and humans have evolved alongside one another. Our interdependence unites us. This is the order and purpose inherent in the great panorama of life. The spirit of nature – dynamically conveyed through the flower essence form of a plant, for instance – provides great benefits for us, as we live, grow and evolve together. Knowledge of, and cooperation with the inner world of nature offers humans a great opportunity to find health and contentment.

After over 3 decades of prescribing flower essences in my private practice, and for myself and family and friends, I wish to share my experience and knowledge of flower essences. The purpose of this book is to give as many people as possible, health practitioners and laypeople alike, an opportunity to understand and experience for themselves the benefits of flower essences. Having provided health counselling for thousands of clients, and taught many courses and seminars about Flower Essence Therapy, I am able to write a book that is very accessible to anyone who has an interest in natural healing, but especially in flower essences. Flower essences help us to cope, navigate life's challenges and thrive. They enable us to heal our bodies, minds and spirits, bringing a better quality of life for us and for those around us.

The book is divided into two main sections. Part 1 gives an overview of the history and evolution of flower essences and an introduction to the subtle energetic dimensions through which they work best. Part 2 answers frequently asked questions about flower essences (and Flower Essence Therapy) and gives comprehensive descriptions of most of the flower essences commonly in use throughout the world today, along with a guide to their selection and use.

PART 1

Flower essences-an overview

Dr Edward Bach

In the early 1930s Dr Edward Bach, a prominent British physician, realised that *emotional and mental factors predisposed most of his patients to the physical ailments from which they suffered.*

Dr Bach felt moved to help his patients in a more profound way than was possible with the conventional treatments available to him at the time. Accordingly, he developed a healing system that could positively influence people on the subtle levels at which illnesses arise. Over a number of years, he put his sensitivity and scientific training into action to collaborate with nature, and so developed his world-

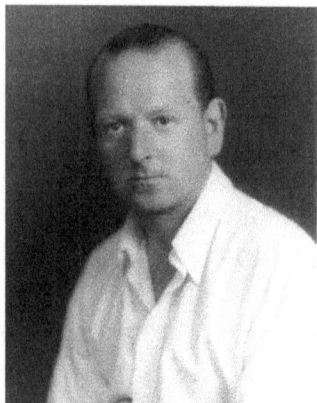

renowned thirty-eight Bach Flower Remedies, selecting five of them to make up the well-known composite mix he called Rescue Remedy. Almost a century since Dr Bach's groundbreaking work, through the great work of other prime movers, the number of flower essences being produced has greatly increased.

Dr Bach was a man attuned to nature, with a remarkable ability to perceive the healing potential of plants. He is credited with discovery of the therapeutic use of plants in flower essence form. In fact, flower essences in general are often referred to as 'Bach Flowers,' which is the name he gave to the 38 remedies he developed. Edward Bach was born near Birmingham in Warwickshire, England on 24 September 1886. As a baby he struggled to survive his first year, and again in his late twenties (prior to 'discovering' his Bach Flower remedies), he experienced further severe illness. Perhaps his early physical fragility was an inevitable consequence of his extreme sensitivity at a deeper level. Being highly sensitive gave him the ability to intuit subtle healing qualities of plants, but it may also have left him more vulnerable psychically and physically to the harshness of city life.

His love of nature displayed itself at a very early age, especially in his great attraction to the Welsh countryside where his family had its roots. Bach's love affair with Wales drew him there again and again, for holidays in his younger days, and later in search of healing plants. Having survived his early years of fragile health, he gained inner strength from this experience of adversity. While still a youngster he developed a reputation for his ability to concentrate on tasks for long periods of time, and would allow nothing to distract his attention or to interfere with his purpose.

He had an overwhelming compassion for all who suffered, whether human, bird or beast, and a love of trees and plants. A natural result of this compassion was his decision to study medicine. After leaving school at 16 he worked in his father's factory in the years 1903–1906. Always a keen observer, he gained much insight into human nature through his study of the behaviours of people around him. At times he found it difficult to continue working at routine tasks, when in moments of inspiration he wished to investigate his insights further, knowing that it was important to respond to inspiration when it occurred. During this period, his study of different methods of healing was confined to times outside his working hours at the factory. His father eventually offered to pay for his training as a doctor, so after matriculating he entered Birmingham University at the age of twenty and completed his medical training in 1912.

Dr Bach always closely observed the personalities of his patients, noticing that people with similar temperaments often responded to the same remedy for a particular physical complaint, whereas those differing in temperament were more likely to respond to a different remedy. Early in his medical practice he became aware of the mind's involvement in health and illness. Eventually he would conclude that 'the personality of the individual was of even more importance than the body in the treatment of his disease' (Weeks 1969). He believed that in order to effect a true cure it was necessary to influence mental and emotional states in a positive way. This belief fuelled his desire to seek out remedies that might bring to bear such positive influences.

It did not take long for Dr Bach to establish a busy medical practice but he became increasingly disillusioned with the training he had received to date, because it did not offer a way to help people in a deep and lasting way. He channelled much of his energy into bacteriological research at the university where, from 1915–1919, he did some great work which is well-documented. In 1918 Bach read the 'bible' of homeopathy – Samuel Hahnemann's *Organon of Medicine* – and was sufficiently impressed to incorporate homeopathy into his medical practice and also to carry out research. It should be noted that like Hahnemann, Dr Bach stressed the importance of a healthy diet, which was rarely taken into consideration by most physicians of his time.

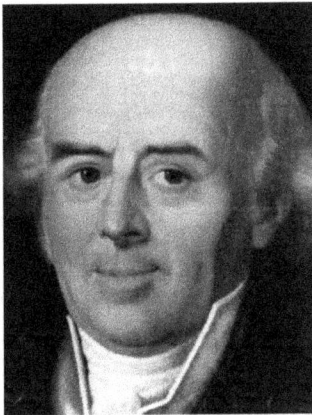

Determined to continue his research in the field of intestinal toxaemia, Bach furnished a small laboratory where he could see his patients and also proceed with his investigations. As a result he developed the seven Bach Nosodes, homeopathic medicines that are still in use today for the treatment of gastro-intestinal problems. Dr Bach was impressed by the gentle and safe action of homeopathy, which uses only minute amounts of medicine and places great emphasis on a patient's mental disposition when prescribing. The Bach Nosodes were derived from seven different bacterial groups which Bach had identified as causes of intestinal toxaemia. After careful preparation in the homeopathic manner, they were administered to patients with great effect. Another indication that Dr Bach was way ahead of his time was his recognition that good gut health is crucial for overall health and wellbeing. This insight has only recently re-emerged as a focus for research and for health practitioners in general. The 'gut-brain axis' as it is commonly called is a subject of much current investigation, because of the strong evidence of its influence on our health – evidence that gives further support to the significance of the mind-body connection, especially as regards our response to stress.

From previous research, Dr Bach had discovered seven distinct human personality types – 'mental' pictures in homeopathic terms – for whom the seven (gut) nosodes were likely to be effective. He obtained spectacular results treating patients with the nosodes according to their temperamental symptoms. In his Harley Street practice in London, Dr Bach became renowned as a homeopath. Although this practice left little time for research, most of the money he made went to fund his unquenchable desire to find plant medicines. Throughout this period of his life he was plagued by ill health but continued to work tirelessly. At one stage, after an operation to remove a gastro-intestinal tumour, his friends and medical colleagues believed he had only weeks to live. The fact that he not only survived but also regained good health only reinforced his belief that if the mind is focused and life is purposeful, recovery and maintenance of physical health can proceed.

In 1928, Edward Bach started work in search of further remedies that would match personality types. One of his many insights occurred while observing fellow guests at a gala dinner party. He suddenly 'saw' all of humanity in terms of a number of types or groups. Soon afterwards, visiting Wales in response to a strong inner urge, he found two plants, Impatiens and Clematis, which he felt displayed qualities corresponding to two of these personality types. Having prepared the plants, he began to use them in his practice, where they proved extremely beneficial. So began a new and profoundly effective system of medicine.

From 1930 onwards, Bach gave up his lucrative Harley Street practice to devote his time entirely to researching flower essences until he had finally developed the full set of 38 Bach Flower Remedies, which stand alone as a healing system in their own right. He died peacefully in his sleep in 1936 at the age of 50, content that he had completed his life's work. The Bach Flower system, with its therapeutic use of plant energies, has had a significant healing impact throughout the world.

There is no substitute for personal experience – like millions of others, I have experienced the benefits of Dr Bach's remedies and many other flower essences. Nearly a century on, word of mouth has undoubtedly been the driving force behind the rapid spread and use of flower essences around the world. No organised marketing campaign was ever required.

Contemporary research and development

Since the time of Bach's ground-breaking efforts, many more flower essences have been produced. Notable contributors include: Flower Essence Services (FES) supported by their research and development body, The Flower Essence Society (also FES); Australian Bush Flower Essences; The Alaskan Project; The Australasian Flower Essence Academy; Desert Alchemy Essences; Bailey Flower Essences; Himalayan Tree and Flower Essences; Amazon Orchid; and Hawaiian Flower Essences, to name a few.

The Flower Essence Society

Alongside the overwhelming anecdotal evidence for the effectiveness of flower essences, there is also a growing body of scientific research and evidence. One not-for-profit organisation at the forefront of flower essence research and development, publication and teaching for half a century is the *Flower Essence Society* (FES), which is dedicated to advancing general knowledge of flower essence therapy and the principles of flower essence science and clinical therapy. FES publishes its research through various avenues including print literature and its website (fesflowers.com) where you can find articles about flower essences, flower essence research, information about training and certification programs and related teaching materials, the FES *International Research Journal Online* and a *Members' Online Repertory*.

The research process conducted by the Flower Essence Society involves many different modalities including field work, botanical studies and general research into plant qualities. One major avenue of research is carried out through what FES calls the *Twelve Windows of Plant Perception* (outlined below and at http://www.flowersociety.org/twelve.htm). A second major avenue features tracking and assessment of case studies and clinical phenomena reported by a worldwide body of thousands of practitioners. The Flower Essence Society has also done some double-blind and single-blind clinical studies (see also my double-blind, cross-over trial of Rescue Remedy outlined below). However, in general, FES, like myself, feels that qualitative research is a 'better fit' for flower essence therapy as it elicits a subjective response from the individual, rather than quantitative/statistical measures (generalised to a population) of alleviation of physical symptoms. Through research collected on each flower essence over the years, FES gradually develops written indications that culminate in the descriptions found in their *Flower Essence Repertory*.

The Flower Essence Society approach supports a belief that we can come to know and appreciate the subtle, trans-physical healing attributes of flower essences by training our senses and thinking capacities in the process of developing a relationship with plants. By consciously extending and refining what we take in with our senses, we can cross the boundary of the physical world of plants and enter into wider dimensions of plant life. This work forms a basis for understanding flower essence qualities and how they affect the human soul. The Flower Essence Society fosters the understanding that our 'ability to hone our perception of plants creates a deep receptivity within the soul – an imaginal field of sensitive awareness – for encountering and being healed by the plant essences that we use for ourselves or select for others' (FES).

Flower Essence Society essences have been developed over five decades through a dynamic, stepwise process involving a great expenditure of resources, especially time and money. I am not aware of any other company or organisation in the flower essence community that sets the bar as high as the Flower Essence Society for this kind of research. The FES Flower Essence Therapy text was my foundational reference book in the early years of practice as a therapist, and is cited in many FES flower essence descriptions throughout this book.

Approaches to plant study

Intuition has always played a vital role in the true understanding of plants, just as it does in understanding the individual for whom you prescribe a flower essence.

It is therefore beneficial to involve yourself in activities that promote its awakening. There are many ways in which intuition can be activated, and one of the most useful and potent is the study and interpretation of *symbols*. Observing and interpreting what is known as the *signature* of a plant (see 'Doctrine of signatures' section) is a good example of symbol interpretation. When we look for a plant's *signature* or *gesture*, we study its outward form in order to understand its inner nature, and in doing so we awaken our intuition. According to Alice Bailey (*Esoteric Healing*, 1984), the study of symbols (as with the study of plant signatures) will produce three effects:

1. It trains us to perceive that which underlies the form (in this case the plant form) and to arrive at a subjective reality.
2. It brings about a close integration of soul-mind-brain. The result is an inflow of intuition and, consequently, an illuminated perception.
3. It puts a 'strain' upon certain unawakened, or at least seldom consciously utilised areas in the brain, and arouses greater mental capacity – the (brow) centre between the eyebrows (the 'third eye') is stirred. In other words, it 'opens doors of perception' and we become better able to realise more of our mind's potential as conscious beings.

Exoteric, conceptual and esoteric studies

We study plants in three ways:

Exoteric study is a study of the plant's external form as a whole: its shape, its lines, its colour and its sectional forms – its arrangements, for instance, in triangles or stars and their mutual interrelation. This involves using our knowledge base/memory. After due study and contemplation of the plant's exoteric form we begin to sense what feelings it evokes, what aspirations it arouses and what dreams, illusions and reactions are consciously registered We can now conceptualise the plant because we have acquired a 'feel' for it.

While signs and characteristics of a plant's outer form and function inform us of the healing potential within it, Michelangelo's creative imagination informed him of the potential of finding the form of David within that 'big piece of marble!' 'I saw a big piece of marble, and in it I saw David, and the only thing I needed to do was to remove the pieces that were unnecessary.' *Michelangelo*

The first 'window of plant perception' identified by the Flower Essence Society (see below) relates to how, when we attempt to sketch a plant, we enter a state of mindfulness that enables us to perceive the essential *gesture* or *signature* of the plant. 'When we capture the "signature" of a plant, our drawing becomes much more fluid and alive, for we have entered into the psychic space of the plant, and we share communion with it' (FES).

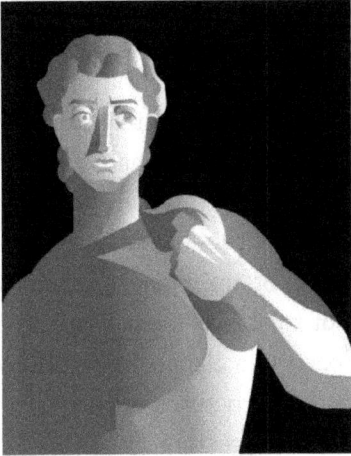

In his book *The Power of Now*, Eckhart Tolle describes what happens in those fleeting moments when, for the first time, we become aware of an invisible added dimension to the world and 'see' the essence, the inner spirit of things. Here he speaks to a woman who experiences the essence of a familiar tree:"You were free of time for a moment. You moved into the Now and therefore perceived the tree without the screen of mind. The awareness of Being became part of your perception. With the timeless dimension comes a different kind of knowing, one that does not "kill" the spirit that lives within every creature and every thing. A knowing that does not destroy the sacredness and mystery of life but contains a deep love and reverence for all that is. A knowing that the mind [alone] knows nothing about. It can only know facts or information [exoteric aspects] about the tree (pg.44)."

Conceptual study arrives at the plant's underlying idea, which may be expressed in a name; or a meaning may emerge in consciousness through meditation; or its significance as a whole or in part may become apparent. This involves the feeling/emotional body and the mind/mental body. When we conceptualise, we articulate our sensitised response to the impact of the plant's qualities. Having studied the plant's form and become aware of its emotional significance and the senses that are aroused, we can appreciate the basic idea of the plant and from there comprehend its esoteric purpose.

Esoteric study allows us to identify the quality and purpose of the plant as it is illuminated by our mind. The brain and mind (the mental body) work in unison to give a mental appreciation of the plant so that we are able to convey its unique message to others

The FES 'twelve windows of plant perception'

The concept of the 'twelve windows of plant perception' was developed by Richard Katz and Patricia Kaminski of the Flower Essence Society as an approach to understanding the qualities of plants. Each 'window' yields a different dimension of information.

While the first forms the basis of our understanding of the plant and additional windows augment this understanding, the wisdom derived is greater than a mere aggregate of the twelve perspectives. The various insights gained must be 're-visioned' and 're-viewed' as a living whole in order to appreciate the essential qualities of any given plant. 'Our imaginal work enables us to ultimately perceive the plant's gestalt or form-pattern, the manner in which etheric formative forces actively create its unique identity' (FES). Systematic consideration of each plant from the full spectrum of perspectives will bring insight into its subtle characteristics.

The first window reveals the *form and 'gesture'* of the plant – qualities that become especially perceptible when we attempt to sketch them. There are innumerable forms and gestures recognisable in all parts of a plant – from root to stem and leaf, flower and fruit (see also the 'Doctrine of signatures' section). For example, flower forms with *cup* and *bell* shapes show differing gestures in relation to the flow of energy. The bell shape can be seen as emptying downwards to the earth while the cup shape lifts to receive energy from above. Many plant essences made from bell-shaped flowers address soul issues that relate to bodily organs or primal emotions that are stored within the 'earthy' cellular structures of the body. They produce essences whose effects are cathartic, stimulating or grounding, enabling the soul to incorporate the physical dimension of life with more conscious awareness.

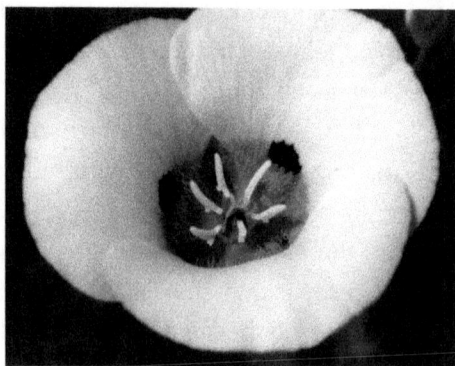

In the case of Angel's Trumpet, the essence brings a conscious awareness that our (earthly) 'time is UP' and helps us to surrender gracefully to being 'born again.' Cup-shaped flowers, on the other hand, open themselves up to receive energy from above – from the heavens and the universe. A good example is the Mariposa Lily (pictured) which prefers rugged and mountainous environments where its beauty emerges out of the rough terrain. Like many members of the Lily family, this flower is connected to its harsh beginnings through shallow roots, and it is able to rise above early limitations to survive and thrive. The flower opens like a *receptive cup filled with an abundance of light and support* – the universe provides what its early life on earth did not.

The second window relates to a plant's *orientation in space and its geometric characteristics*. An example of a plant's orientation in space is the upright, vertical gesture of Sunflower and Mullein plants, which relates to a capacity to impart individualising qualities allowing the 'I' to develop to its full potential. By contrast, plants that engage with the earth by spreading on a horizontal axis possess healing qualities that relate to the social dimension – how the 'I' relates to others. 'Spreading plants that … embrace the earth like the Violet or Lady's Mantle address soul qualities of humility, inclusiveness or the absorption of the individual identity in the larger collective' (FES). The second window also perceives the geometric structure of a plant, especially its flower. The flowers of the Rose Family have a five-pointed star pattern – 'a signature of incarnation.' If we combine that signature with the fact that the root system of members of this family, for instance Wild Rose, grow almost as far down into the earth as the plant's body grows out of the earth, the essence relates strongly to being enthusiastically involved, fully committed and 'well-rooted' in earthly existence. The flowers of the Lily family have six-pointed stars – 'a signature of cosmic harmony' (FES). As mentioned above, Mariposa Lily, for example, can be useful for people who have commenced their life in difficult and disharmonious circumstances. The signature of cosmic harmony reflected in the flower's six-pointed star, combined with its cup shape, indicates that the essence can help such people heal, grow and open up to receive energy from above, and ultimately live in harmony with their surroundings.

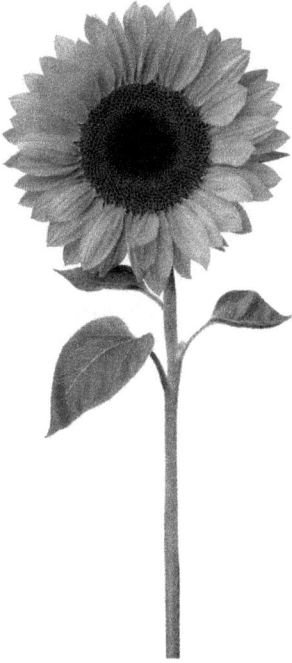

The third window is offered by the plant's botanical family. Botanical classification can give precise information about a plant's properties when prepared as a flower essence and can offer an organising principle for seeing relationships among plants. Plant families provide broad groups that make it possible to study different though related examples and note common themes and variations within the range. For example, within the Lily family (Liliaceae) we find plants that have watery bulbs with shallow roots, simple, linear leaves and star-like flowers that display geometries based around the numbers three and six. These plants evoke the watery origins of life at a primordial stage of the earth's evolution. However, within this broad outline there is also much variation. The fiercely coloured Tiger Lily, for example, is orange with dark spots and has downward-pointing flowers with recurved petals. It is not surprising, then, that its essence is very helpful to people who are overly aggressive, 'fiercely' over-competitive and consequently display 'separatist tendencies' (FES). The Tiger Lily 'separates' itself even from other members of its Lily family. It is not surprising, then, that in my practice I have found it especially helpful for those who experience sibling rivalry. It has a much more active and earthy gesture than, for example, the Mariposa Lily with its creamy-white, bowl-shaped flowers that hover above the earth like the butterfly for which it is named. Tiger Lily helps people develop a greater capacity for cooperation and more of a win/win mentality.

The fourth window relates to the plant's *orientation in time* – its daily and seasonal cycles. The Morning Glory flower opens in the early morning and closes as the day progresses – it is a great essence to help people get back in touch with and benefit from being in sync with their normal, energy enhancing, 24 hour (circadian) rhythms. The California Poppy flower is curled shut in the morning and unfurls as the sun intensifies during the day – the essence opens our hearts up to respond to the real gold in our lives, not just things that glitter. Besides diurnal (circadian) rhythms, we can also examine yearly rhythms. Dandelions burst forth into blossom in the early spring when the tensions of winter come to an end, and its essence helps people to let go and release inner tension. Chrysanthemums hold back until the end of summer or early autumn to produce their flowers, and the essence is particularly helpful in enabling us, in mid-life or even late in life, to expand upon or transcend traditional religious beliefs we have grown up with, so that we can finally become grounded in our own spiritual identity. Better late than never. The life cycle of a whole plant can also offer insights. Perennials, for example, rest during part of the year and may even disappear from above ground altogether, but their essential pattern endures from year to year. Some trees, such as redwoods and olives may live for centuries, and this persistence expresses their qualities of *strength and endurance.* We can also compare the dramatic seasonal responses of deciduous plants with those of evergreens, which are less subject to seasonal rhythms.

The fifth window concerns the plant's *relationship with the environment.* The place where a plant chooses to grow reveals much about it. Sagebrush, for example, grows in the stark simplicity of the desert. It is used as a cleansing and purifying herb, and in flower essence form it helps us to relinquish a false persona in order to be 'in touch with the naked, essential Self' (Kaminski and Katz, 1994). Another example is Penstemon, which inhabits harsh alpine regions above the treeline and can, as a flower essence, help us gain inner strength through confronting adversity. Kangaroo Paw thrives after the environment has experienced bushfires or land clearing. Over time, other long-lived plants crowd out Kangaroo Paw, which is not seen again until the next fire or clearing (White 2008). The plant displays the ability to *quickly adapt* and *fill a niche* in its environment. This reflects how Kangaroo Paw can help 'people who are "green" and socially inept' (White, 2008) *blend better* with and *understand*

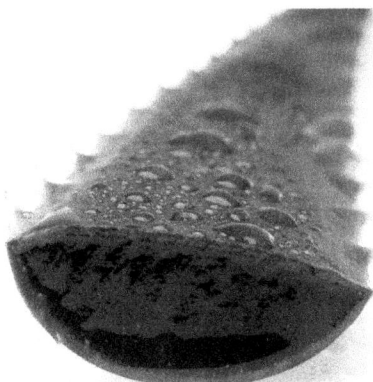

their environment (and the people in it).

The sixth window is accessed via the plant's *relationship to the four elements – earth, air, fire and water* (see also the 'Subtle dimensions' section). Plants live not only in a physical environment but also in one of elemental and etheric forces. The elements form an essential part of many mythologies and represent archetypal qualities: 'Earth is (grounding) solidity; water is (emotional) fluidity; air is (mental) expansiveness; and fire is (creative) transformation' (FES). For example, the strong presence of the water element is clearly recognisable in the Rock Water flower essence. It softens the soul's disposition and creates 'fluidity' and flexibility where previously rigidity/hardness and inflexibility have governed a person's beliefs and behaviour. Frequently two of the four elements are predominant in a plant, expressing a polarity, while the qualities of the other two are less apparent. For example, Queen Anne's Lace (wild carrot) shows a strong earth gesture in its tap root and an airy quality in its finely divided leaves and flowers. As a flower essence it works by integrating the second (sacral) and sixth (third eye) chakras, harmonising sexual/earthbound and psychic energies. Aloe Vera, by contrast, has a strong relationship to fire, evidenced by the hot, dry environment in which it often lives, and also water, as evidenced by the moist gel inside its succulent leaves. These leaves are a well-known soothing remedy for burns, and as a flower essence Aloe Vera is restorative in states of exhaustion and creative 'burnout,' when the passion and creative flow has 'dried up' due to excessive drive and expenditure of energy.

The seventh window allows us to observe the plant's *relationship to the other kingdoms of nature* and the way in which, as a member of the plant kingdom, it coexists with the mineral, animal and human kingdoms. The quality of a plant's relationship to one or more of these kingdoms is an important expression of its inherent character. For example, the Glassy Hyacinth has a special relationship to the mineral kingdom, in that it grows only on thin soil covering dark, volcanic rock. Its essence has much to do with deep transformation and upheaval in the soul. Many plants have a special relationship to the animal kingdom through pollination by insects or birds. For example, Milkweed is pollinated by the Monarch butterfly, with which it has a close, interdependent relationship. It is no wonder that the essence can help people with strong dependencies. The caterpillar eats the Milkweed plant and accumulates alkaloids from the sap in its body, becoming toxic to its predators, even after it has metamorphosed into an adult butterfly. The California Pitcher Plant has a rather unusual relationship to insects – it digests them. This carnivorous plant yields a flower essence that helps us to 'sink our teeth' into the physical world, truly incarnate, and in some cases, even begin to add and better digest a little meat in the diet. Walnut trees have 'an active force which keeps other lifeforms at bay' (Barnard, 2010, pp. 152–53). The tree gives off a fragrance that is pleasant to humans but very unattractive to insects, birds and other plants. Its flower essence helps protect us from outside influences, especially those that lead us away from our own ideas, aims and purposes.

The eighth window relates to *colour* (see 'Doctrine of signatures' section) – a reflection of astral forces which are usually most obviously displayed in the blossoms of plants. However, subtle colour variations may also occur throughout, for example in the bark and stem. Colour is extremely revealing of the inner qualities of a plant and tells us much about its soul qualities and the human emotions to which they relate.

The ninth window involves *fragrance, texture and taste* (see also 'Doctrine of Signatures' section). For example, the soul-impression received from the sweet, even overwhelming, other-worldly perfume of many members of the Lily family contrasts strongly with the pungent aromas of members of the Mint family such as Lavender and Rosemary or the delicate, ethereal scent of Wild Rose or Cherry blossom. The scents of Honeysuckle and Jasmine pervade the atmosphere of a garden; they 'linger on' in the air and in one's mind. Both these plants as flower essences are helpful for people needing to let go of the (lingering) past and become more grounded in the present. On the level of texture, we can think of the formidable thorns of the Star Thistle that give a warning to be careful of how you touch it. The essence helps people who have become 'prickly' and emotionally self-protective to be more generous, inclusive and trusting. By contrast, the silky-smooth petals of Mariposa Lily invite touch and encourage nurturing; the rigid stalk of Yarrow offers strength. In the same way, the smooth bark of Manzanita; the waxy feel of the Waratah flower head; the spongy, liquid Lotus or the rough, hairy leaves of Borage all give information about the plants' essential qualities. The spicy taste of Nasturtium flowers is a surprising contrast to the 'cool' appearance of its round, moist leaves, and this essence 'spices up' and nourishes those who feel mentally and emotionally flat or display a very 'vanilla'

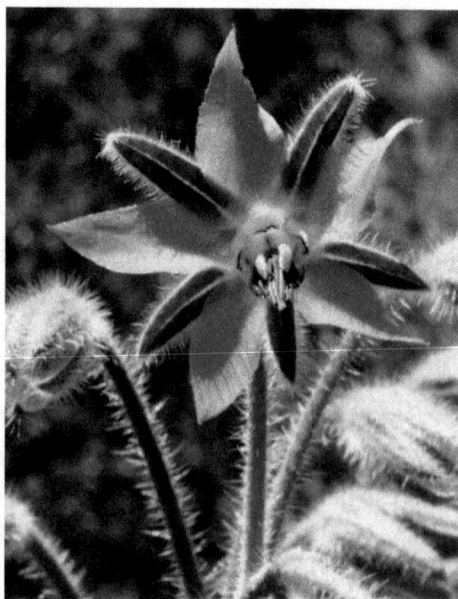

personality! Peppermint leaves give a taste sensation that is both hot (stimulating) and cold (calming) at the same time.

The tenth window is offered by the plant's *chemical substances and processes.* Contemporary science is skilled at analysing the chemical composition of plants. What is usually missed, however, is the energetic processes and qualities represented by chemical substances. (See Rudolf Steiner's *Agriculture Course* for a further discussion of chemical substance and process.) For example, the presence of silica (SiO_2) indicates energetic qualities of light and clarity, as seen in quartz crystals. These qualities can be seen in the fine hairs of the Borage plant or in the needles of Pine and other conifers. A strong silica presence indicates a special relationship to light, and in flower essence form, plants like Borage and Pine can help the soul address certain types of depression and heaviness. Sunflower seeds are rich in Silica also – another property of silica being to help promote and shape calcium deposition in the body. Sunflower essence helps one 'stand up strong,' be true to the inner authority of the

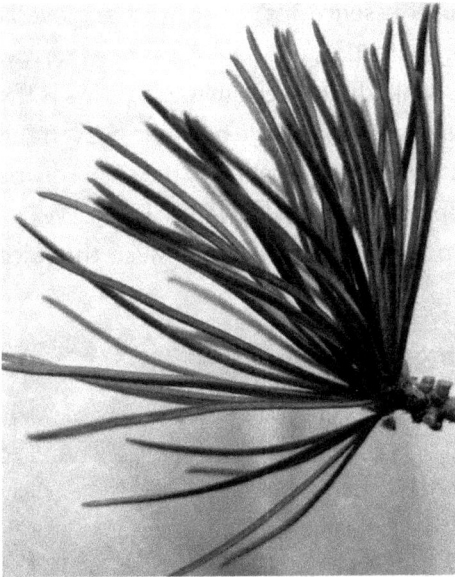

Self rather than to outer authority, and display your real substance. As another example, on a chemical level, alkaloids may be toxic to the physical body but can help to stimulate the astral body. (The degree to which flower essences are diluted makes them completely safe on a physical level.) For example, the family of essences that includes Buttercup, Larkspur, Columbine and Monkshood can help to awaken psychic forces within the soul, reconnect with our inner nature and appreciate our uniqueness and inner beauty.

The eleventh window is revealed by a plant's *medicinal and herbal uses.* We can learn much about plants' subtle effects from their physical healing properties. (This aspect is frequently addressed in the body of this book: 'Flower Essences A-Z'.) As Richard and Patricia from FES put it, 'the soul-healing qualities of the flower essences are like a "higher octave" of the medicinal and herbal healing properties belonging to the plant.' For example, Dill is used as a culinary herb and as a treatment for flatulence, a condition that results when we do not assimilate our physical food. Dill flower essence addresses over-stimulation of the psyche which results in an inability to assimilate sense impressions that should nourish the soul. The bark of the Willow tree is a source of salicylic acid, a natural precursor of aspirin and a well-known remedy for arthritic pain, rigidity and lack of elasticity in the joints. Dr Bach's Willow essence is used for those whose rigidity of soul is expressed through resentment and a lack of emotional resilience. This essence brings flexibility to the soul and a capacity to forgive and rebound from old hurts. Even the branches of the tree display this flexibility and resilience – they are able to bend easily but also re-grow easily when cut back.

The twelfth window relates to *lore, mythology, folk wisdom and spiritual and ritual qualities.* In earlier epochs of human history we experienced a more intimate relationship with the natural world and our relationship with plants was based on an instinctual soul rapport. The remnants of this plant wisdom survive in folklore, mythology, ritual and spiritual teachings about plants. As we strive to rediscover a more conscious relationship with plants, these teachings can offer valuable information and inspiration. For example, the Yarrow plant, *Achillea millefolium*, was named for the Greek warrior Achilles. It was also known as 'Knight's millefoil' and was carried into battle not only for its ability to stop bleeding but also for spiritual protection. This parallels the use of Yarrow essence for those who are overly sensitive and vulnerable and need psychic protection and soul-centering. Yarrow helps stem 'bleeding' on an energetic level. Similarly, in Greek mythology, Iris is the name of the goddess of the rainbow, which symbolises a bridge between heaven and earth, a meeting-place of light and dark and a place of inspiration to the soul. The Iris plant became an emblem of nobility and a representation of heaven on Earth. We use Iris essence to awaken creativity and to help us become open to our Muse, the voice of heavenly inspiration.

The doctrine of signatures

Another approach to plant study which overlaps and resonates with the FES 12 windows of plant perception is that of the ancient 'doctrine of signatures.' The tradition of sensitivity to, and attunement with, the healing qualities of plants is very ancient. Some human beings were more gifted than others in their sensitivity, Dr Edward Bach being such a person.

From ancient times, herbal practitioners and especially the alchemists of the Old World refined the therapeutic uses of herbs by deepening their understanding of the relationship between a plant's *outer form and its inner healing properties.* This practice reached a peak in the 15th and 16th centuries, following on from the work of the herbalist-physician Paracelsus. He is credited with developing a profound understanding of herbal medicine through his realisation that the form of a plant can be understood as an aesthetic representation of its inner soul-life and healing potential. Study of the plant's signature or gesture became known as the 'doctrine of signatures,' relating plant forms to their inner nature and uses. The doctrine of signatures forms the basis from which Western herbal practices developed. These practices continue to have a profound influence on modern pharmacology and

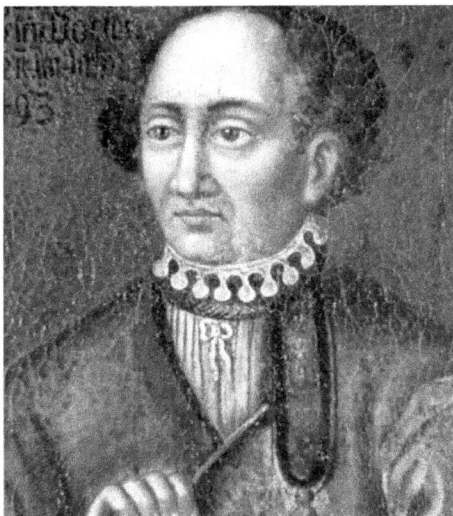

scientific research into plant-based medicines.

Aspects of a plant's signature

A plant's shape, colour, texture, habit of growth, life cycle, preferred environment and evolutionary history can give clues about its healing properties. Taken together, these symbolic clues have come to be called the plant signature. As well as giving insight into a plant's herbal, homeopathic or essential oil qualities, its signature can help us to understand a range of subtle but profound healing potentials which can be accessed through flower essence remedies.

Resemblance

Plants that resemble a *part of the body* are understood to have an affinity for that part. This characteristic is considered through the first window of plant perception.

Mistletoe *(Viscum album)* is a parasitic plant that has traditionally been used to treat problems of the vascular and lymphatic circulatory systems. Its growth resembles a network of capillaries, often with nodular features, and for this reason it has been associated with the lymphatic system. Anthroposophical medicine has taken these characteristics of the plant's signature as an indication of its potential to be used in the treatment for some lymphatic cancers.

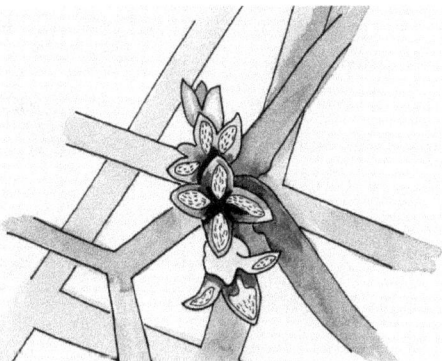

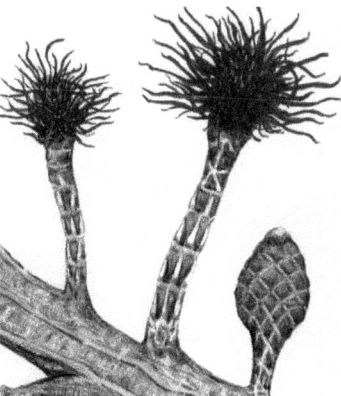

The Australian She Oak *(Allocasuarina glauca)* has a fruit that has been likened in appearance to an ovary. The plant has been used medicinally by Aborigines for female reproductive problems. Ian White, founder of Australian Bush Flower Essences, recommends She Oak flower essence for problems such as infertility where there is no known physiological cause.

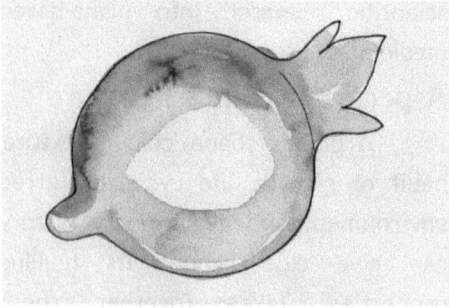

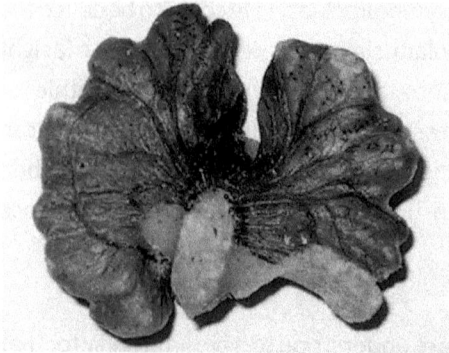

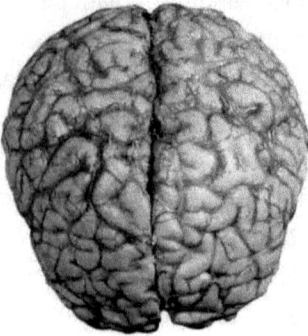

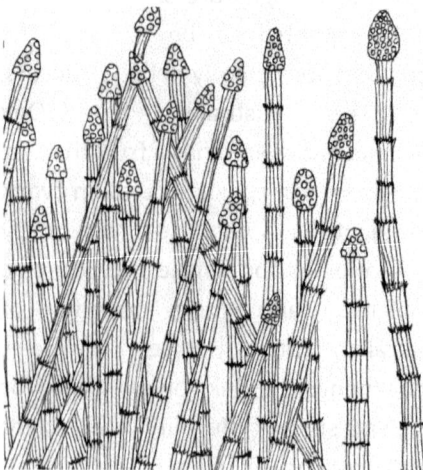

The Pomegranate (*Punica granatum*) has a fruit that resembles a womb in shape. Pomegranate flower essence supports the development of outlets for creative expression, especially for women who experience creative tension between the needs of career and home, and personal and global issues. In addition to its shape, the rich red colour of the flowers and fruit symbolise the strong blood supply to the uterus.

Walnut (*Juglans regia*) gives another good example of 'resemblance'. If you crack open the shell, the kernel inside strongly resembles a brain and is in fact rich in potassium phosphate, which is crucial for proper brain function. Foods rich in this substance should be part of the diet of anyone who has a very 'cerebral' approach to life, whose work is mentally demanding or who suffers from mental fatigue. On another level, Walnut flower essence is useful for people who are going through major life changes and need to maintain mental (brain) strength and not be swayed from following the soul purpose their heart desires.

Horsetail (*Equisetum hyemale*) is used herbally to strengthen hair and nails and to treat rheumatic joint problems. Its finely jointed stems resemble hair shafts. It is rich in mineral silica, known as 'nature's sculptor' because it 'shapes' crude elements of structure – calcium and magnesium – into appropriate form in the body, for example in hair, nails and bones. Silica is vital for the integrity of the spine and other bones and joints. A

THE **ESSENTIAL** FLOWER ESSENCE BOOK

human without silica is a human without 'spine'.

Plants that resemble the *cause* or *manifestation of disease* are also understood to have a potential role in healing. For example, Native Americans use a flower that looks like a deer's eye to treat inflamed eyes and a plant that resembles worms to eliminate worms from the body. Other kinds of resemblances were also acknowledged: for example, Hopi Indians use plants that exude milky juice to promote secretion of milk in nursing mothers and use gnarled wood to treat cramps and convulsions. Resemblances may be subtle and exist on a number of levels, as we will see.

Colour

Colour is a very important aspect of a plant's signature because of the relationship between colours and specific emotional states. Colour is viewed through the eighth window of plant perception.

Red is stimulating – it is associated with the *base chakra* which relates to issues of survival, embodiment and groundedness. It can help us overcome lethargy and activate personal drive and the survival instinct, and it is used by many cultures to represent love, passion and energy. It follows, then, that flower essences made from red flowers are grounding, stabilising, and securing while at the same time they stimulate creative, vital and elemental forces. They enhance qualities of courage, patience and decisiveness and ease frustration and anger.

Orange is a warm and invigorating colour that promotes optimism and creates self-confidence. Orange heals old emotional wounds, making people less withdrawn and more receptive to new experiences. The warming effect of orange eases and relaxes fears around intimacy. It has a cheering effect, providing energy and helping to alleviate physical and mental tiredness. Orange is the colour associated with the *sacral chakra* which relates to creativity and the pleasure principle – sex, food and money. Flower essences made from orange flowers help people to give and receive more easily and achieve balance in intimate relationships. They also assist in procreation and promote the flow of creative energy out into the world, helping people to recognise their value and display their unique 'true colours.'

Yellow stands for the sun and has a cheering effect, encouraging the perceptive faculties and improving interaction with others. It soothes, calms and relaxes, acting as a tonic for the nervous system, helping to overcome exhaustion and apathy. Yellow helps us to 'digest' and assimilate life experiences without being overwhelmed by them, including at the level of physical digestive processes. Yellow is the colour associated with the *solar plexus chakra* and essences made from yellow flowers help us to become personally empowered and autonomous, able to recognise our own inner authority and establish a more harmonious relationship with outer authority.

They help us to be (true to) ourselves so that we can 'shine' courageously, out there in the world.

Green has a balancing and normalising effect. It is the colour of hope, healing, natural immunity and adaptation. Green is the most healing of all the colours– it stands for nature and therefore promotes natural healing and brings calm, contentment and harmony to body, mind and soul. Green is the colour associated with the *heart chakra* and essences made from green flowers can help us to develop unconditional love, forgiveness, compassion and a harmonious group consciousness. As a result of this inner peace and contentment, we are able to create positive relationships with those around us. **Pink** is the secondary colour associated with the *heart chakra* and pink flowers relate to issues of emotional attachment in relationships and 'heartfelt' or passionate involvement in life.

Blue calms, refreshes and relieves pain. It has paradoxical aspects in that it represents both the unconscious and a 'cool and collected' intellectual response. It is the colour of introversion and reserve and also of mental development and knowledge. Blue relaxes and calms and has a positive effect on the nervous system and the over-active mind. Blue relates to the *throat chakra* and the shoulder and neck region. Flower essences made from blue flowers help to promote clear communication, enabling us to be heard and understood, and to discern and attain wisdom through knowledge.

Indigo calms and creates a harmonious atmosphere. It brings about new growth, hope and balance. Indigo stands for creative thought, inspiration, intuition and insight, spirituality, self-knowledge and perception, physical and mental development (because it influences the pituitary gland), and encourages change and personal growth. Indigo is the colour associated with the *brow chakra* or 'third eye' and the influence of indigo and dark blue flowers as essences can help to promote concentration and alleviate mental tension, over-detachment and cynicism. Perception, insight, intuition and peace of mind are enhanced.

Violet promotes concentration and the capacity for logical thought and can have a balancing effect in cases of depression and migraine-type headaches. It strengthens the psyche and helps us access our higher Self so that we feel a sense of belonging to a unified collective consciousness (just as the regular practice of meditation does.) Violet is the colour associated with the *crown chakra* and essences made from violet and purple flowers help us become inspired, sense our soul direction and access divine wisdom and understanding. **White** is a secondary colour associated with the *crown chakra* and white flowers shed spiritual light on the 'subject' (you) – so that you can be a 'clear channel' and achieve mental clarity, clear negative thoughts and emotions and protect against negative influences in your environment.

Shape

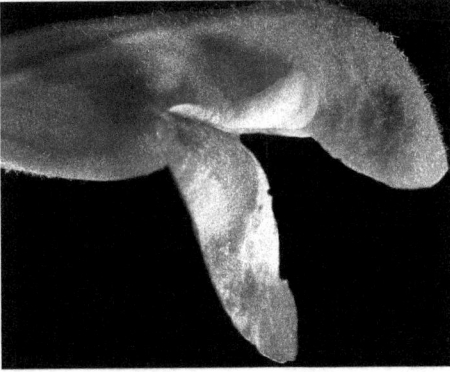

Shape is another aspect of plant signatures and again considered through the first window of plant perception.

An example of the importance of shape in a plant signature is shown by the small flowers of Skullcap *(Scutellaria lateriflora)* which form a distinct hood or cap as the name suggests, and this herb is used medicinally as a remedy for headache and mental tension.

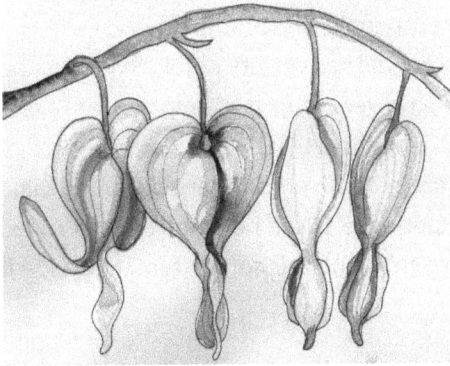

Bleeding Heart *(Dicentra formosa)* has a flower shaped like a pink heart and the heavily-hanging blossoms give an overall impression of downheartedness! In addition, sometimes you can detect a slight furrow down a flower's length – the heart is 'broken.' As a flower essence, it is used for all matters of the heart, especially for loss and a broken heart.

Sunflowers show their silica 'spine' by their upright stance. The seeds are also rich in silica and the plant is used in flower essence form to help bring about a stronger sense of the real Self to people who are very self-effacing, or conversely, for those who spend a lot of time attempting to boost their public persona. It allows them to 'show some spine' – to stand up and 'shine.' Sunflower essence helps both men and women to develop and display positive masculine qualities.

Texture

Texture – the way a plant feels to touch – is another quality that plays an important role in a plant's signature. It is viewed through the ninth window of plant perception. Aloe Vera, Stinging Nettle *(Urticaria urens)* and Comfrey *(Symphytum officinale)* with their spiny and furry surfaces are all used herbally and/or homoeopathically as remedies for the skin. Aloe Vera's herbal value lies in its ability to regenerate damaged or degenerated body tissue, especially as a result of burns. The plant can thrive in dry and hot environments, and according to the Bible (John 19:39), myrrh and aloes were used to embalm the body of Jesus. As a flower essence, Aloe Vera is useful for people who are exhausted or 'burnt out,' especially creatively.

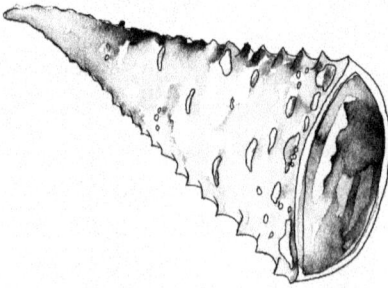

The plant's moist, succulent leaves reflect its ability to soothe and replenish overheated and 'dried up' emotional states (Wells, 2002). As mentioned in the description of the sixth window of plant perception the water element is representative of emotion and fluidity, both so important in the creative process.

Calendula officinale flowers, which have a rich and soft 'fleshy' feel, are used in the treatment of wounds. Calendula flower essence is used to heal and soften communication between people. It is especially useful for 'thin-skinned' types who take offence too easily – and for 'thick-skinned' people who offend others!

Australian Flannel Flower *(Actinotis helianthi)* has velvety petals that have the sensuous feel of silk sheets – and is used as a flower essence to help people to feel more comfortable with what goes on 'beneath the sheets'! It helps to bring a sense of comfort and security for those who experience defensiveness or are uncomfortable in relation to touch and intimate sensual experience. It can help both the so-called 'macho' male and 'butch' female to 'get in touch' with their softer (feminine) side if they so desire.

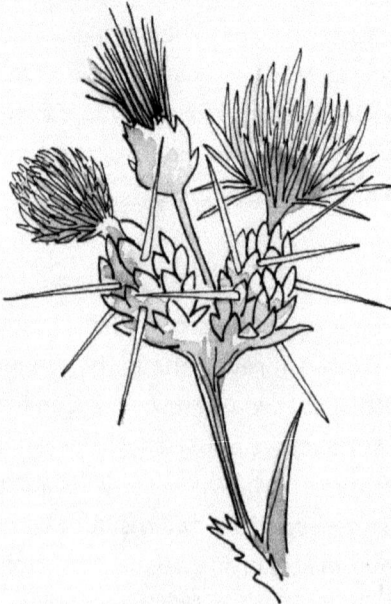

Another good example of texture as signature is given by Star Thistle *(Centaurea solstitialis)*, whose needle-like prickles scream out to anyone who comes near, 'Don't touch me or you'll get pricked!' The flower essence derived from this plant is helpful for people who have been hurt and whose motto is 'Once bitten, twice shy.' It can help them to be less focused on self-preservation so that they don't have to put all their energy into guarding themselves emotionally and/or protecting their material possessions. Star Thistle flower essence can gently 'open' these people to receive the nurturing and emotional nourishment that the universe provides to a more generous soul.

Habit of growth

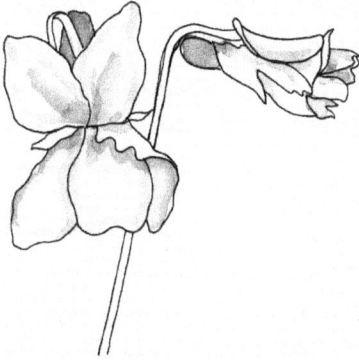

The way a plant grows can give clues to its potential healing qualities and is viewed through the second, third, fourth and fifth windows of plant perception. The growth pattern of Violet (*Viola odorata*) is a good example. Often referred to as 'shrinking violet,' the plant tends to grow low, hugging the ground and often appearing to hide under taller plants. Their attractive odour is often noticed before you can see them. Violet flower essence is helpful to people who are shy about expressing sensitive, artistic aspects of their nature, especially if they believe that they may be ridiculed or taken advantage of. When I look at the form of this flower, I see a head that is bashfully bowed.

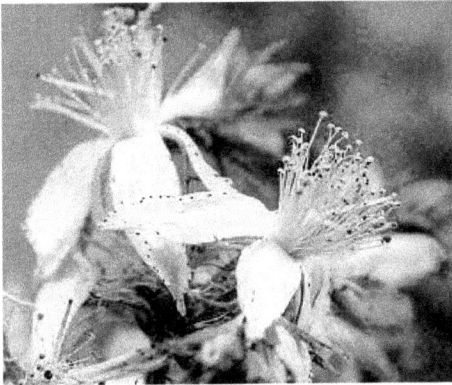

In bloom, the flower of St John's Wort *(Hypericum perforatum)* presents itself to the sun with petals bent backward, appearing open and vulnerable.

The plant's receptive posture allows it to absorb fully and deeply the strengthening and life-supporting rays of the sun. As a flower essence, this plant assists people who feel too 'open' and vulnerable, especially when this is reflected in repeated experiences of disturbing and fearful dreams. When the emotional and etheric bodies have lost integrity and their boundaries have become weakened, disturbing thought forms can create anxiety. The bright yellow, clearly defined petals of St John's Wort are like the little sun of individual selfhood that radiates from the solar plexus of a healthy person, untroubled by shadowy influences. These flowers show that it is possible to be open to the universe and yet fully retain our identity in this incarnation.

Red Clover (*Trifolium pratense*) grows in masses – no wonder the flower essence helps people to remain calm if they are susceptible to mass hysteria and/or become 'panicky' in large crowds.

The Australian Silver Princess tree grows with a spreading, open canopy and this openness allows plenty of light to filter through. The flower essence allows inspirational 'light' to filter 'down' to consciousness, providing direction and guidance.

Environment

The environment in which a plant lives can tell much about its potential therapeutic use. Horsetail (*Equisetum hyemale*) and Hydrangea (*Hydrangea arborescens*) grow on the banks of clear ponds and free-flowing streams, and both are used as diuretics or as therapeutic aids for shifting indurated deposits in the body, such as calcium in the joints.

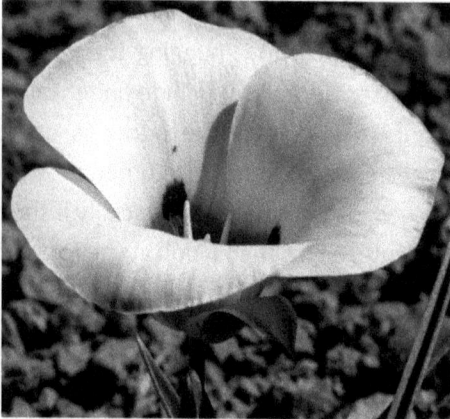

Mariposa Lily (*Calochortus leichtlinii*) grows in harsh and rocky mountainous terrain, emerging out of inhospitable-looking ground to display itself unashamedly, its flower cup receptive to the sun and the healing energies of the universe. As a flower essence, Mariposa Lily is used to heal the 'mother-nurturer' within us, allowing us to nurture ourselves in ways we may have missed or been unreceptive to during the crucial early stages of mother-child bonding. Like the beautiful and resilient flower that blossoms despite its harsh environmental beginnings, a person deprived in some way of love and emotional sustenance as a baby can still grow and blossom, safely opening to receive the universal love they require.

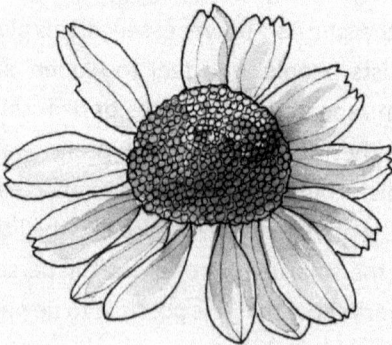

Of course, many plants combine two, three or more of these aspects in their signature, as we have already seen when discussing the shape and colour of the Pomegranate. For example, Chamomile (*Matricaria recutita*) is used for treating digestive problems that have a nervous origin. The signature begins with the yellow colour of the flower's centre, which relates to the *solar plexus chakra*, the energy centre concerned with how we physically and emotionally digest experience; in addition, the pattern of the flower heads resembles the stomach's secretory cells. The centre of the flower protrudes, symbolising emotional swelling or 'overwhelm'. Chamomile flower essence has helped to settle many an overwrought child and adult.

THE **ESSENTIAL** FLOWER ESSENCE BOOK

Perceiving the signature of a plant is a process that comes naturally for some, while others need to develop their capacity. The doctrine of signatures states that the external world bears the stamp of its internal counterpart – this is analogous to what the celebrated Swiss psychotherapist Carl Jung said of the relationship between the body and mind – that they are just different sides of the same coin. The signatures of plants have been tested by trial and error over many thousands of years, as common sense combines with experience to enable us to make use of the healing potential in their Nature. As humans evolve and healing needs change, history has shown that certain plants come to the fore while others recede. (The same pattern can be seen in the history of diseases, which arise when conditions suit them and then recede to be replaced by others caused by new virus variants, for instance, that are better adapted to newer conditions. This occurs irrespective of human intervention.) Vibrational energies of certain flowers and plants accommodate themselves to our needs and become more relevant to the next stage of development. Carl Jung coined the term 'synchronicity' for this experience of meaningful coincidence. Here we see the synchronous emergence of a human need and a plant with healing qualities which meet this need. We can become attuned to appropriate plants when the need emerges and the time is right.

In describing this subtle human-nature co-evolution, Einstein's analogy, which likened scientific progress to climbing a mountain, also holds true – each time we advance up the mountain our new vantage point allows us to 'see' wider and further, while not dismissing what we already have come to know from a lower vantage point. As consciousness evolves we experience a wider perception of the (natural) riches offered.

Some clinical trials

In the scientific world, double-blind, placebo-based trials are commonly used as a method of verifying claims regarding the traditionally-acknowledged healing qualities or therapeutic properties of plants. As mentioned earlier, the Flower Essence Society has carried out some such trials, and I was also involved in conducting research of this kind at Victoria University; and the results were significantly better than what would be expected from placebo alone. Here are some results of a few of the many placebo-based trials that have been carried out.

1. Double-blind placebo based study – Bach Flower remedies

OVERVIEW

- Three groups – placebo, four-remedy mixture, seven-remedy mixture (100 participants)
- Used psychological tests, POMS (Profile of Mood States), measuring self-awareness, self-confidence, wellbeing, etc

- Tested at beginning, 3 weeks and 6 weeks after remedies

RESULTS
- Efficacy of Bach Flowers demonstrated (4 & 7 remedy groups showed significant improvement)
- 7 remedy group, however, also had more of a tendency to drop out – further research warranted

(Weisglas, M., "Bach Flower Essence Research: A Scientific Study", *The Flower Essence Journal*, 1 (1980), 11-14)

2. Single-blind Bach Flower study

OVERVIEW
- Participants select 'most appealing' image of Bach Flower
- Participants given placebo or remedy (participant unaware of what they were given – 'single blind')
- POMS questionnaire given to participants at start and after 3 weeks taking remedies

RESULTS
- Significant POMS score differences between placebo and treatment
- Efficacy of Bach Flowers demonstrated, further research highly recommended

(Plemming and Redenbach, 1995. Swinburne University, Melbourne)

3. Double-blind cross-over placebo based trial

While working towards a Masters in Health Science by Research at Victoria University under the supervision of Dr Damian Ryan and Dr Barry Nester, I conducted a double-blind, placebo based, cross-over trial with the Bach Flower combination *Rescue Remedy*. For me, it was a labour of love. The 'cross-over' aspect of the trial involved giving the *same* person both placebo and Rescue Remedy and comparing the effects. This is the procedure that is followed in situations where each person's response is very *subjective*. (For example, it is used in pain management trials – there is no point in comparing how a substance affects the pain of two different people, because everyone has a different pain threshold so it is necessary to give each individual both the substance and a placebo.) My Bach Flower trial compared how a person responded to a placebo against how the same person (after a break) responded to *Rescue Remedy* and vice-versa. The cross-over approach offers a ready-matched 'pair' situation, which is particularly useful when the endpoint is a subjective assessment by the participant because it allows a comparison of the two treatments.

As mentioned previously, the FES researchers feel, as I do, that qualitative research is a 'better fit' for flower essence therapy as it tends to take into account the subjective response of individuals, so it was important for me to apply a cross-over approach in the trial.

The trial for each participant was conducted over seven weeks. Each received either *Rescue Remedy* or the placebo for the first three weeks, followed by a one week 'wash-out' period without taking either mixture. After the 'wash out' period, they were 'crossed over' and allocated the placebo mixture if they had previously received the *Rescue Remedy* and vice-versa. As in all double blind trials, neither I nor the participant had any knowledge of what was in the bottles they were given (placebo or *Rescue Remedy*). I, the experimenter, followed a pre-coded numbering system for the mixtures so was also 'blind' to their status when they were given to participants.

OVERVIEW

- Investigating the influence of Rescue Remedy (RR) on mood state in females (aged between 18 and 40 and taking no medication)
- POMS questionnaire at start, after 3 weeks (followed by a 'wash out' period of one week), after 4 weeks and after 7 weeks
- 40 participants randomly selected to take placebo and RR in the first or last 3 weeks

RESULTS

- Significant POMS score differences between placebo and RR treatment (with 4 participants removed)
- Most significant POMS score differences between placebo and RR treatment when 'tension/anxiety' scores isolated
- Significantly better POMS scores after RR in participants who took placebo in the first 3 weeks

(Wells, 2002)

4. Double-blind cross-over placebo based trial

An article in *Callx: International Journal of Flower Essence Therapy* (FES, 2001) presented the findings of a series of studies conducted to determine the clinical efficacy of flower essences on the treatment of mild to moderate depression. Five clinical outcome studies are presented, each lending evidence towards understanding the clinical effects of flower essences on the treatment of depression.

'Results of these studies were measured using the Beck Depression Inventory

(BDI) and the Hamilton Depression Scale (HAM-D). A time series analysis of the data was conducted using an ANOVA (analysis of variance) for repeated measures' (FES, 2001).

Four of the studies were conducted by therapists sponsored by the Cuban Ministry of Public Health. The first study examined over 100 patients with half of them completing the therapy. These patients were tracked over a five month period, the outcome of which indicated a significant reduction in depressive symptoms. The second and third studies involved 20 subjects and were conducted over a 2 month and three month period respectively. Both studies showed significant reductions in the BDI total score of 76–77%. The fourth study involved 24 cases over a three month period and significant reduction in depressive symptoms was observed in the first two months. These figures stabilised at a 60–80% reduction during the third month.

The fifth study was a multi-site clinical trial conducted in the United States (Cram, 2001b). There were twelve depressed subjects in a one month baseline followed by 3 months of treatment that involved usual care (what was already in place) along with flower essence therapy. A 50% reduction in depression scores followed the introduction of flower essence therapy. This significant clinical change was maintained over a period of 3 months until the completion of the study.

While none of these trials utilised a randomised control group, the findings of these five studies strongly supports the effective administration of flower essences as an adjunct to facilitating resolution of mild to moderate depression.

HUMAN/PLANT CO-EVOLUTION – a positive human-nature conspiracy

*From time immemorial, plants, animals and humans have evolved alongside one another. The spirit of nature serves us, while we in return pay homage to nature in **a selfless conspiracy to live, grow and evolve together.** Here lies the order and purpose inherent in the great panorama of life. Knowledge of, and cooperation with the inner world of nature offers humans their greatest opportunity to find happiness (from Spiritual Unfoldment, White Eagle 1998).*

The integral relationship between nature and humans was established from the beginning. Evolution of plant life and human life are to a great degree mutually dependent on each other for progress. In other words, we need each other whether we like it or not, or more to the point, whether we appreciate it or not. Because of this intimate, subtle relationship, plants respond in sync on a macrocosmic level to the collective human psyche. On a microcosmic level too, individual plants respond to the needs of individual humans (in a specific environmental niche, for instance). The relationship is co-dependent, in this case in a positive way! Individuals also notice and respond to those plants that meet their individual needs, and visual recognition plays a big part in their response. This is one of the reasons I incorporated a process in my consultations many years ago which I refer to as the 'Flower Affinity Test.'

The Flower Affinity Test is an extremely useful tool when used in the context of a healthy working alliance between practitioner/therapist and client, based on empathic understanding, non-judgement and mutual respect. The 'test' involves showing clients a range of photos of specific flowers, taken in a way that accentuates their 'signature' expression. I only give clients a brief moment to look at each photo and ask them to choose the ones that stand out and are aesthetically pleasing to them. I usually say: 'Choose whichever ones give you a good feeling, and a "warm fuzzy" sense response, the way you respond to music you like, even before you recognise who the artist is or what instruments they are playing.' I originally conducted the Flower Affinity Test with children when their parents brought them in for a consultation, because the children were generally able to choose their favourite three or four flowers easily and spontaneously, from up to seventy or eighty photos quickly presented one by one. Often, when I described the qualities of the chosen flower essences, the parent(s) would say, 'Oh, that is so spot on!'

I eventually summoned the courage to try the test with adults – some can be very sceptical at first – and the results were immensely helpful. At the very least they provoke in-depth discussion, but usually they provide an accurate reflection of the emotional and mental state of the client. I also find the test is a great way to focus in on the areas and issues in a client's life that they will be most receptive and comfortable talking about and working on, and I believe there are two reasons for this. Firstly, clients feel empowered because they have made their own choices, rather than having me tell them what's best for them. Secondly, their choice of flower essences reflects what they're already subconsciously grappling with, so they are more receptive and comfortable about discussing feelings and issues that are familiar to them on some level.

On average, I conduct the test with around 2/3 of my clients. I am not at all dependent on it but find it a very useful tool. In-depth interviewing, active listening, empathic understanding and counselling are still essential in a consultation and are ultimately the most powerful in helping both client and therapist to work together to choose the most appropriate flower essences.

The strengths and vulnerabilities of our bodies and minds provide the freedoms and limitations that help us to experience life lessons, uniquely our own, and achieve personal growth and ultimately the free expression of the spirit. Life's struggle involves learning to live with one's unique and individual incapacities. As Clint Eastwood was heard to say in one of his films, 'A man's got to know his limitations.' Life's reward is discovering the profound qualities of the transpersonal Self that transcends individuality and connects to a world beyond conventional space and time. The more conscious we become of our relationship with all other life forms at the deepest (soul) level, the more aware we are that there is no such thing as splendid isolation; there is in reality no separation between the various forms of life, for all are interdependent and all create one harmonious whole.

From ancient times to the present, the struggle with the limitations and incapacitating effects of our cumbersome physicality has driven the spirit to achieve greater refinement. This is how we evolve as individuals. The physical body's boundaries are there to be exceeded by a developing mind that continually broadens its horizons. Ken Wilber's book *No Boundary – Eastern and Western approaches to personal growth* (2001), expresses the belief that we are here to experience the ultimate metaphysical secret – that there are no boundaries in the universe. Boundaries are illusions, products of the way we try to map and edit our reality. They may help us to get a sense of our own territory but reality is not so confined. All such boundaries and personal territories are permeable to the human-nature connection. If we don't understand this we will continue to face environmental crises that inevitably become human crises.

Plant forms have established working allegiances with human nature, successfully supporting humans in areas of healing and spiritual growth. Philosophers such as Plato and spiritualists such as Rudolf Steiner speak of legendary paradises where past civilisations constructed vast settlements that blended with nature. Gardens were created in which houses were built from the living material of plants and trees. (It is no surprise then, and a very welcome development, that many buildings are now being constructed with plants and nature incorporated into their design.) All facets of life were considered sacred and every activity, whether building a house, facilitating healing or administering government, had a psychic dimension and a spiritual context. According to these legends, ancient peoples could build a dome by causing plants and trees to intertwine artfully and form a waterproof canopy, fully integrated with the environment. They created from nature and felt totally integrated within it; boundaries between people and the natural world were permeable. Flower essences and other types of vibrational healing allow us to experience this type of interaction with the plant world via 'permeable' boundaries, providing a medium for gentle, respectful and mutually beneficial exchange on physical and more subtle levels.

Over time we have moved away from rituals of communication and cooperation with nature, in favour of scientific and technological advances, especially in the use of genetic engineering. While modern science has helped transform the world in many marvellous ways we would be wise to take heed of the words of Rudolf Steiner warning us of the responsibilities and perils associated with these technologies.

Our consciousness is re-awakening to realms beyond the purely material, as witnessed by the upsurge of interest in subtle approaches to healing, the steady refinement of methods used in medical science and the increasing interest in the mind's power and influence on medical outcomes. Our capacity as individuals to respond to the subtle dimensions of life is growing. Herbal medicines – the most material way of conveying a plant's healing qualities – were the main remedies used for thousands of years and they are still effective today. Over the past 2000 years, though, we have also become increasingly sensitive and responsive to the less material and more energetic qualities of plants. All forms of healing, conventional and unconventional, have gradually become more refined and/or subtle – or at the very least, less crude – in their practices and applications.

A good example of this development of human sensitivity to less material energetic forces over the centuries can be seen in our broadening appreciation of the herb Yarrow. As mentioned earlier, White Yarrow (*Achillea millefolium*) is named for its use as a wound-herb after the warrior Achilles and the soldiers of ancient Greece. Carrying it on their persons as they marched into battle, soldiers used it both internally and externally to help stem bleeding and were enabled by it to fight on despite their wounds. Today's use of Yarrow as a flower essence or vibrational remedy also aims at stemming bleeding – but on a subtle-body level rather than a physical level, for those who, as a result of oversensitivity and susceptibility, are easily 'wounded' by negativity, such as excessive radiation, in their immediate environment. The flower essence Yarrow helps to seal and protect subtle body boundaries – the aura – in a way that parallels the herb's action in sealing and protecting the physical body's boundaries by stemming bleeding.

Generally we are only just beginning to re-establish our conscious connection with the natural 'internet' as it vibrates powerfully in collective cyberspace. Some of us are just beginning to tap in, some are permanently connected, while others are ignorant of, or at least oblivious to its influence. Fortunately, the more we ignore it, the more it won't go away! We manifest our differing degrees of awareness of this human-nature alliance in many different ways. One obvious way is the rapid emergence in recent times of 'green' groups who set out to protect a threatened natural world. A beautiful conspiracy between humans and nature has always existed. We are beginning to acknowledge it once again in a more tangible way, and this conscious recognition will add further impetus to our common purpose – the mutual evolution of all individual life forms on this Earth toward their place in their heaven!

Holistic health

Humans have co-evolved with and alongside other life forms in a process in which all are linked, by the energies in and around us – the universal life energies that encompass, animate and nourish us. We are much more than sophisticated machines to be repaired when broken, or complex bio-computers occasionally in need of re-programming. This holistic understanding that *a human being is a system of energetic forces that is more than the sum of its physical structures and biochemical activity* is not new. Many religions have recognised and referred to the life force or soul in their doctrines. The ancient concepts of *chi, prana* and *vital force* describe the energy that animates all living matter.

A deficiency or disturbance in life energy can lead to stress in the physical body, thus lowering resistance to disease. At the present time, the awareness of the concept of life energy has been devalued in favour of measurable material phenomena. Scientific paradigms that currently organise our understanding of the world rely predominantly on physical parameters, shifting the focus well away from anything more subtle. Phenomenological evidence for the existence of life-energy forces is rarely given any scientific attention (positive or otherwise), although some quantum physicists have recognised *the illusion of matter and the infinite divisibility of the atom* in conceding that if we follow matter to its most fundamental components, eventually we are left with pure energy.

Physical structures are fundamental to life, but if we look only at physical systems, we ignore the forces that animate them. Kaminski and Katz (1996) use the analogy of trying to understand the images on a television by analysing its parts,

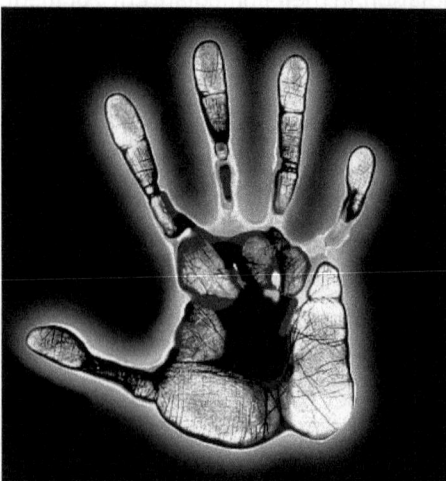

without recognising the electromagnetic energy field that carries the broadcast signal. The electromagnetic fields with which we are so familiar in the electronic age do provide a useful analogy in order to comprehend the energy fields of living beings. However, it would be a mistake to try to explain life just in terms of the physical energies of electricity and magnetism. Etheric life energies have their own distinct qualities, characteristics, shapes and forms. They envelop the physical body and can be said to constitute the etheric body, which distinguishes the living from the non-living.

Two health modalities that are well-established today – Homeopathy and Traditional Chinese Medicine (TCM) – recognise and address human etheric energy fields. In terms of numbers of people treated, TCM and Homeopathy are second only to Western allopathic medicine. What distinguishes Homeopathic remedies (including Tissue Salts) from conventional medicines is that some of them are so physically dilute that any direct biochemical influence is attenuated or eliminated, while their energetic forces are enhanced. This is achieved through a potentisation process involving rhythmic succussion that accompanies each stage of dilution. The remedies then impact, not only the physical body, but also the body's energy fields according to the Law of Similars. This principle holds that a substance which causes a particular set of symptoms in large doses will stimulate the body to heal that same set of symptoms when taken in a (minute) homeopathic dose. Thus, Homeopathy acts as a catalyst to rally the vital forces to engage in the healing process. Acupuncture is an ancient medical science in which tiny needles are inserted along vital energy pathways called meridians. Acupuncture is used successfully to treat all sorts of ailments affecting physiological systems by adjusting and toning the human energy field.

Subtle dimensions – the body as a system of energy fields

Having developed the concept that we are a vitalistic system of energy fields, we can explore the intricacies of these subtle dimensions more deeply. Human physical and mental health and wellbeing results from the integration of all levels of our multidimensional anatomy, which takes progressively more subtle forms, from the physical body to the etheric, emotional, and mental bodies.

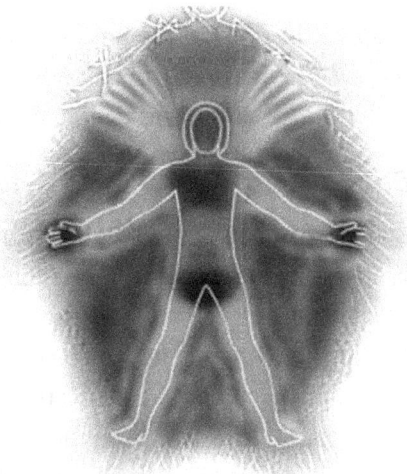

In this section each of these levels will be discussed in turn, examining ways in which they relate to one another to form a whole. Recognising the existence of the etheric body as a field of life energy is the first step to gaining an understanding of human subtle anatomy – the structure and function of energy fields that extend beyond the physical dimension. Many who engage in religious contemplation accept the existence of a soul. According to multidimensional understanding, the subtle anatomy, interacting with the physical body, provides the soul with a 'vehicle' on life's journey. True health, wellbeing and contentment are found when this vehicle operates at its optimum so that the soul can be sensed and its purpose can become manifest in this life. Then we become aware of our true vocation, doing what we do best and feel best doing, whatever that may be.

Some analogies may help to describe how the subtle energy bodies relate to one another to form an integrated whole. If we took a bucket and filled it to the top with large rocks to represent the physical body, we might naively say that the bucket is full. However, we could fill the spaces around the rocks in the apparently-full bucket with small pebbles and stones: this would represent the etheric body. Further, we could refill the spaces that are left around the pebbles with sand to represent the mental body, and then refill the whole bucket with water, representing the emotional body. Hence the bucket is filled with elements that range from the very crude to the very subtle. The various dimensions of our being coexist in the same way. The structure of a house provides another analogy for the organisation of the subtle being. First the foundations are laid and the framework is established, representing the physical body. The bricks and cement that bind the structure together to give it form and function represent the etheric body. Decoration, colours, furniture etc give the house its character and feel, and this represents the emotional body. The mental body could be represented by the original concept, plan or architectural design of the house.

Before we investigate the subtle bodies individually, it must be stressed that they are in fact inseparable and never operate as single entities. Our whole being derives its existence and function from the constant interaction and integration of physical and subtle bodies. They constantly intertwine, overlap and diverge, only to quickly merge again. However, in order to understand and work with the subtle anatomy, it is necessary to conceptualise the subtle bodies as distinct and separate aspects of our whole being.

The body that is easiest to identify (and identify with) is the physical body We can see it, touch it, manipulate it and, obviously, damage it. Nobody needs to be convinced of its existence. The medical establishment of today is fixated on the physical body, and medications target its dense anatomy – by necessity in a relatively crude way. From a multidimensional viewpoint, however, symptoms of illness pertaining to the physical body are seen as symptoms of dis-ease or imbalance at more subtle levels. Complete and permanent improvements in health and wellbeing can only be achieved by remedies that facilitate healing at these other levels. While palliative health care is useful, humane and important, treatments aimed only at the physical level tend to modify symptoms rather than influence deeper causes of illness.

The etheric body

If we wish to influence health more profoundly, the next closest level to the physical body is found in the etheric body. At different times the etheric body has gone by other names, such as the 'electro-physical' body or the 'bio-energetic' body. The etheric body is the energetic template that guides the growth, development and function of the physical body. Dis-ease may appear in the etheric body days, weeks and even months before it becomes manifest in the physical body, but is often felt at the etheric level just prior to its initial physical manifestation. For example, many of us experience the feeling of 'coming down with something' the night before actual cold or flu symptoms appear in our bodies. If the most astute medical physician examined us at this stage, he or she would not detect any illness at the physical level. And yet we feel 'off' and we know where it leads – we wake up physically sick, having first felt dis-ease at the etheric level.

Distortions, disruptions, dis-ease or weakness at the etheric level eventually show up in the form of illness in the physical body. Conversely, just as we may feel 'off' at the etheric level before becoming physically ill, we may also become healthy on the etheric level before the physical body becomes symptom-free. This is especially so when vibrational medicines such as homoeopathic remedies, which act on the etheric level are used to treat long term physical illness. When the etheric body is treated successfully using appropriately prescribed vibrational medicines, improvement begins with the person reporting that they 'feel much better in themselves' despite the fact that some physical symptoms remain. These physical symptoms soon start to disappear but even while they persist, the person may have a much more positive outlook with regard to their illness and a sense of inner wellbeing. Low potency homeopathic remedies, especially in the form of Tissue Salts, have a direct impact not only on the etheric body but also the physical body. This makes Tissue Salts therapy practical and effective as a treatment for short and long term (ie acute and chronic) health issues.

Energy pathways and directions of flow called meridians in the ancient discipline of acupuncture exist at the etheric level. Acupuncture is a healing modality which has been accepted by many in the West because it actually works, despite the fact that it confounds Western medical paradigms! However, much positive scientific research into TCM is gradually 'winning over' the medical fraternity. Acupuncture treats disease states that have their origins in stagnation and imbalance of etheric energy. By improving the pattern laid down by the etheric body, acupuncture improves the physical body's future health. Spontaneous healing through natural self-recuperative powers can also occur at the etheric level. Many migraine sufferers report that symptoms occur at the end of a period of stress and that after the pain

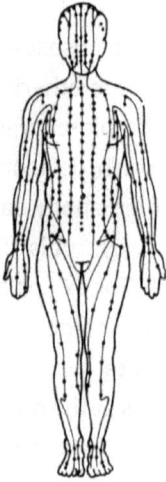

has eased, they feel more relaxed and at peace for a time. (I can vouch for this having been a previous sufferer!) After enduring a head cold without suppressive intervention, many people say that their head feels clearer and that they feel mentally relaxed and energised. In these situations, our innate healing capacity brings about a 'shake-up and clean-out' at the etheric level. Equilibrium is re-established through a process in which a natural and manageable healing crisis is experienced at a physical level (in the form of migraine or head cold symptoms in the examples given above). Soon after this brief crisis, if things are allowed to run their natural course while resting, re-establishment of better health in the etheric body is reflected in the physical body's renewed vitality.

Images of the etheric body can be obtained through a procedure known as Kirlian photography, which produces images that look like photographic negatives. A Kirlian photograph of a leafy twig, for example, whose leaves look perfectly healthy and unblemished to the naked eye, might show one leaf that has only a vague outline. This shows that even though the leaf looks outwardly healthy, its vague outline in the Kirlian image is an indication of dis-ease at the inner, etheric level. Visible signs of this disease would start to appear at the physical level within a day or two, when the leaf might start to lose colour and moisture and would fall from the tree. The Kirlian photograph has let us 'see' serious disease or weakening at the etheric level, soon to be followed by disease at the physical level. The phenomenon of 'phantom limb' can be explained in terms of etheric effects that can be felt at a physical level. When someone has suddenly lost a limb through injury or amputation, they often report that they still 'feel' the non-existent limb. This sensation is not a figment of the imagination but rather a fragment of etheric orientation – at a physical level the body still registers (or

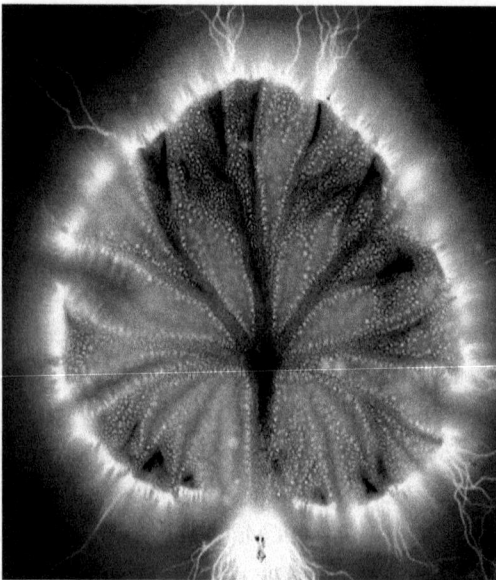

'senses') the slowly receding etheric aspect associated with the lost limb.

Anaesthesia is a procedure that can influence the subtle anatomy, temporarily dislocating the etheric body from the physical body. Subjective sensations, including pain, are intricately associated with the etheric body, which has its most immediate influence on the physical body via the nervous system. (The emotional body, on the other hand, exerts most of its influence via the endocrine system.) Once an anaesthetic takes effect, no pain is felt, because the etheric and physical bodies are no longer integrated so as to permit the full range of physical sensations. Unfortunately, after this dislocation has been achieved, the subtle anatomy may take time to reintegrate, or in some cases, may only partially reintegrate. Many people feel 'out of it' or 'not quite right' for days, weeks or even months after an anaesthetic, which has an effect on the subtle anatomy similar to traumatic shock. Only when the subtle bodies settle back into a stable configuration can they function in unison, allowing the healing process to progress efficiently. It should be noted that the Bach Flower Remedy, Star of Bethlehem, and/or homoeopathic or flower essence forms of Arnica have a special role in helping the subtle anatomy re-establish equilibrium after trauma and shock (including anaesthesia).

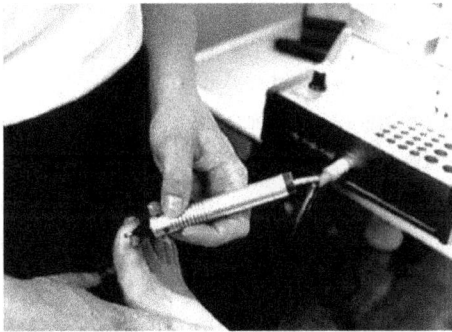

In recent times, instruments such as the Vega machine have been developed to help carry out bio-energetic evaluations of a person's etheric state, assisting a practitioner to make an assessment and track health progress at this level.

The emotional body

The next level of the subtle anatomy is the emotional body (often referred to as the astral body), which is the subtle body that conceives, generates and reflects emotions. In terms of the human race as a whole, the emotional body is the one that most urgently needs attention, as the high level of violence in many societies testifies.

We are often victims of our emotions, overwhelmed by their intensity, responding to impulses by blindly lashing out or 'losing it' in relationships or other life situations. At these times, we experience ourselves and our emotions as separate from the person we regard ourselves to be most of the time. Such states occur when the emotional body is not integrated with the rest of our subtle being. The emotional body is the most 'badly behaved' of all the subtle bodies and needs the most nurturing and guidance via the higher mental body. The aim of this guidance is not to suppress or get our emotions under control (although that is the ultimate result), but to direct them into avenues where they can work with us rather than against us or anyone else. Integration channels the energetic charge – the passion of emotion – into areas of our lives that bring the most fulfilment. A sporting analogy may help make sense of the process of integration. If you're a golfer, your success depends on how skilfully you swing your golf club. There are many aspects of the swing that must be considered simultaneously – head down, knees bent etc – and if one aspect is out of sync with the others, the whole swing is thrown out, affecting the shot's direction and distance. To make a successful shot, many facets of self-awareness need to be integrated. When this is achieved the swing functions 'naturally' and effortlessly, and the ball is placed exactly where the player wants it.

For a player who achieves integration, everything comes together to achieve their purpose in golf – and for some golfers this is the same as their purpose in life! But alas, one facet or more of a golf swing usually fails to integrate with the others and the standard of play is affected. This is especially the case if the intense (emotional) frustration felt from a few bad previous shots interferes with the any of the many facets of self-awareness required to make the next good shot. In the same way, our lives go off course and lose direction when one facet of our subtle anatomy gets out of sync with the rest. The emotional aspect is the culprit more often than any other, because it creates its own separatist agenda, temporarily distracting us from our purpose (like the desire for a chocolate biscuit when we are dieting to achieve the goal of losing weight). Our task is to integrate emotions so that they serve rather than hinder personal growth and what we want to achieve in our lives.

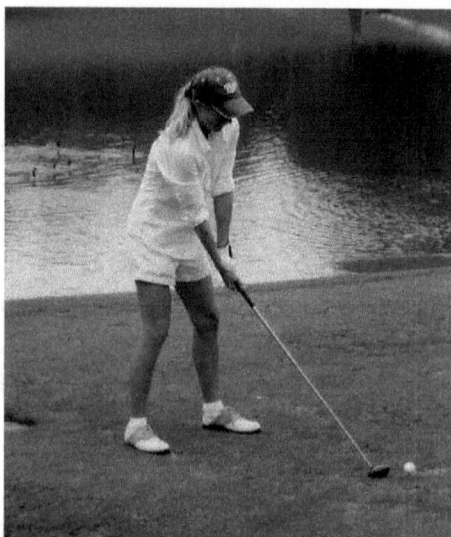

The emotional or astral body goes 'wandering' in the dream state while we sleep. Symbols and visions are conveyed to consciousness from more subtle levels via the astral vehicle. When people take flower essences, which directly influence the emotional body, they commonly report a heightened awareness of their dreams, and sometimes have a sense that they are dreaming more often and more vividly. Dreaming is a very important process in the maintenance of overall wellbeing, providing at the very least a natural form of stress release, and suppression of dreaming should be avoided if possible.

Depression and other emotional disturbances have their origins in the emotional body and its relationship with the subtle anatomy as a whole. The healing process involves allowing emotional imbalances to 'work their way out' from the emotional body via the

THE **ESSENTIAL** FLOWER ESSENCE BOOK

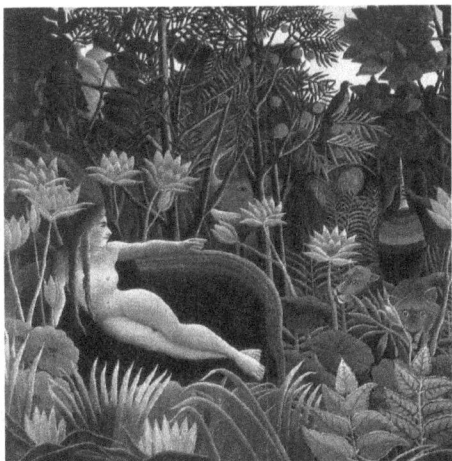

etheric level to the physical body where, as discussed earlier, they may manifest as some kind of physical illness or 'healing crisis' before resolving themselves. This process can take anything from minutes to years. As a natural therapist, I often see people whose anxiety and emotional distress is ameliorated by the onset of, for example, a skin eruption, a mucus discharge, a migraine, a bowel episode etc. It is almost as if we have come to earth to dump our spiritual toxic waste and so refine ourselves as a whole. The body is the final processing station for this toxicity, which then discharges into the environment. We are certainly on the right planet at the right time to work on issues such as efficient and respectful waste-disposal on personal and interpersonal levels as well as environmental ones.

In the face of recent scientific evidence, especially in the area of psychoneuroimmunology, it seems indisputable that emotions and attitudes have a profound effect on health. Research has shown that depression and long term emotional stress suppresses the immune system – the system that is responsible for our natural defences against illness. For example, it has been shown that when a partner in a long-standing relationship dies, the incidence of the other partner becoming seriously ill within the next two years is far greater than normal. In this instance, *unresolved* grief, which is dis-ease at the level of the emotional body, eventually manifests as disease at the physical level. Most of us have experienced the connection between prolonged stress and illness, whether it manifests as a head cold or something more severe. When dis-ease at the emotional level finally impacts on the physical body, the immune system temporarily gives way. The restful 'time out' created by an episode of sickness often makes it possible to gain a fresh and healthier perspective after the healing crisis has run its course.

The mental body

The emotions we experience act like cement that binds and sets our thoughts and beliefs, which occupy the next, more subtle level of being – the mental body. *The state of the mental body reflects the quality of our thought patterns and characteristic attitudes or personal mindset.*

The mental body houses our fundamental beliefs about ourselves – our concept of Self. These beliefs have profound effects on our total experience of life and therefore on our health and wellbeing. Negative thought patterns and beliefs reside in this domain, predominantly at a subconscious level, but our conscious behaviour gives us clues to their existence and nature. For example, 3-year-old Johnny keeps asking questions while his father is trying to concentrate on a job in his garage workshop. Johnny just wants to feel involved and helpful to his Dad. Alas, Dad sees him as a pest and keeps telling him to get out and stop getting in the way. Young Johnny hides his sense of rejection and eventually walks away, unable to express the deep hurt he feels at not having his fundamental needs met, of being accepted, loved and connected. This experience can become ingrained at the level of the mental body. The emotional pain generated by repeated rejections stays with him and becomes consolidated as a belief that he gets in the way all the time and doesn't fit in anywhere and/or that his fundamental survival needs won't be met. The painful emotion associated with the experience(s), if not processed to some degree naturally in time and/or in therapy, will undermine many of his life experiences going forward. Powerful emotional experiences become deeply entrenched in belief structures about life and our identity and self-concept.

Our fundamental beliefs shape our identities, and we often defend them with our lives.

The chakras

The chakras are energy centres that form an integral part of the body's subtle energy system. There are seven chakras located along the length of the spine and in the head. Each person's energy is refined and directed over the course of a lifetime via the successive unfolding of these energy centres. The chakra system gives further insight into multi-dimensional anatomy, including the condition of the physical body, and as we will see in this section, can deepen our understanding of how to prescribe flower essences effectively.

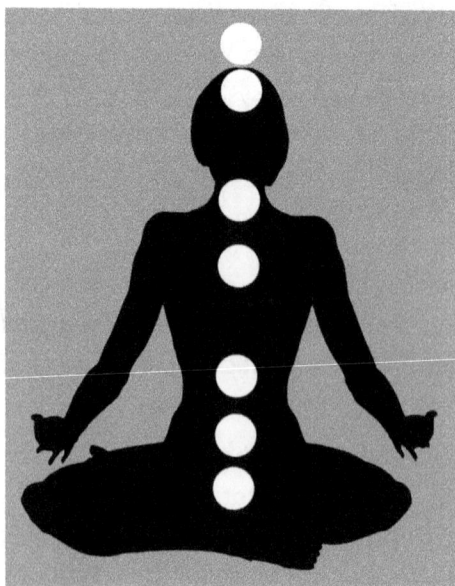

The chakras exist at the etheric level as 'transformer' points where threads of energy cross one another. Alice Bailey (1984) describes them in the following way:

'Within the human etheric body there are to be found seven major force centres which are in the nature of distributing agencies ... providing dynamic forces and qualitative energy to man. They produce definite effects upon his outer physical manifestation [body] through their constant activity.'

Each chakra relates to specific physical, emotional and mental aspects of the multidimensional anatomy. Energies pass through each chakra the way traffic passes through a busy intersection. Anyone who remembers the aerial view of a traffic jam in the opening sequence of the original Dick Tracy cartoon will have an insight into what the solar plexus chakra looks like under stress!

Psychics and/or 'sensitives' describe the chakra centres as being like a series of discs or wheels, each containing a particular number of petal-like segments. As particular states of consciousness associated with a chakra develop, these 'petals' begin to unfold. In their usual order of development, the seven centres are: the base chakra, the sacral chakra, the solar plexus chakra, the heart chakra, the throat chakra, the brow chakra and the crown chakra.

- The base, sacral and solar plexus chakras relate to *intra*personal, 'I'-centred aspects of being.
- The heart, throat, brow and crown chakras relate to *inter*personal relations with the rest of the world – 'you'-centred aspects of being.

Of course, inward-directed (intrapersonal) facets of consciousness affect the outward-directed (interpersonal) facets and vice versa. Let's see how this works in practice. A newborn child operates very much from the base chakra level. This chakra's energies are concerned with personal survival: gaining physical and emotional nourishment (eating) and carrying out waste elimination (pooing) are understandably of prime importance at this time. If these needs are adequately met it becomes possible, as we mature, to consider the needs of others, and when they become as important to us as our own needs, heart chakra consciousness has been activated.

Underdevelopment or overdevelopment of intrapersonal chakras has a bearing on interpersonal development and vice versa. For example, an individual may have highly evolved throat chakra capacities, with a resultant ability to communicate in a very 'technically correct' manner, giving detailed descriptions and word-perfect, textbook recitals when speaking. Unfortunately, they may also be dead boring if there is inhibition at the level of the sacral chakra, which relates to self-esteem and the unique creative 'flavour' of one's expression and contribution to the world. The colour, warmth and individuality that results when the sacral chakra is freed to exert its dynamic influence can dramatically change both the presentation and the presenter's sense of fulfilment. As an example of how flower essences work to positively affect the sacral chakra, Trumpet Vine flower essence helps to integrate an individual's unique and colourful energy into their verbal communication.

Ideally, the chakras open at a comfortable pace as part of each person's evolution, and consciousness develops to the degree appropriate to each chakra so that we are psychologically prepared to deal with the natural 'awakening' of chakra potential. In reality, however, this process is often disordered or interrupted. For example, let's say a young child is given (and accepts) responsibilities greater than would normally be expected of someone their age – perhaps being asked to mind their difficult-to-manage younger brother or sister on a regular basis. If the influence of the interpersonal chakras is very strong, they may seem to cope with the added responsibility – and as a result they may be promptly given more responsibility. Unfortunately, what this child really needs is to throw a few tantrums, misbehave occasionally and generally have more time behaving like a kid, in totally irresponsible bliss. To develop fully, a child needs to be given space and opportunity to 'free up' the lower and more self-centred intrapersonal chakras. If this does not happen, a six-year-old going on forty may find that they are responding to everyone else's needs, losing touch with the ability to fulfil needs of their own. If allowed the freedom of irresponsibility (within reason!) for a good part of early childhood, they have a better chance of knowing how to take on an appropriate degree of responsibility later in life, sharing responsibility in relationships for instance.

Over-emphasis on academic achievement at too early an age can also contribute to unbalanced development. The focus on higher chakras associated with academia and structured learning may raise a young child's awareness in a way that results in bypassing or neglect of developmental needs intrinsic to the lower chakras associated with emotional and social development.

Mind-altering drugs, from sugar to LSD, can also force a premature opening – a 'space invasion' of the heart, throat, brow and crown chakras – before an individual's ego-consciousness has reached a level that can comfortably accommodate suddenly expanded perspectives. Violent awakening to realms potentially associated with these chakras can, at the very least, be emotionally and mentally painful. At worst, for a person not psychologically prepared, such an awakening can put at risk a mind made fragile by newly heightened sensitivity.

The chakra system forms a network through which body, mind and spirit interact holistically. Body-mind connections can be studied by relating aspects of consciousness that pertain to each chakra to areas of the body conditioned by that chakra, giving insight into psychological processes that may have a bearing on physical illness. Of course, because chakras work together to form each individual's energy network, we cannot take one chakra out of its context among the others. Although for the purposes of study we look at the chakras individually, we must continually remind ourselves that it is their condition relative to one another that is of prime importance. We cannot influence one chakra without simultaneously influencing all the others.

I will use the analogy of a company that runs a factory. The crown chakra can be likened to the general manager, the brow chakra to the directors, the throat chakra to a factory-floor manager, and the heart, solar plexus, sacral and base chakras can be likened to the factory workers. All are vital to the proper running and success of the company. A general manager inspires by creating a vision for the direction of the company. Ideally, the directors synthesise and focus energies and resources generated by the factory unit to move the company towards realising that vision. In reality, however, they are often distracted by the floor manager who is having difficulty dealing with everyday problems arising on the factory floor.

For example, problems with personal relationships (intrapersonal chakras), problems with morale and motivation (heart chakra) interfere with production, distracting the general manager from creative envisioning of a prosperous future for the company, ultimately affecting its viability.

Often our life direction and purpose, as sensed by the crown chakra, is put on hold or clouded when lower chakras fail to work together in harmony. When working harmoniously with one another and with the higher chakras, the personality, represented by the lower chakras, can provide the energetic impetus to fuel the fire and generate resources that help realise one's true purpose in life. A balanced and harmonious relationship must be established between all chakras, just as in the factory a harmonious relationship must be established between personnel and management.

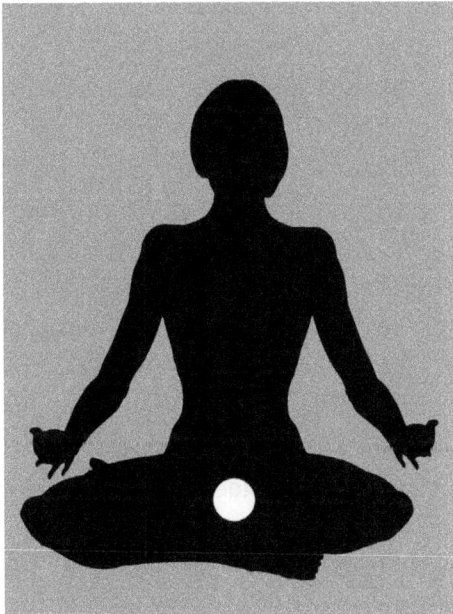

The energy of the **base chakra** is associated with the will to be – our instinct for survival and self-preservation (or lack thereof). Often called the root chakra, it is located at the base of the spine and esoteric teachings associate it with life energy and vitality, describing it as having four *red* petals. It is understood to be the origin of the kundalini energy – the fire of life, or chi as it is known in Chinese medicine. The base chakra functions to keep us 'earthed' so that our energies are focused, enabling us to fulfil our daily and life-long purpose under the guidance of deep consciousness accessed via the crown chakra. In a person whose development is proceeding well, base and crown chakras operate in a relationship that is more and more synergistic.

The *sacral chakra*, located in the area just below the navel and described in esoteric teachings as having glamorous, *red-orange* petals, governs sexuality and procreation but also vitality and personal creativity. It is the chakra that absorbs most of the impact of shock or trauma, especially that which is experienced during childhood. Often the 'memory' of an experience, in the form of congealed (primary) emotional 'charge,' remains entrenched in the sacral chakra. This may contribute to maladaptive behaviour aimed at avoiding re-experiencing the unresolved emotional pain, and/or may lead to inhibitions in behaviour, not only around sexuality but also in areas of creative endeavour. The sacral chakra adds uniqueness and colour to self-expression, and nurtures our ability to relate intimately with others. In personal development, the practical realism associated with the sacral chakra's impulse to bring projects into material existence works synergistically with the visionary idealism associated with the throat chakra.

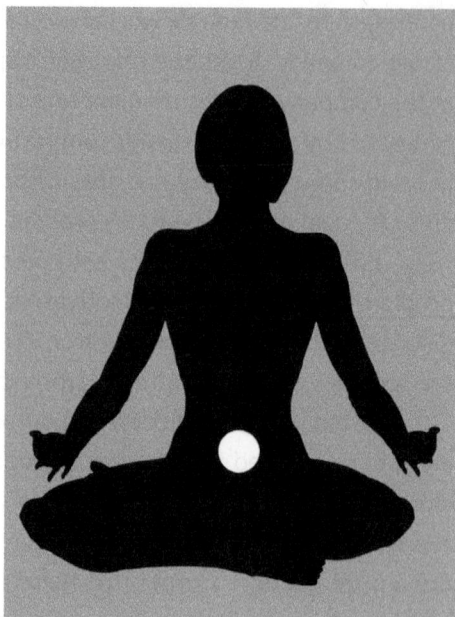

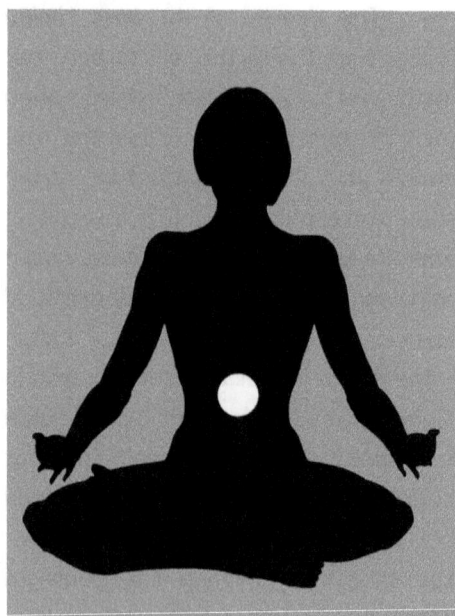

Moving up the body and out into the world, we find the *solar plexus chakra*, located just above the navel and below the chest. It has twelve petals and is associated with the colour *yellow* and all its qualities. This yellow, 'solar' aspect of the chakra highlights its relationship with how we 'shine' as an individual in the world. It represents the point of transition between intrapersonal and interpersonal aspects of self and so its condition reflects internal experiences of the world outside. Metaphors about 'digesting' life and 'taking it all in' are extremely appropriate here, as the solar plexus chakra governs the physical organs of digestion.

The *heart chakra* is situated at a point midway between the shoulder blades. It has twelve petals and the colour primarily associated with it is *green*, representing 'free space' and natural immunity, both on a physical level (this chakra governs the thymus gland) and on an emotional level. Its secondary colour is *pink*, the colour

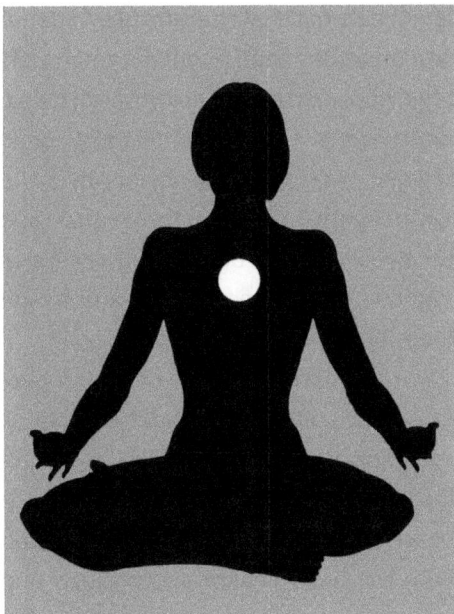

of love, and in particular, love of life and attachment to it. Heart disease and auto-immune diseases occur in epidemic proportions in the world today. The Theosophical explanation is that this is a manifestation of the energetic turbulence created by a shift of emphasis, from solar plexus consciousness to the style of consciousness that belongs to the heart chakra.

This shift is occurring both individually and collectively. When development of the base, sacral and solar plexus chakras is complete, our self-centred emphasis shifts and the more inclusive outlook of the heart chakra becomes the predominant influence in our dealings with the world. What we are seeing at present is an oscillation of energy back and forth between the heart chakra and the solar plexus chakra on a global scale. The world is aspiring to the heart chakra's level of consciousness, where individuals work for the good of all, not just the survival of self. Under the positive influence and protection of the heart chakra, we can empathise with and understand the problems of others (rather than merely sympathising, to everyone's detriment). From the space of unconditional love we can really offer help without dumping our fears and expectations on others.

Further up, at the front of the base of the neck we come to the **throat chakra** in all its sixteen-petalled, *sky-blue* brilliance. The condition of the throat chakra reflects how well we communicate our needs to the world so that the world can best support those needs. The creative aspect of Self is transmitted from the brow chakra, where it is conceptualised, to the throat chakra, where, acting in balance with the sacral chakra, creativity is vitalised and implemented. Using the house-building analogy, you could say that the brow

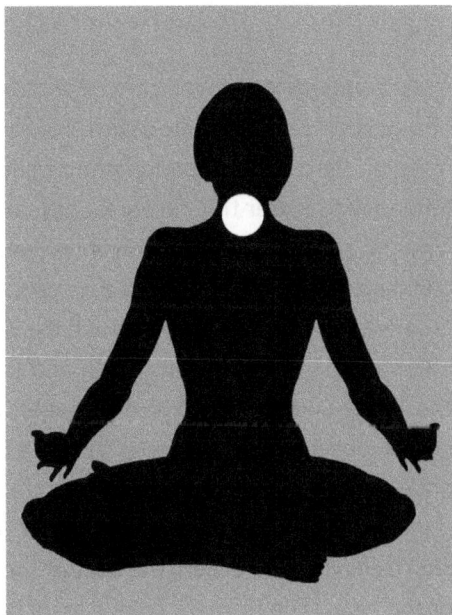

chakra conceptualises the architectural design; the throat chakra drafts plans so that the design can be 'read,' while the sacral chakra organises finance, building materials and expert trades persons required to bring the whole structure into physical being. Just as the thyroid gland has a strong influence over the major glands below it, so the throat chakra, conditioner of the thyroid gland, plays a managerial role over the energies of the lower chakras. If a person has an overly influential throat chakra, it will dominate and suppress – 'micro-manage' – the expression of the chakra energies below it. This is often the case with a more controlling type of personality and people in close relationships (work or family) with these types will feel stifled.

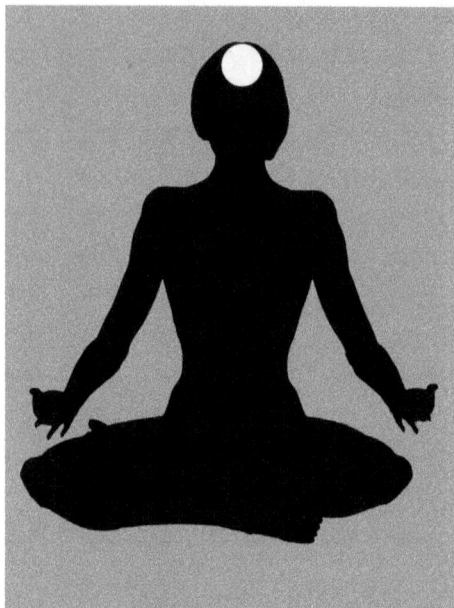

The **brow chakra**, or 'third eye,' said to be composed of ninety-six petals radiating a *deep-purple/indigo* colour, is located above the bridge of the nose between the eyes. Qualities associated with the brow chakra are intuition and insight, soul realisation and the ability to 'see' behind and beyond the superficial. Development of imagination and even clairvoyance occurs under the influence of brow chakra consciousness, as does the ability to concentrate and to relax mentally. The sinuses are conditioned by this chakra and sinus problems often reflect not only physical congestion but also congestion at a mental level. Brow chakra dominance or over-control of chakras below it leads to suppression by the mind of aspects of Self associated with chakras 'below the navel.' Because of its reliance on rational, 'hard science' explanations of life and its phenomena, Western society has a tendency to foster this cerebral approach which characterises current brow chakra consciousness. It's not that we should give desires generated by the lower chakras a completely free rein but a balance does need to be achieved between the dynamic creativity of the lower chakras and the discipline and guidance of the chakras above. The struggle between emotional and mental aspects of consciousness – between the heart and the head and between qualitative and quantitative approaches - can be observed everywhere. When a balance is struck the outcome is tolerance, understanding, growth and wisdom.

Finally on our chakra tour we come to the 'thousand-petalled-lotus' or **crown chakra**, also called 'the seat of the soul' located at, and just above, the crown of the head. The primary colour associated with the crown chakra is *violet* and the

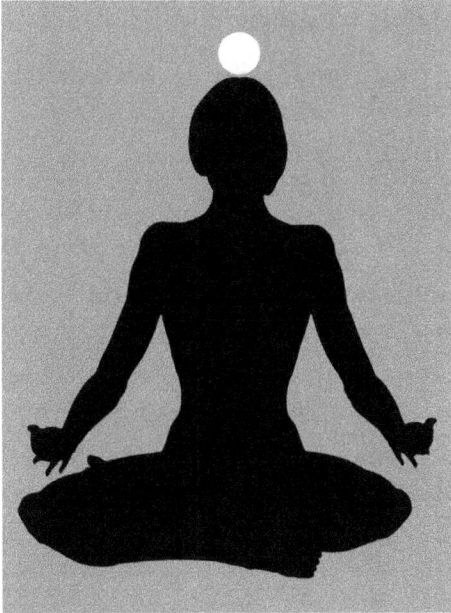

secondary colour is *white*. It is strongly integrated with the brow chakra and as we evolve as individuals the two chakras work more and more in harmony.

Just as the pineal gland receives and responds to light from the environment, so the crown chakra, which conditions the pineal gland, receives and responds to spiritual light and inspiration from the higher realms of our existence. A person with an inhibited crown chakra may lack direction, motivation and/or purpose in their life – there is often a feeling of being alone, disconnected or even marginalised. A person with a crown chakra that is overactive relative to the others may be highly self-motivated, with a strong sense of purpose and direction, but may lack tolerance and understanding of the people they are unsuccessfully trying to direct! Creative inspiration, a sense of oneness and unification with the universe, and a resulting desire for selfless service are qualities that characterise balanced crown chakra consciousness.

As we have seen, each chakra relates to issues that carry a powerful emotional charge: the will to survive; the desire to create; the capacity to shine in the world; the capacity to love unconditionally; the capacity to communicate; the capacity to focus; the capacity to be inspired. In this way, states of consciousness exert an indirect but constant influence on physical health. Disease results when there is inadequate, distorted or excessive energy flowing through one or more chakras, each of which is associated with, and acts to condition, a specific endocrine gland and certain organs and tissues. Imbalance of energy initially affects how we feel, and this is followed by changes in endocrine secretion, consequently manifesting as disease of organs and tissues.

Because of its groupings of associated mental and physical conditions, the chakra system can assist, alongside other guiding indications, in the prescription of specific flower essences. Emotional states provide pointers to possible physical consequences, and conversely, physical symptoms can give clues to underlying emotional states. As Carl Jung stated, 'The body and the mind are just two sides of the same coin.' Flower essences can be grouped and prescribed according to their potential influence on states of mind and/or physical symptoms that characterise energy disturbances in a particular chakra.

Chakras and related flower essences

On the understanding that each chakra is associated with a specific endocrine gland and certain organs and tissues where imbalances manifest as disease, I will now discuss specific ailments associated with specific chakras. In this section of the book, many individual flower essences are grouped according to their strong relationship with a particular chakra.

Base chakra

The base chakra is located between the legs and has its dynamic core in the coccyx or tailbone at the base of the spine. This chakra's sphere of influence includes the adrenal glands, kidneys, ureters, urethra, bladder, the whole spine and particularly the lumbar area, and the external genitalia and associated erogenous zones. Our most basic instincts, drives and passions are sourced in the potent energetics of the base chakra and strongly influence the function of related organs and glands. Their state and function reflect the state of dynamic balance or imbalance within the base chakra.

Let us look at some physical disorders that relate to imbalances at the level of the base chakra. They involve the spine, especially in the lumbar area, the kidneys, bladder and adrenal glands. Low blood pressure can result from insufficient energy flowing through the base chakra. This in turn can reflect a lack of will, drive or motivation in an individual, whether they are conscious of it or not. Low blood pressure may also relate to a temporary 'withdrawal' from life, a loss of passion and enthusiasm, in which case the heart chakra is equally involved.

An over-activated base chakra may result in an overstimulated adrenal gland, which may cause high blood pressure. Often people with this imbalance act and feel extremely busy, with too much to do and too little time to do it in, and are therefore constantly agitated. The stimulated adrenals have them ready for action but unfortunately they are often 'all dressed up with nowhere to go,' or 'driven with nowhere to drive,' so that eventually, if they don't address the problem, they become adrenally fatigued, often to the point of exhaustion and burnout.

The base chakra 'grounds' each of us in this life, and represents, at a deep level, our will to be here. When life is physically threatened, the adrenal glands, under the influence of the base chakra, respond by releasing adrenalin into the blood to prepare the body for action. The body responds to adrenalin by making available more blood to muscle tissues of the limbs so that the body is prepared for fight or flight. This 'fear, fight or flight' mechanism has saved lives since the dawn of time in circumstances of physical challenge but it may also shorten our lives when it takes the form of stress syndrome. In medical science adrenalin injections can be used successfully as a last-ditch effort to save a life in some cases of collapse, and cortisone, also secreted by the adrenals, is used in the treatment of life-threatening conditions such as extreme (anaphylactic) allergic reactions and asthma. In these examples a person's life is at stake, and this is the realm of the base chakra.

Total physical collapse requiring adrenalin use is an extreme example of the withdrawal of base chakra energies; a less extreme example is that of a person who is simply not 'grounded', and is lacking drive, focus and the capacity to concentrate. The need for cortisone is an extreme example of how an over-energised base chakra over-reacting to life or trying so hard to save it, can actually put life at risk! A less extreme example of base chakra over-stimulation may be seen in the person who is impatient and easily angered, trying to live as much life as possible and to achieve desperately important goals. If the high achiever in you is gradually taking over your life to an unsatisfactory degree, you might like to re-evaluate your priorities (and think about using some of the flower essences listed in this section).

On a global scale, collective imbalance in the base chakra is reflected in power battles that lead to high levels of aggression and violence in our societies. Stress or its absence indicates what state the base chakra is in. Drive, motivation and the desire to be a 'high achiever' reflects a base chakra flexing its muscles, and the same is true of 'hyperactivity' in children. Wherever we encounter red in the world there will be an associated stimulation of the base chakra, whether it is the red in the restaurant décor stimulating our appetite for food or the red in the 'red-light' district stimulating our sexual appetite. A study was carried out in Melbourne, Australia by a car insurance company to investigate the car colour most involved in accidents – and guess what? It was red! It just goes to show that there is a lot of 'bull' in all of us-especially when our personal space in threatened. A world full of balanced base chakras will be a world full of self-motivated people, peacefully working towards a common, fulfilling purpose. Perhaps reading about and using the following plants as flower essences will help bring the realisation of such a world a little closer.

Flower essences with a special affinity for the base chakra

As well as being the most important way a plant attracts and communicates with human beings (refer also to my Flower Affinity Test description), colour is very important to the doctrine of signatures in terms of the qualities it conveys, helping us to make connections with human chakras and their characteristic colours. Related to the base chakra, red's stimulant qualities are helpful to people when their basic survival skills need to be aroused, especially during times of stress. This principle is vividly illustrated at both herbal and flower essence levels in red peppers and hot chilli (*Capsicum* species). Red Clover (*Trifolium pratense*) flower essence and the Australian Bush Flower essence Waratah (*Telopea speciosissima*) also show the stimulating effect of red for those who feel consciously or unconsciously that their personal survival is under threat. The reds and purples of such herbs as Echinacea

(*Echinacea purpurea*), Burdock (*Arctium lappa*) and Sweet Violet (*Viola odorata*) can easily be related to their life-sustaining roles as 'blood cleansers' although their action may be described these days in a more 'sophisticated' way.

Some flower essences for base chakra imbalances

- Aspen
- Cayenne
- Indian Pink
- Love-Lies-Bleeding
- Mountain Pride
- Red Chestnut
- Scarlet Monkeyflower
- Waratah
- Californian Pitcher Plant
- Cherry Plum
- Fuchsia
- Lady's Slipper
- Macrocarpa
- Red Clover
- Trillium
- YES formula

Sacral chakra

The sacral chakra is located at the base of the lumbar spine just above the pubic bone, from the back to the front of the body. It influences and conditions organs, glands and tissues associated with the reproductive system. These include the ovaries, uterus and fallopian tubes in the female and the testicles and prostate in the male. The sacral centre determines the intimate relationship between the feminine and masculine forces within an individual. It influences the nature of our intimate relationship with self and others – the affection felt for self and others, our sense of value of self and others and our social urges.

Our urge to unite with others in society is generated by the sacral centre. On Earth, this urge to blend or 'instinct towards unity' (Bailey 1984) first seeks physical union in the form of sex (which has its source in our innate urge to (re)unite with the divine). Sexual relations enable the most intimate physical contact and so our sexual nature and the condition of all organs, glands and tissues associated with our sexual being are influenced by the state of our sacral centre. According to Alice Bailey (1984) the sex organs, in their relationship with the sacral centre, represent 'the creative aspect, the fashioner of the body.'

An individual's unique creative expression in the world, only possible when a deeply intimate relationship exists with oneself, has its dynamic source in the same aspects of our being as does the longing for intimate sexual interaction with another. That energy source or focus is the sacral centre. The female uterus represents the feminine principle; metaphysically, it is regarded as the seat or home of the sense of creativity in a woman. We find the sacral chakra's core in this area, seated directly in the centre of the sacrum, through which the most intimate emotions are sensed and experienced. On a physical level, the uterus provides the immediate environment for encouraging and nurturing the growth of a human being – the ultimate expression of creativity in the form of procreation on Earth. Within each menstrual cycle the uterus is prepared to receive a fertilised ovum and nurture and nourish the foetus.

Physical health problems affecting the female reproductive organs and the menstrual cycle may reflect fundamental or more current issues concerning creative expression in life. Are you able to nurture the growth of your own ideas? Do you have creative outlets in your life that support the initiation, nurturing and release of thoughts and ideas that are important to you? Problems with one's menstrual cycle could also reflect a struggle for acceptance of the feminine within the self. Any rejection, denial or resistance to the feminine may manifest in problems in the uniquely female area of the female reproductive organs. This may be relevant, for instance, to the driven, 'high achiever' who resents 'that time of the month' with a passion, believing it responsible for leaving her unable to function at her optimum.

The prostate represents the masculine principle. This gland secretes a thin, milky, alkaline fluid that 'packages' sperm and assists its flow and reception by the ovum for which it vies with other sperm. A male encountering problems with the prostate or with fertility might need to consider how he asserts or 'markets' himself – issues which relate to his level of self-esteem and self-worth. If a man is dealing with physical impotence, he may be wise to reflect on how 'potent' he feels generally and whether he may feel powerless to some degree in his work environment or his relationships. Masculine energy being what it is, many men respond to this experience by adopting a compensating persona, for instance an overt display of bravado. The underlying low self-esteem – a characteristic associated with an out-of-balance sacral centre – plays a strong role in the development of problems of impotence and sterility, which can further lower self-esteem – a vicious cycle. Working on improving self-esteem and self-worth is crucial, as well as treating the physical problem.

The sacral centre relates very closely to the etheric body in that they are both strongly implicated in what precedes physical manifestation. The sacral centre is described by Bailey (1984) as the 'predisposing agent towards physical generation,' and the etheric body, as discussed previously, provides the pattern or energy template for 'draughting' plans for growth, reproduction and birth. Etheric and sacral energies work together dynamically in the development of the template for a child's future health and have a significant influence on inherited health issues. The function of the sacral centre is therefore crucial in the first seven years of life. From a health perspective, Rudolf Steiner identifies this time as the best opportunity we have in our life to 'clean the slate' and create permanent change for the better. Otherwise we may consolidate inherited predispositions to certain types of illness. This depends to a large extent on individual karma but also on health approaches chosen for the child during these formative years. For example, suppressive treatments designed solely to oppose the symptoms of illness with no regard to the root causes and how these symptoms relate to the whole person, often only serve to perpetuate and consolidate the deeper imbalances that lie behind the outward expression of disease. On the other hand, health approaches that recognise and seek to understand the natural wisdom behind the production of certain physical symptoms provide the opportunity for, and often facilitate, resolution of a child's inherited constitutional health weaknesses.

The impact of emotional, mental and physical shock is experienced mainly through the sacral centre by human beings whether in the womb, as infants or as children. Because of its strong influence on the etheric body during the formative first seven years, a traumatised sacral centre can have a significant effect on future health and wellbeing. We should never treat the emotional impact of any childhood experience lightly and always take every opportunity to avoid or repair any emotional damage that can result. Star of Bethlehem (a component of Rescue Remedy) and Arnica flower essences, which have special affinities for the sacral chakra and solar plexus chakra, are great healers when one has experienced trauma or shock.

Our sacral centre also directly influences how we manage our 'material' appetites relating to food, sex and creature comforts associated with the 'pleasure principle' (Jacka 1990). Money is intimately connected with food, comforts and possessions and often, unfortunately, with sex. It 'can be thought of as crystallised energy or prana and is directly related to the sacral centre.' Therefore, there is a strong relationship between sacral activity and our ability to attract and manage money. It is not so much about how much or how little money we possess, but about our relationship with money and how rich we feel within.

The state of our relationship with money also reflects much about how we value ourselves and what value we put on our own contribution to the world. In other words our self-worth is directly related to the state of our sacral centre. When there is over-activity of the sacral centre, energies become too easily dispersed and unable to be properly contained or elevated to be creatively expressed through the throat chakra, the higher counterpart of the sacral chakra. What often results is 'excessive sexual activity, an excessive emphasis on material values, and a general squandering of money' (Jacka 1990). As we grow personally we learn to manage, guide and direct these energies better.

As the throat centre becomes more active, 'the energies of the sacral centre are drawn upwards and regulated by the throat centre to provide the physical means for expressing our mental creativity and for grounding our plans and ideas' (Jacka 1990). The mind then becomes more and more influential in directing physical reactions and occupies itself more with purpose and meaningful fulfillment.

From a global point of view, we can observe changes in activity of the sacral centre of particular populations, like a pendulum swinging from one extreme to another. England's Victorian era reflected a generally inhibited sacral energy, while later the pendulum swung back towards promiscuity, with accompanying epidemics of venereal disease such as genital warts, herpes, and of course HIV/AIDS. The pendulum, necessarily, has to some degree swung back, but not to Victorian extremes. We no longer have to go as far as covering the legs of furniture to preserve modesty but codes of sexual conduct do include a new 'covering' device – the condom. And because of better sexual education, more understanding of monogamy's potential joys and satisfactions has made faithfulness to one person more attractive.

We can see the swinging pendulum of sacral influence operating within the world economy too. The high-flying, 'sacrally-stimulated' entrepreneurs of the early 1980s were easily able to attract and accumulate money and possessions. They were swept along by a tide of activity in the sacral centre of the population as a whole until the economic collapse of the late eighties brought about their demise. So began a much more conservative and restrained time under the influence of the throat chakra, as its inhibiting and controlling relationship with the sacral centre reasserted itself.

Gross imbalances in global wealth and resources are a result of distorted sacral energies in the world. Weather imbalances are also associated with acute disturbances in the sacral dynamics of a population. The swinging pendulum of sacral energy operates in all of us, every day. We just have to look at our relationship with food, as we move from a period of overindulgence to one of total abstinence or dieting and back to overindulgence. We are always seeking moderation, a balanced approach to life and its pleasures, a way of living that reflects a balanced energy state in the sacral centre and a balanced relationship between the throat and sacral centres.

Finally, glamour, whether psychic or materialistic, is an expression of the attractive quality of the sacral centre, its ability to 'magnetically' attract admiration, resources and other Earthly goods. We see this quality displayed clearly in entrepreneurs, film stars, sex symbols, gurus etc. But many people blinded by glamour have been painfully reminded that 'all that glitters in not gold.' Californian Poppy flower essence is one of nature's best contributions to helping us better understand glamour and avoid being 'sucked in' by the illusions it can create. Glamour can serve a great purpose too – for example, it often brings soulmates together through mutual attraction. After the initial infatuation wanes, learning and personal growth can begin in earnest and in time, you develop in yourself those attributes you initially fell in love with in your partner. If this doesn't happen, your partner may become a constant reminder of qualities that you admire and never managed to attain. The psychoanalyst Carl Jung and those influenced by his work have written extensively on this phenomenon.

Flower essences with a special affinity for the sacral chakra

Orange relates to the sacral chakra and the emotional warmth and hospitality that is generated by that centre. Think of the feeling we get when we are greeted by the orange flowers of Calendula (*Calendula officinalis*) outside someone's door. As a flower essence, Calendula helps to bring warmth to our communication with others. The brilliant orange-gold flowers of Californian Poppy (*Eschscholzia californica*) also indicate its usefulness in bringing emotional centring, stability and 'coming home' to our hearts after searching beyond ourselves. It is said that along the Californian coastline, sailors once used the brilliance of these flowers on the hillsides as beacons to guide their course.

The Tiger Lily (*Lilium humboldtii*) has orange flowers with brown spots and is used as a flower essence to balance feminine and masculine energies, especially when masculine forces dominate. This plant is also used homoeopathically to establish better feminine hormonal balance, as in cases of inflammation, pain and prolapse of the female reproductive organs. The sacral chakra conditions our experience of intimacy and this extends to the reproductive organs through which intimacy is expressed. Consider the over-use or abuse of orange by the so called 'orange people' and their blind worship of their guru – glamour in action – see Californian Poppy for help! Plants that relate to the sacral centre mostly have flowers in shades of orange or gold. Another less frequently occurring flower colour associated with the sacral chakra is earth-brown, the colour that results from combining red and green. The flower of the elm tree is red and green and its flower essence has a strong affinity with the sacral centre.

When we become dissatisfied or disillusioned as a result of an obsession with the Earthly pleasures of the sacral centre rather than seeing them as a means to an end, or when we are faced with a catastrophe brought on by sacral excesses, 'we start to use the mind more actively to search for meaning in life' (Jacka 1990). If such a crisis has not occurred earlier, mid-life often brings with it a state of mind receptive to this kind of serious contemplation. The original colour of Chrysanthemum was golden-brown and its flower essence is often helpful to people going through a midlife crisis, especially around dissatisfaction with a materialistic focus that lacks meaning for the soul.

Some flower essences for sacral chakra imbalances

- Alpine Lily
- Calendula
- Calla Lily

- Billy Goat Plum
- Californian Poppy
- Canyon Dudleya

- Crab Apple
- Elm
- Indian Paintbrush
- Larch
- Oak
- Pomegranate
- Star of Bethlehem
- Sweet Chestnut
- Trumpet Vine
- Dogwood
- Hibiscus
- Kangaroo Paw
- Nasturtium
- Pine
- She Oak
- Sticky Monkeyflower
- Tiger Lily
- Willow
- Chrysanthemum

Solar plexus chakra

The solar plexus chakra is located inside and on the front and back of the body just above the navel. It passes through the diaphragmatic hinge between thoracic vertebra twelve (T-12) and lumbar vertebra one (L-1). Yellow is the colour associated with the solar plexus and all yellow plants and flowers have a special affinity for it. The solar plexus chakra energetically supplies and conditions all the organs and tissues of the gut area including the stomach, liver and gall bladder, pancreas and spleen. (In conjunction with the brow chakra, it also conditions the nervous system.) All physical digestive complaints relate to the condition of the solar plexus chakra. This in turn relates to how we are coping with or 'digesting' life experience. If we easily assimilate what we need from our experience of life and eliminate or 'let go' of what we don't need, we are inwardly calm and attuned to our 'gut' feelings and are able intuitively to flow with life. We possess a 'vague sense of knowing' (Brennan 1987) or intuition that allows us to sense our purpose in the moment.

The state of the solar plexus chakra very much reflects the condition of the intrapersonal chakras below it. Their condition is expressed through the solar plexus, which shapes the individual personality and the persona projected out into the world. The solar plexus is a reflection in the personality of the 'heart of the sun … the central factor in the life of the personality' (Bailey 1984) for most people. By facilitating the outward expression of the personality through our life and work, the solar plexus can act as a 'great clearing house' for the energies derived from the centres below the diaphragm. All our feelings and desires, from the crude to the subtle, are focused in the solar plexus, ranging from basic appetites to our desire for recognition, prestige and status, or just to be like someone we admire. The relationship between the solar plexus and the astral (emotional) plane is strong as it receives all the emotional reactions and desirous and impulsive energies from within and without. 'Mankind, through its individual and also through the collective solar plexus, is being subjected to almost unendurable pressure' (Bailey 1984). We are 'under fire' from all directions

– from fellow human beings, from the media, from geopathic and environmental stresses, from everywhere!

The solar (sun) plexus relates to how we, as individuals, 'shine.' When we are happy and content with who we really are, we become comfortable with living and openly displaying our real Self to the world. This issue of who we really are is foregrounded most dramatically during early adolescence in the second half of the 7–14 year age period. At that time emotional (astral) body development occurs, bringing greater personal accountability for our responses to life experience and our behaviour. It is interesting that in many cultures, children are thought to begin to become morally responsible for their actions at seven years of age, and seven year cycles are thought to mark significant turning points throughout life. The seven year Saturn cycle in astrology is a case in point, as Saturn represents the principle of learning and acquisition of wisdom from difficult life experience. It metaphorically holds up a mirror to us, especially during our 28th year. Each seven years of the Saturn cycle can reflect the development of a more responsible relationship to oneself and self-actualisation through honest confrontation with fears that inhibit personal growth and awareness.

A heightened sense of self-responsibility, especially during our teens, is accompanied by a need to manage feelings and desires. We develop our own inner authority over basic urges, especially those fascinating new desires of a sexual nature. As we grapple with the development of inner authority, we usually also have significant encounters with outer authority – most often our parents. What goes on without is a reflection of what happens within, and 'without reflects within' is the catch phrase for the solar plexus as our intrapersonal self ventures out into the interpersonal world. Acknowledgement of this projection of self onto the environment and its ability to mirror what is happening within is the key to personal responsibility and self-determination.

'All emotional disturbances, conflicts, suppressions and neuroses are connected with imbalances in the solar plexus' according to Jacka (1990) and Bailey (1984). The period between 7–14 years of age is therefore crucial for consolidation of integral emotional aspects of our personality. If we negotiate our teens well it can save us a lot of time (and money!) that we might otherwise need to spend in therapy and lot of hardship in our adult relationships.

On a global scale, mass hysteria associated with sporting events, rock concerts, political rallies, teenage peer groups, media frenzies over fear of disease etc relates to the state of the collective solar plexus. Our ability as individuals to be emotionally discerning and exercise choice over how strongly we are affected by the emotional atmosphere depends on the state of this centre. If we lose our ability to make good choices and find ourselves 'sucked in' by peer or group pressure, overwhelmed by the emotional 'heat of the moment,' this is a reflection of solar plexus imbalance. The increasing emphasis on personal growth and integration therapies, counselling and psychotherapies is a global response to a need to better direct and guide our emotional nature, rather than suppressing or releasing it indiscriminately. This work will enable our healed emotional nature to work better for us individually and for the good of mankind.

The solar plexus and heart centre have a special relationship at an individual level, evidence of which can also be seen from a global health perspective. Digestive complaints at the individual level are rampant, reflecting strong solar plexus imbalance, which in turn creates problems for the heart chakra directly above. The energies of the solar plexus centre have to be directed to the heart centre as we develop personally, just as the energies of the sacral centre have to be directed to the throat centre, as there is a strongly interactive feedback relationship between the chakras in both cases.

As polarisation shifts from the solar plexus to the heart and oscillates between the two, there has been an upsurge of nervous, digestive and heart problems throughout the world. The transference of accumulated solar plexus energies to the heart centre can cause serious difficulties and this is why so many people today die of heart disease. 'In the long cycle of soul life and experience, this is of relatively small moment; in the short cycle of the individual ... it is of great difficulty and oft of tragedy' (Bailey 1984). It is interesting to note that as heart disease has reached epidemic proportions we have begun to focus more seriously on the type (and amount!) of food we eat and the role it plays in increasing our risk of heart disease. In other words, by watching our diet, lifestyle and stress levels we are inadvertently focusing attention back on the state of our solar plexus. By 'cleaning up our act,' the shift of settled and integrated energies of the solar plexus to the heart centre can take place more easily and less dramatically.

Proper digestion and assimilation of life experience results in the acquisition of wisdom and higher knowledge. This in turn leads to acknowledgement, acceptance and expression of our individuality and autonomy. The state of the physical organs of digestion can provide insights into the manner in which we may be digesting and assimilating our everyday life experiences. The purpose on a physical level of the digestive system is to filter foodstuffs by converting them into simple constituents which can be easily absorbed and assimilated into the blood and utilised by various tissues. On a metaphysical level, the digestive process reflects our ability to filter life experiences by converting them into recognisable constituents that can easily be absorbed and assimilated into our being, and then utilised and responded to, according to our personal requirements and life purpose.

Flower essences with an affinity for the solar plexus chakra

The colour yellow in plants, especially when displayed in their flowers, reflects a connection to the qualities of the solar plexus and has an innate ability to influence it positively. Sunflowers stand up to four metres tall and project the radiance of their yellow flowers into the world without reserve. This energy is strong and upstanding but most of all it is itself. Being yourself and standing up for your spiritual Self are the qualities conveyed by this plant and the colour yellow. These qualities also reflect a balanced solar plexus.

Some flower essences for solar plexus chakra imbalances

- Agrimony
- Arnica
- Buttercup
- Chaparral
- Dandelion
- Evening Primrose
- Golden Ear Drops
- Goldenrod
- Hibbertia
- Madia
- Mullein
- Rock Rose
- Scleranthus
- Snapdragon
- Sunflower

- Aloe Vera
- Black Eyed Susan
- Chamomile
- Corn
- Dill
- Fawn Lily
- Golden Yarrow
- Gorse
- Hornbeam
- Mimulus
- Mustard
- Sagebrush
- Scotch Broom
- St John's Wort
- Tall Yellow Top
- Tansy

Heart chakra

The heart chakra is located between the 4th and 5th thoracic vertebrae at the centre of the chest. It conditions the heart, thymus gland and circulatory system including arteries, veins, capillaries and the lungs and breasts. It also governs the arms and hands in conjunction with throat chakra. The thymus gland is part of the endocrine system that is integral to the immune system, especially in producing T-lymphocytes – the white blood cells that provide protection through natural immunity against immune system challenges. Interest and research has focused on the role of the thymus gland in recent times because of the increase in auto-immune diseases such as HIV/ AIDS, cancer and other serious infections not controlled effectively by conventional medicine.

The primary colour associated with the heart chakra is green and its qualities relate to personal space, protection, natural resistance and immunity to negative influences in one's surroundings. The heart chakra's secondary colour is pink and its qualities are at the other end of the spectrum from green, relating to generous and unconditional giving of 'space' to others, and to letting go and unconditional love. Disorders that stem from heart chakra imbalance are heart problems including cardiac arrest, congestive heart failure, valvular dysfunctions, circulatory problems, high and low blood pressure (the base chakra influences blood pressure also) and lung ailments. Heart centre imbalance, in conjunction with other factors, influences the development of immune deficiency syndromes such as HIV/AIDS, cancer, lupus, scleroderma and rheumatoid arthritis.

The heart chakra is the higher octave of the base chakra and in this sense represents unconditional love for all life, which goes far beyond but is still inclusive of self-love (base chakra). It also transcends the qualities of the solar plexus related to personal love. When there is someone we love so much that we feel the importance of their life and wellbeing as keenly as our own, we are experiencing life through our heart centre. An obvious example is the way we place the lives of our children before ourselves. The heart centre relates to empathy – the ability to identify with, understand and enter into the heart of all beings, without taking on their state of mind or condition (thus the heart's radiant, natural immunity). The heart chakra confers the ability to 'walk a mile in another's shoes' and appreciate what another person feels and experiences without being brought down or undermined by it. Judy Jacka (1990) tells us that 'the radiance of the heart augments the aura and provides immunity ... from the negative conditions of people with whom we live, work and serve.' This is distinct from sympathy (associated with the solar plexus) which creates over-identification – 'For God's sake, get better for my sake!' – which results in psychic and emotional exhaustion. As healers (and lovers) we need to be aware of this.

The heart centre is the dynamic generator of group awareness and community involvement, giving us the ability to respond to group (community/world) need. Our heart's compassion provides the incentive to help. In the course of personal growth and development that occurs through serving the community and the world, the heart centre draws up energies from the solar plexus, thus integrating the emotional/feeling nature more and more with the mind. The mind, inspired by our higher nature, becomes increasingly the director of our personality. In meditation we aspire to reach a conscious state of pure reason and intuition which occurs when we commune with the collective mind. Most of us catch just a glimpse of this during meditation or at other times in our daily lives when we briefly get that crystal clear and inspirational sense of what needs to be done and the best way to do it. A deep understanding and feeling for what is right for our life is associated with a balanced heart chakra.

From a global perspective, groups or individuals who respond with service to a particular need in the environment are strongly under the influence of the heart chakra. Red Cross, the Salvation Army, groups that work towards environmental repair by clearing pollution, replanting trees, saving animals etc, groups involved in feeding the starving, educating and healing those in need are all under the guiding influence of the heart chakra. Sometimes the solar plexus takes over in individuals belonging to these groups when personality differences, individual power struggles ('politics'!) or over-emphasis on financial gain compromises the initial and true purpose of the group. Nevertheless, even with mixed motives that blend heart and solar plexus activity, these groups still transmit love energy to varying degrees. If the group is to survive the test of time, as for example the Red Cross and Salvation Army have done, the selfless qualities of the heart chakra need to prevail over self-centred (ego-driven) qualities often associated with the solar plexus.

From an esoteric perspective our stage in the development or evolution of human consciousness is in transition between that of the self-centred solar plexus and the selfless heart centre. As individuals our concerns oscillate between individual ambition and community welfare, personal gratification and unselfish giving, and between conditional and unconditional love. The unprecedented rise in heart disease and related problems further emphasise this subtle movement. This is the physical manifestation symptomatic of a collective energy shift. The frantic pace of life, which some refer to as the 'quickening,' will, hopefully, give way to a new inner and outer sense of peace and contentment.

Traditional Chinese Medicine's outline of the states of mind associated with physical states of the heart are relevant here:

Qualities associated with a healthy heart
- Mental clarity
- Good orientation
- Enthusiasm, happiness
- Alertness, awareness
- Joyfulness

Qualities associated with an unhealthy heart
- Vagueness, dullness, apathy
- Confusion, disorientation
- Disembodied and unconscious states

Flower essences with an affinity for the heart chakra

Both green and pink flowers signify the presence of heart chakra qualities and connections in a plant. Foxglove (*Digitalis purpurea*) with its pink flowers is used homoeopathically for many heart conditions and as a flower essence it assists us to 'follow our heart' and remain focused on its long term goals and aspirations. The colour green reminds us of the plant kingdom and the 'heartfelt' sense of personal space, protection and immunity from harm that we can sometimes sense when surrounded by growing plants. The green flower of Walnut (*Juglans regia*) produces a flower essence that improves natural immunity (protection) on all levels of our being. In homoeopathic form, this plant is used to treat skin conditions, and the skin can be seen as a source of information about our natural immunity to stressors in our surroundings, giving us clues about how we are reacting to what is happening around us.

Some flower essences for heart chakra imbalances

- Bleeding Heart
- Californian Wild Rose
- Cosmos
- Crowea
- Echinacea
- Holly
- Mallow
- Mariposa Lily
- Nicotiana
- Pink Yarrow
- Quince
- Shooting Star
- Sweet Pea
- Walnut
- Wedding Bush
- Bottlebrush
- Centaury
- Flannel Flower
- Lotus
- Manzanita
- Pink Monkeyflower
- Quaking Grass
- Red Grevillea
- Sturt Desert Pea
- Vervain
- Wild Rose
- YES formula
- Zinnia

Throat chakra

The throat chakra is located between the 7th cervical and 1st dorsal vertebrae. It conditions the thyroid gland and the mouth, tongue, pharynx, larynx, trachea, bronchial tree, upper lungs, lymph glands, shoulders, arms and hands. Imbalance in the throat chakra can lead to problems in the thyroid gland. The main hormone produced by the thyroid is thyroxine which regulates many metabolic activities in the body. An overactive thyroid resulting from an overstimulated throat centre speeds up metabolism in general. In extreme cases this can lead to weight loss, accelerated heart and pulse rate, high blood pressure, nervousness and restlessness. On a subtle level, this can occur when mental energies are frustrated and unable to find creative expression in the environment, becoming bottled up and turned in on themselves.

We find ourselves 'all dressed up with nowhere to go', busy but not getting anything done.

An underactive thyroid resulting from underactivity in the throat centre leads to a slowing of metabolism, weight gain, general sluggishness in mind and body, dry skin and hair and energy depletion. One can feel stifled and repressed as if there is no way out. All avenues seem blocked and there are no creative outlets. There can be a sense of hopelessness. In mid-life many of us experience these feelings. Inspiration is needed to open oneself up to new and fresh possibilities in life – a new perspective. Iris flower essence is a classic remedy to help in this situation.

Asthma, recurring bronchitis and throat infections reflect energy imbalances in the throat chakra. Congestion in the lymphatic system, especially around the throat and upper chest area is also indicative of 'congestion' in this chakra.

The throat chakra has a close relationship with the mental body in that it develops as the individual develops mentally and creatively through the ages of 14 to 28. (It is interesting to note that most study is undertaken within this time frame.) An 'old dog can still learn new tricks' later but this period is the optimum time to acquire knowledge and learn how to think and evaluate. As the mind develops, the energised throat chakra becomes a dynamic generator for planning and design – in writing, music, landscaping, creative living etc – while sacral chakra energies provide and attract the physical resources – money, energy, time, entrepreneurial support etc – for expression and manifestation of your plan in the world.

When there are imbalances between the throat and sacral chakras at an individual level, we see impractical idealists (throat chakra is over-energised and dominant) or short-sighted entrepreneurs (sacral chakra is over-energised and dominant). Impractical idealists have plenty of good ideas and thoughts that unfortunately are not put into practice and so never come into fruition. Short-sighted entrepreneurs may make a lot happen but have not properly thought it through and as a result are not prepared for the consequences of their actions. The first stage of our spiritual journey in life is marked by the transmutation of energies from the sacral to the throat chakra – occurring from the pre-teenage years, through the teenage years to adulthood. During this time we begin to develop control and direction of our physical appetites for food, sex and comfort. The pendulum can swing between strict dieting and food bingeing, celibacy and promiscuity, and on another level, between the ability to use our mental energies for self-gratification or for altruistic and spiritual purposes. The increasing activity of the throat chakra draws up energy from the sacral chakra for use in planning and structuring creative pursuits. Thus physical appetites for food, sex and comforts are re-channelled and regulated rather than suppressed. A so-called 'creative lifestyle' can be achieved in the true sense of the word.

From a global perspective the implications of a human race with more activity at the throat chakra level is seen in the advancement of communications technology. Radio, telephone, television, satellites and of course computers have dramatically advanced our ability to disseminate knowledge and extend communications throughout the world. We can now aspire to the education of the masses and ultimately the development of each individual's full creative potential.

Flower essences with an affinity for the throat chakra

The colour blue resonates with the throat chakra and expresses the same qualities. This centre conditions the thyroid gland, the lymph glands, the bronchioles and upper respiratory tract and structures involved in speech. Hyssop (*Hyssopus officinalis*) is used as a herb for respiratory problems and the flower essence made from the purple-blue flower can be helpful for those who have trouble letting go of the past, especially when feelings of grief and guilt have been suppressed. In Traditional Chinese Medicine grief is associated with the lungs. When you are feeling deeply 'blue' and discouraged and/or grieving, the essence made from the blue flowers of Borage (*Borago officinalis*) can help lift your mood to one that is more light-hearted, cheerful and positive.

Some flower essences for throat chakra imbalances

- Baby Blue Eyes
- Cerato
- Forget-Me-Not
- Iris
- Morning Glory
- Vine
- Borage
- Chicory
- Hound's Tongue
- Larkspur
- Rock Water
- Yerba Santa

Brow chakra

The brow chakra is located above the bridge of the nose and between the eyes, and for this reason it is also known as the 'third eye.' The glands and tissues conditioned by the brow chakra include the lower brain, the eyes (especially the left), the sinuses, the nervous system (with the solar plexus) and the pituitary gland. The brow chakra and its physical counterpart, the pituitary gland, supervise and regulate the chakras and endocrine glands below.

The most common physical ailments associated with a brow chakra imbalance are sinus congestion and associated headaches, nervous tension and migraines. Disorders of accommodation in the eyes, especially long and short-sightedness, are indicative of brow chakra imbalance – a reflection of how we accommodate different perspectives or struggle to 'get our head around' issues that we 'see' in our lives. Other disorders stemming from a brow chakra imbalance can include endocrine imbalances resulting from an overstimulated or understimulated pituitary gland.

The brow chakra synthesises, regulates and focuses lower chakra energies associated with our individual personality. As we develop and mature we have a choice about whether to direct the focus of these energies into self-centred ambition or more altruistic purposes or both. When working in unison with the crown chakra – our connection with our higher Self – the brow chakra can utilise the energies of our lower chakras – the personality – to become the means of distributing spiritual energies in the world. It works something like this: the brow chakra receives an idea via the crown chakra which in turn receives its inspiration from 'above on high'; the throat chakra organises this idea conceptually into a practical plan which will direct and guide the use of energies from the chakras below.

The brow chakra is the seat of our imagination and abstract ideas and so represents the highest form of creative intelligence. In this sense, we are only limited by our imagination. The nervous system is governed by the brow centre and solar plexus in conjunction. When you are intuitively able (through the brow chakra) to follow your 'gut' or feeling sense (through the solar plexus chakra) you will make the best decisions and be able to find and follow your true path in life. You remain calm and at peace. The 'head' (representing the upper chakras) and the heart (the lower chakras) are working together in harmony. When 'heart and head' find balance, the nervous system remains strong and at ease.

From a global point of view, integrated and coordinated personalities can be found in all walks of life. Often the media likes to feature ambitious and successful people who are able to follow a particular life purpose, intention or goal. These people are often driven initially by self-centred ambition but find that the achievement of ambition is not as fulfilling as expected and a feeling of emptiness and meaninglessness follows. 'In many cases this coincides with personal crises and with the development of the heart chakra as the person develops a more inclusive viewpoint of life' (Jacka 1990). They then become more part of the global brow chakra force, formed by world servers and healers, allowing the world to become a better place.

Flower essences with an affinity for the brow chakra

Dark blue and indigo colours in plants relate to the brow chakra, which conditions the way we think and 'see' things, whether calmly and clearly or in a way that is 'stressed' and without clarity. Lavender (*Lavandula officinalis*) is used herbally and as an essential oil and flower essence to calm an overactive mind and ease headaches that result from associated muscular tension. Lavender flower essence can assist in developing a meditative approach to everyday life – the hallmark of a balanced brow chakra – by helping the mind let go of unwanted thoughts and trust what lies ahead. (It eases headaches that stem from a 'head aching to go the way of the heart' and the nervous tension resulting from this struggle and associated worry.) Brow and crown chakras are closely connected, as is shown by the Elder tree, whose blossoms are used herbally to help clear the head and sinuses during colds. The colour of the purple-black berries signifies the Elder's relationship with the brow chakra, while the clusters of small white flowers sitting flat and receptive to the heavens show its affinity for the crown chakra.

Some flower essences for brow chakra imbalances

- Angelsword
- Chestnut Bud
- Honeysuckle
- Lavender
- Penstemon
- Self-Heal
- White Chestnut

- Blackberry
- Clematis
- Jasmine
- Olive
- Purple Monkeyflower
- Star Tulip
- Wild Potato Bush

Crown chakra

The crown chakra is located on and immediately above the crown of the head. The glands and tissues conditioned by it are the pineal gland, the upper brain and the right eye. Descartes originally regarded the pineal gland as the seat of the soul. Later, as knowledge of physiology and biology developed, it came to be regarded as a mere evolutionary relic until its role in hormonal regulation was recognised. We are learning more and more about the importance of melatonin, the hormone produced by the pineal gland during the hours of darkness. Melatonin has an inhibitory effect on the growth and maturation of the sex organs until puberty. Certain types of psychological depression (Seasonal Affective Disorder) can occur as a result of low melatonin levels due to lack of sunlight in winter. The reception of light (via the optic nerve) is a critical factor in the balance of pineal secretion. Excess light suppresses secretion and upsets the 24 hour (circadian) biorhythms of the body – poor lifestyle, lack of sleep and jetlag have this effect. The pineal gland operates through the hypothalamus and pituitary gland to regulate the circadian rhythms of endocrine activity in the body.

Our spiritual will flows through the crown chakra. This can enable us to comprehend at some level our best and most Self-fulfilling life path – the one that fits into the 'bigger scheme of things.' The crown chakra receives spiritual light or grace – inspirational energy – from 'above on high,' just as the pineal gland functions through a regulated reception of natural light. The crown chakra completes and refines the synthesising activity of the brow chakra. It directs 'gathered up' energies into the service of our soul's purpose and aspirations. This process, when fully developed, is a reflection of the crown and brow chakras working in perfect harmony. The resulting energy field has been sensed and portrayed as a 'halo' around the head of spiritually developed individuals.

The base and crown centres have a special relationship. The base chakra has the ability to ground us and provide drive, passion and energy (the fuel) so that we can act on inspiration we receive through the crown. The crown chakra is our most direct connection with the 'big picture' and a vision of where we 'fit in.' The base chakra is responsible for 'plugging us in' to life energy so that we can take action towards achieving our vision. As this relationship between base and crown chakras develops, most of us oscillate between directed energy and a lack of direction and motivation. When we do 'get it together,' we feel energised enough to achieve goals and fulfil our burning desires. A good rapport between crown and base chakras allows an individual's soul purpose to become manifest.

The primary global implication of the crown chakra is the movement from chaos towards order by following spiritual direction. This will occur as more and more individuals find purpose and fulfilment in their vocation and so devote their life to service in some creative way. This is happening in the arts, religion, science, healing and all walks of life.

Keywords for a balanced crown chakra:
Creative imagination; mystical instinct; sense of spiritual unity; grace and charm; co-ordination, fluidity, overview and perspective; direction and purpose; a meditative approach; wisdom; idealism and selfless service; broadening of perception.

Keywords for an unbalanced crown chakra:
Over-critical and intolerant; martyred self-righteousness; overly objective; constant day-dreaming or preoccupation; negative attitude; sense of alienation; boredom and lack of inspiration; confusion; oversensitivity.

Flower essences with an affinity for the crown chakra

The colours violet, purple and white in plants, especially when displayed in their flowers, reflect a connection with the qualities of the crown chakra and an ability to influence it positively. For example, the sharply-pointed Filaree flower bud transforms into a beautiful, well-rounded flower. The violet colour of the flower relates to the crown chakra, the 'overseer' of our lives. This reflects the flower essence's ability to help people gain a wider perspective – an overview – when they are worried or stressed over minor details and petty concerns. From the other end of the spectrum, the violet flower of Impatiens is useful for people who have an overactive crown chakra. These people know where they want to go but mere Earthlings keep getting in their way! Impatiens flower essence helps balance the crown chakra with the base and heart chakras to bring a sense of tolerance and connection, through the recognition that although we are all on different paths we are all heading to the same destination!

Some flower essences for crown chakra imbalances

- Angelica
- Deerbrush
- Fairy Lantern
- Garlic
- Impatiens
- Peppermint
- Rosemary
- Shasta Daisy
- Water Violet

- Angel's Trumpet
- Easter Lily
- Filaree
- Heather
- Mountain Pennyroyal
- Queen Anne's Lace
- Sage
- Silver Princess
- Yarrow

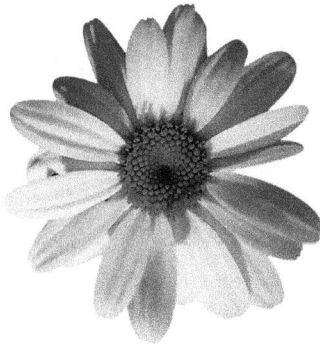

PART 2

An A–Z of flower essences

Introduction

This section contains:

- answers to frequently-asked question about the flower essences, including information about prescribing and dosages
- detailed descriptions of many well-known flower essences
- brief descriptions of further flower essences
- a flower essence selection guide

Refer to the descriptions of emotional states listed in the selection guide to find the best match with your current feelings. Then turn to the flower essences recommended for each emotional state and choose those with a personality profile that provides the best match for you.

About the flower essences – FAQs

This section is intended both as an introduction for the novice and as clarification for more experienced users of flower essences. Basic questions about the essences are answered, drawing primarily on my own many years' experience as a practitioner, and also on experience and feedback gained from participants in the courses I teach and from flower essence producers and colleagues and fellow-writers in the field.

What are flower essences and what can they do?

Flower essences come in a bottled, liquid form and are taken orally a few drops at a time. They are completely naturally derived and are made directly from specially selected flowers, picked at the time in their blooming that will give them greatest potency and healing power. After the flower infusion process is complete, only a trace of the material substance of the original flower (approximately 1/6000) remains in the potentised liquid, rendering it completely safe and non-toxic.

Flower essences act as a catalyst for positive inner transformation. They can, through raising self-awareness, assist us to transform our most negative states – fear, uncertainty, loneliness, oversensitivity to outside influences, despondency – into the corresponding positive states of courage, clarity, independence and peace of mind. They can help us develop self-esteem, assertiveness, self-reliance and self-discipline, and above all, spontaneity and warmth in relationships. Working with flower essences is like cooperating with nature to gain emotional security, health and wellbeing. Like blossoming flowers, we can open up to a fuller understanding and appreciation of ourselves, others and our world.

Flower essences are nature's soul food. The right flower essence will touch you in a special way, helping you get back onto your right path in life. After taking flower essences, many people experience a subtle shift within, which marks the change to better health and a more positive outlook on life. They experience a higher level of wellbeing and vitality, their mind is clearer and they gain a new lease on life. Flower essences can help you transform your life after long-term stress at work or in the family, when experiencing relationship problems, or after a significant loss, exerting a gentle but powerful and positive influence. With flower essences you have the tools to help yourself and others on all levels of being – physical, mental, emotional and spiritual. My personal experience and many years work as a therapist support Dr Bach's belief that emotional and spiritual health is essential for physical health. Often clients say: 'I've got this (physical) problem and I know stress makes it worse!' Appropriately chosen flower essences help them to cope better with their stresses and strains, gaining a better life perspective and a deeper sense of wellbeing. Overall improvement in health and vitality flows on from this better state of mind.

How are flower essences made?

The most common method of flower essence preparation was devised by Dr Bach and is called the Sun Method. Briefly, this involves sprinkling recently-picked blooms over the surface of pure spring water in a crystal bowl (see below). The bowl is left out in full sunlight for a specified period of time, after which the flowers are removed from the bowl. The remaining sun-potentised liquid is combined with an equal amount of brandy – a natural preservative. This liquid is often referred to as the Mother Tincture. The Stock Bottle is prepared by putting two drops of Mother Tincture in a small bottle filled with pure brandy.

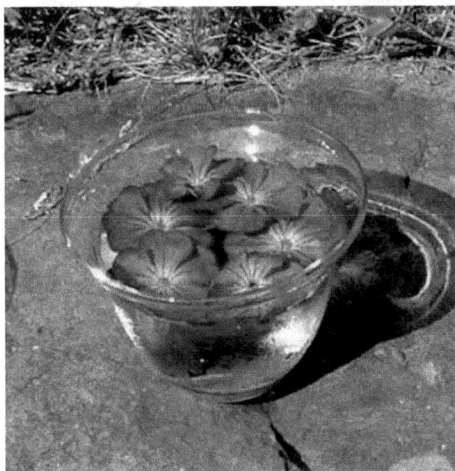

Stock liquid may be used medicinally by taking two drops under the tongue four times a day. Single or combined flower essences are also made from Stock – four drops to a 25ml bottle, for example, containing spring water and approximately ¼ brandy or vodka or pure ethanol (or vegetable glycerin or apple cider vinegar) to act as a preservative. This is called 'dosage strength,' to be taken six drops at a time, four times daily.

The sun method

- *Flowers float on spring water in bowl in full sunlight = Mother Essence Water*
- *Mother Essence Water (decanted impregnated spring water–flowers removed) + 50% brandy = Mother Tincture*
- *2 drops Mother Tincture in brandy = Stock*
- *Dosage Bottle = 4 drops Stock in 20 ml spring water and 5 ml brandy*
- *Dose = 6 drops from Dosage Bottle into mouth, generally 4x daily*

Dr Bach also used a Boiling Method to prepare some remedies. It is a similar process to the Sun Method, except that instead of being exposed to the sun, the plant material is boiled.

How do I take flower essences? Are they safe?

Flower essences are taken orally, either directly onto the tongue via a glass dropper or in a small amount of water which is sipped slowly. As previously mentioned, the ideal frequency of dose is four times daily. In acute cases, such as after an accident or other trauma or for 'pre-performance nerves', the essences may be taken much more frequently (even up to every 5 minutes for half an hour or so, if required).

We are most susceptible to the healing influence of flower essences at bedtime and on arising – at these times we are usually most relaxed and therefore most receptive. Also, during sleep we process much of the day's stress and receive insights from the unconscious. The two other doses should be spread apart across the day as evenly as possible – just before lunch and just before the evening meal are good times.

Other times that are ideal for taking flower essences are: while having a bath (they may also be put in the bathwater); after meditation and relaxation practices; during therapy or any other time you feel particularly relaxed, secure and receptive.

Do flower essences produce any side effects?

Flower essences are extremely safe. There is NO possibility of a toxic effect, because the physical amount of plant substance in the remedy is minute. Infants, children, the elderly and even pets respond positively to well-chosen flower essences with absolutely no side effects like those sometimes experienced using pharmaceutical drugs. In a very few cases there may be a heightened awareness of a particular feeling, for example while grieving, and only when a person is *ready*. One may briefly be more aware of feelings of sadness in the process of letting go of grief. This is a natural and positive experience, easily managed by adjusting frequency of dose to suit individual needs. Most people accept the process and quickly move on to a more peaceful state of mind.

Flower essences never suppress feelings but help us gain a broader perspective that enables us to better acknowledge and cope with genuine emotional reactions to life experiences.

How do they work?

The best way to understand how flower essences work is to use them yourself. This is a subjective experience and there are as many descriptions of how they work as there are people using them, and that's a lot!

Selective sensitivity response

This idea is my humble contribution to the body of flower essence experience. It can be summarised in the following way.

The inherent life force unique to each flower essence is captured and preserved in liquid form. This liquid acts as the medium between plant and person. If someone has strong similarities to the personality profile of a particular flower essence, they will be sensitive to it. This means that the distinctive life-force pattern of the flower will act as a blueprint for change, especially on the emotional level. The selective sensitivity response can be compared to the way different people respond favourably to hearing particular music or seeing a particular painting, or even to wearing particular clothes. Everyone has a unique and absolutely valid response.

By taking flower essences one develops a raised awareness, not only of the aspects of self that are interfering with one's quality of life but also of one's potential for changing those difficult aspects for the better. Of course we are free to choose what we do with this awareness; no change is forced upon us by the flower essences. We are simply offered a glimpse of our full potential.

Prescribing

Anyone can prescribe flower essences. They are totally safe and effective natural healers that are easy to understand and administer. As mentioned earlier, Dr Bach's original intention was that flower essences should be easily accessible to all. Naturally, the more familiar one becomes with the remedies through personal experience and study, the more effective and proficient one becomes at prescribing for oneself and others. For over 75 years, professional health practitioners and lay people have been prescribing the flower essences for themselves and for family, friends and pets.

It is always reassuring to remember that flower essences have a natural, in-built safety mechanism – if you choose a remedy that is not appropriate, the worst effect it can have is absolutely NO effect.

How long do I need to take the essences?

This depends on the nature of the problem. A long-term problem – one that first manifested in early childhood for example – is unlikely to resolve overnight. A flower essence may be taken for some months and then after a pause they may be taken again for a time as different aspects of the problem gradually resolve and new insights are gained. On the other hand, a more recent emotional upset may require only a few doses of the appropriate flower essence to give significant relief.

The length of time one needs to take a flower essence depends entirely on the nature and depth of the issue being addressed.

After having a good response to a flower essence, there may be no need to take it again for years, if ever – there is no need to continue after the problem is resolved.

How many flower essences can I take at one time?

Research results and my own experience as a practitioner indicate that the ideal number of flower essences to take at one time is between one and four. (However, Rescue Remedy and YES formula (FES) each comprise five flower essences and will be considered elsewhere in the book.)

It appears that taking more than four flower essences** simultaneously may make them less effective in proportion to the increase in number (refer to 'Clinical trials' section in book). This may be because, in taking more than four remedies there are too many issues to manage at once. The subtle influence of each essence becomes diffused and so has less effect or the effect is more superficial. When this happens, people may stop or just 'forget' to take the essences after a shorter period than prescribed.

** Where they have been chosen specifically for an individual (this does NOT refer to pre-formulated combinations designed for specific emotional states and/or conditions).

How do I self-prescribe?

If the negative qualities described as being addressed by a flower essence correspond to the way you are feeling NOW, then taking the remedy will give you a great opportunity to make profound positive changes in your life. As long as your state of mind and feelings closely resemble the main issues described for the essence, they do not need to match the flower essence qualities in every detail.

The key to choosing the most appropriate flower essence for yourself lies in ascertaining what you feel at this moment – your current state of mind.

Matching how you feel now with the descriptions of flower essences' emotional states will direct you to the essence most beneficial to you. Often it is easy to relate a flower essence to your past experience but I want to stress the importance of choosing according to present feelings, rather than from an intellectual analysis of your personal life-history.

> We are 'guided from within outwards ... every external motion, act, gesture, whether voluntary or mechanical, organic or mental, is produced and preceded by internal feeling or emotion, will or volition, and thought or mind ... no outward motion or change ... can take place unless provoked by an inward impulse, given through one of the three functions named.' (Blavatsky, 1888)

How do I prescribe for someone else?

> You prescribe for someone else in the same way that you would prescribe for yourself. You must ascertain the other person's current feelings, attitudes and state of mind. From this information you can choose appropriate flower essences for their use.

Asking others to disclose their feelings is something that should be done with great sensitivity. You should also respect their choice not to reveal their feelings, no matter how desperate you may be to prescribe the flower essences for them. Vervain (Bach) is an excellent remedy for anyone wishing to prescribe for all who cross their path. Often we can help others more by changing our own reactions than by forcing them into changes we think they need. In other words, it may be more productive to take an appropriate flower essence ourselves!

The flower essences A–Z

In this section there are comprehensive descriptions of flower essences produced by four different groups or organisations: Alaskan Flower Essences; Australian Bush Flower Essences; Bach Flower Essences; Flower Essence Services (FES).

Alaskan Flower Essences

Lake Minchumina is the largest lake in the interior of Alaska and is located in the geographical center of the state. In this pristine wildflower paradise, the late Steve Johnson began preparing the Alaskan Flower Essences in 1983. He founded the Alaskan Flower Essence Project in January of 1984 to coordinate preparation and research into new flower essences from this extensive and unique ecological region. I am very grateful to Steve, whose wonderful work provided the research and written material that was my original source of information on the healing qualities of these flower essences (see www.alaskanessences.com).

My descriptions of Bunchberry, Cassandra, Icelandic Poppy, Lavender Yarrow and Opium Poppy in the Supplementary Flower Essences section of this book include the abbreviation **Alask** after the plant's botanical names to indicate that these are Alaskan Flower Essences.

Australian Bush Flower Essences

Ian White is the driving force behind the Australian Bush Flower Essences. His excellent book, *Australian Bush Flower Essences*, was my original source of information and formed the basis of my understanding of this group of essences before I began to use them regularly in my practice as a therapist. I feel forever grateful for the marvellous contribution he has made and continues to make to flower essence therapy. His book gives comprehensive descriptions of the plants, their healing properties as flower essences and the intuitive ways he was drawn to these plants in the first place.

The abbreviation **Aus** indicates that the following essences belong to this group: Angelsword, Billy Goat Plum, Boab, Bottlebrush, Crowea, Flannel Flower, Hibbertia, Kangaroo Paw, Macrocarpa, Paw Paw, Red Grevillea, She Oak, Silver Princess, Sturt Desert Pea, Tall Yellow Top, Waratah, Wedding Bush, Wild Potato Bush; the Supplementary Flower Essences section includes Fringed Violet, Jacaranda.

Bach Flower Essences

For more information on the Bach Flower Essences (see also the earlier section on Dr Edward Bach) go online to the Bach Centre website (**www.bachcentre.com**) which also gives information on accredited courses run by the Centre. The work of Julian Barnard is also outstanding in the field of this group of essences, building on the foundation provided by Dr Bach. This insight and experience is available via the *Bach Flower Research Programme* (**www.edwardbach.org**) and can be found in Julian and Martine Barnard's book *The Healing Herbs of Edward Bach: an Illustrated Guide to the Flower Remedies* (1988). This book has had a significant influence on me and how I view the plants and I thank them sincerely for it.

The abbreviation **Bach** is used to indicate that the following essences belong to this group: Agrimony, Aspen, Beech, Centaury, Cerato, Cherry Plum, Chestnut Bud, Chicory, Clematis, Crab Apple, Elm, Gentian, Gorse, Heather, Holly, Honeysuckle, Hornbeam, Impatiens, Larch, Mimulus, Mustard, Oak, Olive, Pine, Red Chestnut, Rescue Remedy[TM], Rock Rose, Rock Water, Scleranthus, Star of Bethlehem, Sweet Chestnut, Vervain, Vine, Walnut, Water Violet, White Chestnut, Wild Oat, Wild Rose, Willow.

THE **ESSENTIAL** FLOWER ESSENCE BOOK

Flower Essence Services

The history and philosophy, work and achievements of the Flower Essence Society and Flower Essence Services, headed by Richard Katz and Patricia Kaminski, have been recognised previously in the 'Contemporary research' section of this book. FES divide the flower essences into three different categories and differentiate between them as follows:

1. Essences included in the *Flower Essence Repertory* (indicated by abbreviation FES)

Flower essence descriptions in this category are based on indications gathered from two to three decades of clinical reports (and this research continues to grow in depth and refinement – it is far from static). Descriptions in the *Repertory* reflect original research carried out by the Flower Essence Society.

The FES *Repertory* has been my foundational source of information in relation to this group of essences and has formed the basis of my understanding. From this foundation I have prescribed FES essences in my practice for the last 30 years.

Essences in this first group belonging to the FES *Repertory* are indicated using the abbreviation **FES** and include the following: Aloe Vera, Angelica, Angel's Trumpet, Arnica, Baby Blue Eyes, Basil, Black Eyed Susan, Blackberry, Bleeding Heart, Borage, Buttercup, Calendula, Californian Pitcher Plant, Californian Poppy, Canyon Dudleya, Cayenne, Chamomile, Chaparral, Chrysanthemum, Corn, Cosmos, Dandelion, Deerbrush, Dill, Dogwood, Easter Lily, Echinacea, Fairy Lantern, Filaree, Fuchsia, Garlic, Golden Ear Drops, Golden Yarrow, Goldenrod, Hibiscus, Hound's Tongue, Indian Paintbrush, Indian Pink, Iris, Larkspur, Lavender, Lotus, Madia, Mallow, Manzanita, Mariposa Lily, Morning Glory, Mountain Pennyroyal, Mullein, Nasturtium, Nicotiana, Oregon Grape, Peppermint, Pink Yarrow, Pomegranate, Pretty Face, Quince, Rabbitbrush, Red Clover, Rosemary, Sagebrush, Saguaro, St John's Wort, Scarlet Monkeyflower, Scotch Broom, Self-Heal, Shasta Daisy, Shooting Star, Snapdragon, Star Thistle, Sticky Monkeyflower, Sunflower, Sweet Pea, Tansy, Trillium, Trumpet Vine, Violet, Yarrow, YES formula, Zinnia; and in the 'Supplementary flower essences' section: Black Cohosh, Evening Primrose, Fawn Lily, Forget-Me-Not, Lady's Slipper, Love-Lies-Bleeding, Milkweed, Mountain Pride, Mugwort, Penstemon, Pink Monkeyflower, Poison Oak, Purple Monkeyflower, Queen Anne's Lace, Sage, Star Tulip, Yellow Star Tulip.

2. Essences for which FES have published information but which are not yet included in the FES Repertory (indicated by abbreviation FES-RL)

Currently, the FES *Range of Light* kit is in this category. It was made publically available some years ago from a selection of research remedies for which FES had received sufficient reports to move them forward from group 3. These indications were first published for members on the FES website so that FES could continue to receive reports and feedback. As understanding continued to clarify, a brochure and separate kit were created and sufficient indications have now been received for inclusion in a forthcoming edition of the *Repertory* (although they will be identified as being still in the research category so that practitioners know the insights are new and in development). **Once again, the FES brochure and website were my original source of information about these flower essences and formed the basis on which I have prescribed them in my practice over the last decade and more in some cases.**

Essences in this second group are indicated using the abbreviation **FES-RL** and include the following: Almond, Lemon; in the 'Supplementary flower essences' section: Alpine Aster, Blazing Star, Californian Peony, Californian Valerian, Cherry, Chocolate Lily, Columbine, Corn Lily, Explorer's Gentian, Fireweed, Glassy Hyacinth, Green Cross Gentian, Hawthorn, Hyssop, Joshua Tree, Lady's Mantle, Lady's Slipper, Lilac, Milkweed, Monkshood, Mountain Forget-Me-Not, Ocotillo, Red Larkspur, Redwood, Rue, Tall Mountain Larkspur.

3. Remedies produced by FES for which research is inconclusive or not substantive enough for publication (indicated by abbreviation FES-res)

This third category includes 'research remedies' which appear to hold healing promise or which practitioners have requested FES to carry. (From time to time FES eliminates flower essences for which they have never received significant reports and no longer carry them. Others they continue to carry in the hope that they will be able to 'flesh out' their healing properties in a manner that is coherent and reliable enough to move them forward into group 2 for use and research by FES members. I hope I am making at least a small contribution to this cause!) Within this group are many sub-categories – for instance FES may discuss certain preliminary indications in seminars or a specialised group of practitioners may work with certain promising remedies (for example animal healers or those who work in the hospice movement or midwifery and so forth).

For this category, my understanding has been informed by FES materials, my own herbal and homeopathic knowledge, personal research and experience in my practice as a therapist, and information provided by other flower essence producers, practitioners and students. During three decades of practice I have gathered experience of the healing qualities of these essences but agree with FES that their descriptions remain open-ended and in need of further refinement. Please take this into consideration when reading my descriptions, especially those

included in the 'A–Z' section of the book.

Essences in the third group are indicated using the abbreviation **FES-res** and include the following: Apricot, Coffee, Cotton, Foxglove, Harvest Brodiaea, Nectarine, Onion, Pansy, Passionflower, Wallflower, Watermelon; in the 'Supplementary flower essences' section: Comfrey, Daffodil, Fig, Grapefruit, Hops, Jasmine, Orange, Pear, Pennyroyal, Petunia, Prickly Pear Cactus, Skullcap, Squash (Zucchini), Stinging Nettle, Thyme, Turk's Cap.

How to use the A–Z section

Each entry is listed under its common and botanical names and these are followed by a description of the personality type that responds best to the flower essence under discussion (see 'Selective sensitivity' from 'About the flower essences – FAQs' section).

Features of flower essence descriptions include:

Key words/phrases: These are used to describe the **negative state** addressed by each essence and the **positive state** that is restored by taking the essence. Individuals seeking healing through flower essences need to match their current state of mind and emotions to the description of the negative state that is addressed. This makes sense on several levels, since, for best results, we need to acknowledge and 'own' a negative state of mind before we can transform it into its positive counterpart. In this section, direct quotes from Kaminski and Katz's FES *Flower Essence Repertory* and are followed by the abbreviation **(FES)**.

Plant signature: In the opening paragraph of each description, I often refer to the personal signature (or gesture) of the flower using the doctrine of signatures (see Part 1), giving key features of its signature in italics.

Characteristic 'personality' or 'state of mind': Many of the flower essences are described in detail, outlining qualities that come together to form a distinct, recognisable *core personality*, with *traits* and *issues* that can be identified. For people who show a 'classical' close match with these traits and issues, the flower essence will act as a constitutional remedy that is useful for a wide range of mental and emotional symptoms.

Other flower essences are described less in terms of a personality profile and more in terms of their usefulness in addressing *a state of mind that is commonly experienced by many people*. In other words, the same flower essence can help many different people facing the same emotional challenges or suffering from a similar state of mind. These flower essences are often used for briefer periods until the specific state of mind or emotion has improved. In such situations the flower essences work rapidly, as they have been selected for a fleeting emotional state rather than for who show a 'classical' close match with these traits and issues, the flower essence will act as a constitutional remedy that is useful for a wide range of mental and emotional symptoms.

Other flower essences are described less in terms of a personality profile and more in terms of their usefulness in addressing *a state of mind that is commonly experienced by many people*. In other words, the same flower essence can help many different people facing the same emotional challenges or suffering from a similar state of mind. These flower essences are often used for briefer periods until the specific state of mind or emotion has improved. In such situations the flower essences work rapidly, as they have been selected for a fleeting emotional state rather than for the personality as a whole.

Benefits of taking an essence: This section explains the benefits to be gained from taking a particular flower essence. If the core issues of the flower essence relate to you, though not necessarily in every detail, then taking this essence will help you feel better and give you the opportunity to make far-reaching changes in your life. Where appropriate, a case history is included to further illustrate how the flower essence can help in daily life.

Physical imbalances: To date, the physical problems that can be addressed by using the flower essences have not been extensively explored. However, since it is clear that mental and emotional distress and imbalance creates the preconditions for physical illness, it follows that flower essences have a powerful role to play in supporting physical wellbeing. I believe that we cannot be cured without reference to the subtle aspects of our being. I have included this section because I have a passion to discover the preconditions that contribute to illness. Under this subheading are descriptions of:

- General and specific *physical problems encountered most commonly in those who responded well* to the flower essence under discussion, as I have experienced them in my practice as a therapist.
- What I have learned from experience about body systems most likely to be affected in certain personality types *according to esoteric law*, especially related to the chakra energy centres.

Over the years, experience gained in the first area has validated the insights of the second. These connections will continue to be made as we all become more enlightened about the subtle links between mind and body. *Never choose a flower essence on physical symptoms alone*, although symptoms may be used to confirm a choice based on personality type. Physical manifestations arising from a mental and emotional state are very likely to improve following a positive change of mind.

Common uses: This section describes a group of *specific situations* in which the flower essence may be useful. It is best not to choose a flower essence on the indication of a specific situation alone. They are intended as key points in an overview of the remedy, quick references to steer you towards an appropriate choice or towards a better understanding of the full remedy picture.

Complementary &/or similar flower essences: Flower essences listed in this section are those I have found to be appropriate for use:

- *In conjunction with* the flower essence being discussed: They may complement it by covering a different facet of the pattern or their closely related qualities may reinforce its action. The overlap and the differences can create a synergistic effect, where components enhance each other in the way that those of *Rescue Remedy* or *YES formula* do. OR
- *As an alternative* if it fits the emotional pattern more accurately.

Supporting the changes: This section explores *ways of enhancing the healing action of the flower essence and supporting the positive changes that occur in response to taking it.* By developing certain life skills and engaging in appropriate activities and therapeutic techniques, we can maximise our response to the essences. Also included are suggestions for making the most of opportunities to support externally the positive internal changes that are happening. Possibilities for self-nurture during periods of vulnerability that sometimes arise when change is occurring at a deep level are also discussed.

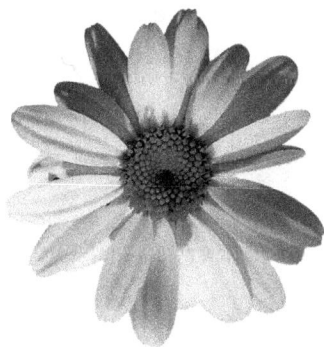

Agrimony

Agrimonia eupatoria (Yellow / Bach)

Positive state

Integration of life's light and shade – inwardly at peace
Honest expression of feelings

Negative state

Repression of sadness – inwardly tormented
Social 'mask'

Agrimony grows vertically from a small rosette of leaves at its base. It bears upright spikes of tiny yellow flowers that stand above the surrounding grasses and give it the common name of *'Church Steeples'*.

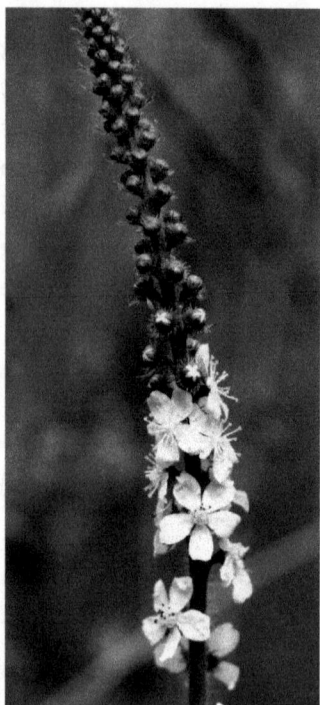

As a flower essence, Agrimony makes it possible to face, release and *rise above* painful personal *'demons'*. Dr Bach described Agrimony as a beautiful plant that had a church-like spire with seeds like bells. Agrimony's upright, spear-like growth trajectory symbolises an individual's solitary path and single purpose in *aspiring to higher levels*. Just as a church steeple rises high above its surroundings, the Agrimony person seeks to *transcend the pain and turmoil* of everyday life and tries to hide and contain the painful twisting and churning of their *gut feelings*. The plant is strongly linked to the *solar plexus* or feeling centre through its *yellow* bloom which, before it opens, resembles a *clenched and twisted claw*. When the flower opens it exposes its full and true self to the healing rays of sunlight. People taking Agrimony flower essence are also enabled to *open up* so as to release internalised pain and become more receptive to their surroundings. Then they can experience a *genuinely joyful* engagement with the world.

The Agrimony personality

Through personal growth and development we can elevate our consciousness into the natural positive Agrimony state. However, in the negative Agrimony state, we may escape or hide from reality behind a facade of high spirits (often assisted by drinking spirits!) or joviality. The Agrimony person finds it difficult to share their full experience of life with anyone else.

Agrimony people fear the consequences of exposing their true feelings to others. We are not all comfortable with what we believe to be our darker side and some of us go to great lengths to avoid uncovering it, hiding real feelings behind an easy-going, cheerful facade. We believe that if we reveal our true feelings, they may provoke rejection and contempt in others. We spend the whole day attempting to stay 'above it all', suppressing inner pain and worry that haunts us. We go to the movies, bury ourselves in books, plan the next holiday or overseas trip or drink and socialise till all hours of the night, often the life of the party. It is only when we are alone, perhaps in bed without the distractions of the day that the pain emerges and demands our full attention.

Benefits of taking Agrimony

Agrimony can help free us from societal or self-imposed emotional bondage, so that we can be comfortable about expressing honestly what we feel and who we really are. We don't have to pretend we are happy when we are not. A true feeling of cheerfulness comes very naturally to the Agrimony person when he or she can also give vent to other emotions. All aspects of the self are seen and accepted in a new light by one who is outwardly fully expressed, and therefore inwardly contented.

Possible physical imbalances

The body often expresses what the mind cannot. In the case of the Agrimony person emotional toxicity may manifest in some form of physical toxicity. Digestive disorders are common, arising from a 'suppressed gut' reaction to the world – the liver, in particular, suffers when feelings are suppressed. The digestive tract may be literally churning and knotting in the attempt to control inner 'felt' reactions.

Common uses

For disguised inner torment and worry; for insomnia from worry; for addictions and dependencies in the Agrimony type; for fear of intimacy and intense emotion; for escapism – into movies, travel, drugs etc; for the withdrawn teenager; to feel better about oneself; to help open up the heart to the world and to give protection and support in the process

Complementary &/or similar flower essences

Baby Blue Eyes, Boab, Buttercup, Californian Poppy, Chaparral, Fawn Lily, Fuchsia, Goldenrod, Golden Ear Drops, Lady's Slipper, Mullein, Nicotiana, Pink Monkeyflower, Sagebrush, Sunflower, Tall Yellow Top

Supporting the changes

- Study the Jungian concept of the Shadow.
- Maintain a healthy diet and lifestyle. Choose exercise and activities that are vigorous and extraverted rather than passive. Gentle and natural detoxification and liver-cleansing diets are worth considering. Get professional guidance if unsure.
- Until you are confident, avoid social situations where you feel under pressure to perform in some expected way. Seek out environments and people that make you feel comfortable to just be yourself.
- Say what you feel!

Almond

Prunus amygdalus (Pink/white / FES-RL)

Positive state

Independent – personally empowered
Balanced growth on all levels of our being

Negative state

Dissenting – feels oppressed and powerless
Stunted (repressed) development on one level

Almond has white flowers tinged with *pink*. The colour pink represents the *heart/ life* chakra and *white* represents the *crown* or *spirit/consciousness* chakra. When working in harmony, these two centres help to bring about *balanced and coordinated growth* on all levels of being. Another signature which emphasises Almond's influence on balanced/coordinated growth is the appearance of flowers a long time before the leaves in young almond trees. Almond flower essence can be particularly helpful during periods when there is *splinter growth* in one area and *stunted (repressed) growth* in another. For example, a teenager may mature to adulthood physically but on other levels – emotionally and mentally – still lacks maturity. This can create dissension in the mind of the teenager when they feel that they are 'all grown up' in so many ways, and yet their parents, who recognise a lack of maturity in other ways, still feel it necessary to place some limits on the teenager's freedoms for their own safety.

Another example of stunted growth is the adult who develops and becomes able and competent in many areas of life but overall remains far from fully self-realised due to significant emotional repression, as a consequence of, for instance, early childhood trauma. I believe this is a complex example of what FES describe as *'obstacles to proper growth.'* Modern research into *psychoimmunophysiology* has confirmed the serious effects of *repressed feelings* associated with life experiences, especially associated with feeling *disempowered and impotent* in one's capacity to modify or resolve experiences and their consequences. If an emotional issue is *'eating away at you'* from inside, there will always be something happening on the outside to increase its appetite. Serious illness can become a real possibility over time. Almond flower essence can help broaden our perspective of Self and enable us to take the first step towards holistic healing by *confronting inner demons* that are obstacles to our growth. It is interesting to note here that Naturopathy (originally referred to as the Nature Cure) is based on a fundamental premise which states that 'it is not the germ, it is the soil' that predisposes us to disease. In other words, it is primarily individuals' states of health and wellbeing that influence how susceptible they are to disease in their environment.

The Almond personality

The person who requires Almond flower essence usually has a deeply suppressed need for independence. Their dependence, up until now, may have prevented or 'stunted' aspects of their development. Kaminski and Katz (2008) describe the possibility of 'imbalances or lack of integration in physical and mental aspects of development.' In my practice I have observed that people who respond well to Almond flower essence often express *dissent* that can no longer be ignored. They feel that something or someone else has 'got them over a barrel' – too long have they been submissive; now they have a desire to take control of their own life and destiny and any obstacle to personal independence must be removed! We may feel this in relation to a boss, supervisor or the 'powers that be' or at home towards a domineering partner or parent(s). The rebellious teenager with 'attitude' can be a prime candidate for Almond flower essence. (Once you get over the hurdle of getting them to take it they'll thank you for it in some indirect way!)

Benefits of taking Almond

Almond helps us change our ATTITUDE to life circumstances and develop a more mature and responsible outlook. In other words, we start to 'grow up' with the integration of what, until now, have been delayed aspects of our personal development. Just as Almond oil can help moisturise and regenerate layers of our outer skin, this essence can help us nurture and generate new growth in levels of our inner being, so we become more 'comfortable in our skin.'

I treated a young woman who was currently feeling oppressed in her life. Her parents were immigrants with very strong traditional religious beliefs that belonged to their native country and the traditions of the past – she felt caught between cultures. Her friends were allowed much more freedom and she resented not being allowed to join their outings and functions. This situation caused much friction with her parents and she felt 'too angry to talk to them properly'. Almond flower essence helped her to lose some of her resentment so she was able to present her point of view calmly and clearly, without bringing any additional 'heat' to their discussions. In this way, she took a much more 'mature' approach to the situation – which did not go unnoticed by her parents. She acknowledged and respected her parents' beliefs and was able to negotiate a compromise that gave her a greater sense of freedom and independence.

Possible physical imbalances

As a therapist, I have found that a significant number of people who respond well to Almond flower essence experience skin complaints of an inflammatory nature, in particular eczema and other rashes. It seems that this is partly due to a repressed, 'heated' or 'angry' reaction to a predicament they find themselves in. It's as if things have really 'got under their skin'!

Common uses

For TEENAGERS with attitude; for people feeling resentful of their dependence on others; for 'dissension in the ranks' and feelings of powerlessness; when physical, emotional, mental and spiritual development are out of sync, producing 'stunted growth' at some level; to take the reins in one's life; to contact your inner (spiritual) authority; to develop autonomy

Complementary &/or similar flower essences

Angelsword, Blackberry, Bottlebrush, Cayenne, Chestnut Bud, Cosmos, Deerbrush, Fairy Lantern, Forget-Me-Not, Iris, Lady's Slipper, Lotus, Manzanita, Mullein, Red Grevillea, Sagebrush, Self-Heal, Sunflower, Tansy, Violet, Wallflower, Walnut, Willow

Supporting the changes

- Accept some positions of responsibility – even voluntary ones – where the 'buck' stops with you. Learn how it feels to have to delegate responsibility.
- Practise setting goals – short term and long term – to achieve what you desire.
- Be patient, and then speak up when the time is right.
- Look without and dream, but more importantly look within and WAKE!

Aloe Vera

Aloe vera (Yellow to orange-red / FES)

Positive state

Regenerated and rejuvenated
Creative/life force 'juices' flowing again

Negative state

'Burned-out' feeling (FES)
Overworked and creatively 'dried up'

Aloe Vera is found in many cosmetic products such as shampoos, skin creams and gels. Aloe's value lies in its ability not only to *regenerate* damaged or degenerated body tissue but also to *preserve and protect* against damage and degeneration. According to the Bible (John 19:39), myrrh and aloes - possibly Aloe or a closely related species – were used to embalm the body of Jesus. Traditionally, gel from *Aloe vera* leaves has also been used for the treatment of burns. Records from the first century AD tell us that the fresh juice was commonly used for external application to heal wounds, bruises and irritations. In modern medicine, fresh *Aloe* juice is employed as a salve for radiation burns.

Aloe Vera has adapted well to a harsh hot and dry environment. Survival of the fittest through *adaptation* to the environment is the cornerstone of evolution. People who push the boundaries and have created life situations for themselves that go beyond their adaptive capacity can often benefit from Aloe Vera flower essence – after *harsh reality* has finally hit home! Herbally, Aloe Vera enhances the function of the skin, which acts as a buffer between the external and internal environments, shielding us from the outside and sealing in internal moisture. The plant's moist, succulent leaves, filled with a jelly-like pulp, signify a strong and enduring presence of water, the element associated with emotion in both folklore and modern psychotherapy. Aloe Vera flower essence has the ability to soothe and replenish the *emotional element* in an individual, avoiding a shrivelling of the *etheric body*. Aloe leaves are tough and have serrated edges that can cause lacerations – this signature

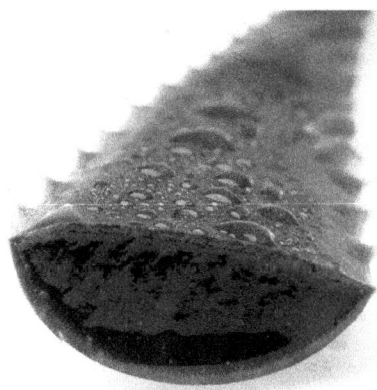

reflects the plant's ability to *heal* such lacerations or tears in the skin. Aloe Vera flower essence can help *repair* the integrity of the aura – our dynamic 'skin,' which when damaged, can bring about many emotional and nerve-related disorders

The Aloe Vera state of mind

Aloe Vera flower essence is extremely useful for people who are exhausted or burnt out from stress and overactivity. They have become depleted and 'dried up' emotionally and creatively and may have great difficulty adopting and adapting to new and healthier behaviours and habits.

Benefits of taking Aloe Vera

When you are feeling physically, mentally and emotionally exhausted, especially as a result of forcing the completion of creative work or straining for creative inspiration, consider the benefits of Aloe Vera. Over-striving can make you ignore your emotional and physical needs, neglecting food, rest and social contact in order to accomplish your goals. Kaminski and Katz (1994) explain how this attitude 'cripples [our] ability to experience life in a heart-felt way, impoverishing the feeling life, and draining the body of vital energy.' Aloe Vera can restore nerves frayed by overzealous living and help you to experience life in a heartfelt way.

The emotional body is often likened to water or fluid and it dries up when we 'burn the candle at both ends' or abuse our internal creative forces. Our creativity, ideas and inspiration are often described as being related to the fire within. The analogy of a pot boiling dry is appropriate when it comes to emotional burnout – the fire element consumes the water element. Aloe Vera flower essence replenishes the water element and brings back to balance the fire and water aspects of the psyche.

Possible physical imbalances

Physical and emotional 'burnout' is associated with the need for Aloe Vera flower essence. One feels exhausted and depleted on all levels.

Common uses

For 'burnout'; for creative block; to help revitalise, nourish and rejuvenate; to restore balance between the fire (energy/drive) and water (emotion) elements; to help the 'workaholic' gain perspective and balance in their life; to help adapt to better and more healthy behavioural patterns; for rejuvenation

Complementary &/or similar flower essences

Arnica, Chaparral, Cherry Plum, Dill, Echinacea, Forget-Me-Not, Hornbeam, Indian Paintbrush, Indian Pink, Nectarine, Olive, Lavender, Macrocarpa, Morning Glory, Nasturtium, St John's Wort, Vervain, Wild Potato Bush, YES formula

THE **ESSENTIAL** FLOWER ESSENCE BOOK

Supporting the changes

- Rest and take time out! Get some sleep before midnight on a regular basis.
- Give yourself space and time for creative pursuits. The best inspiration comes naturally and without effort.
- Meditation and relaxation methods will be helpful.
- Nourish your nervous system with nervine herbs (such as Avena, Skullcap or Passionflower), Vitamin B supplements and foods rich in this vitamin.

Angelica

Angelica archangelica (Greenish-white / FES)

Positive state

Feeling safe, secure and guided
A real sense that 'someone's looking after me'

Negative state

Feeling insecure and 'cut off' (FES)
Vulnerable; without inner guidance

The name Angelica suggests the *'guardian angel'* status that is often attributed to this plant. Herbally, it has traditionally been viewed as *protecting* against disease and poisons as well as malignant spirits and witchcraft. Its strong connection with the 'other side' is further enhanced by the *ghostlike* or *otherworldly* appearance of the flowers and stems after blooming.

Angelica's pungent, sweet smell and taste make its candied stalks perfect for decorating cakes and puddings, while the whole plant is a warming expectorant for colds and flu (Allardice et al 1994).

The leaves and flowers of Angelica consist of a vast array of complex extensions which are also *multifaceted*. This signifies its relationship with the complex network of the nervous system and its ability to help coordinate and *enhance communication* between all dimensions of the human being – none are left in *isolation*. The *white and green* colours of the flowers relate to the balanced relationship/ connection created between the *crown* and the *heart* chakras, grounding the spirit and allowing *higher guidance* to be communicated to our *everyday*

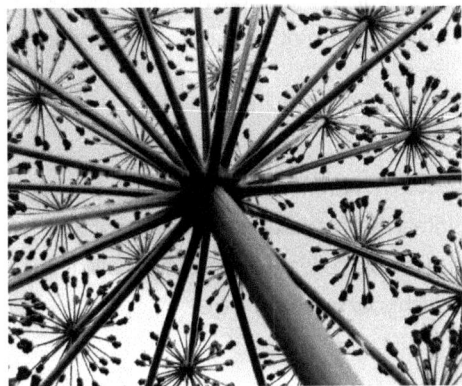

consciousness. This more open channel to our higher Self can help us sense better our connection to angelic forces, allowing us to experience a subtle sense of benevolent guidance throughout the day. This results in a lighter and more contented, meditative state, which in turn attracts (to its 'light') further benevolent support from our guardians in the angelic realms.

Angelica flower essence helps us to feel secure in our inner guidance, bringing clearer insights into aspects of personality and everyday problems.

The Angelica state of mind

When we are vulnerable and without spiritual support, Angelica flower essence can help us feel more secure. We may have lost the sense of a benevolent presence watching over us. We may even feel as if our lifeline has been severed on a spiritual level. Sometimes we come to a point in life when we believe it would be constructive to embark on self-exploration to find out what really 'makes us tick', then lose our nerve once we start to delve. Professional support – outer guidance – should be considered in this situation but Angelica can also help to take the edge off anxiety by providing a sense of inner guidance and comfort.

Benefits of taking Angelica

Taking Angelica flower essence can help us reconnect with the being who looks over us – whether it be our God, our higher Self, a guardian angel, spirit guide, soulmate or deceased relative or loved one – who we feel inspires and guides us at crucial times. Kaminski and Katz (1994) tell us that, through 'a living relationship with the angelic realm, the human soul receives guardianship and guidance in daily affairs.' Angelica can help us tap into the faith and trust that gives us strength and calm self-assurance, without letting us become reckless or overconfident.

Possible physical imbalances

The psychological sense of lack of protection can lead to a general lack of natural immunity and defence at a physical level. Research confirms that fear of 'catching something,' for instance, can undermine your natural resistance. The overproduction of cortisol – the stress hormone – suppresses our natural immune reaction. In these cases, Angelica flower essence, taken in conjunction, will enhance other natural treatments to boost the immune system.

Common uses

For feeling vulnerable and isolated on a subtle level; for a sense of being 'too open' and unguarded on an energetic level; to help the integrity of one's aura or subtle anatomy; for clearer insight; for support through major life passages – birth, death, important rituals, mid-life and menopause, major surgery etc; to 'touch base' with your guardian angel!

Complementary &/or similar flower essences

Arnica, Angel's Trumpet, Aspen, Forget-Me-Not, Fringed Violet, Garlic, Golden Yarrow, Mimulus, Mountain Pennyroyal, Oregon Grape, Queen Anne's Lace, Red Clover, Shooting Star, St John's Wort, Star of Bethlehem, Yarrow, YES formula

Supporting the changes

- Enhance your physical wellbeing with good nutrition and natural health care.
- Read about people whose faith has got them through adversity and troubled times.
- Practise meditation to tune up and tune in to your higher Self.
- Trust in your SELF!

Angel's Trumpet

Brugmansia candida   (White / FES)

Positive state

Surrendering to the path of least resistance – 'the watercourse way'
Letting go, to enable comfortable inner transformation (re-birth)

Negative state

Fear of losing control (and life)
Resistance to inner change

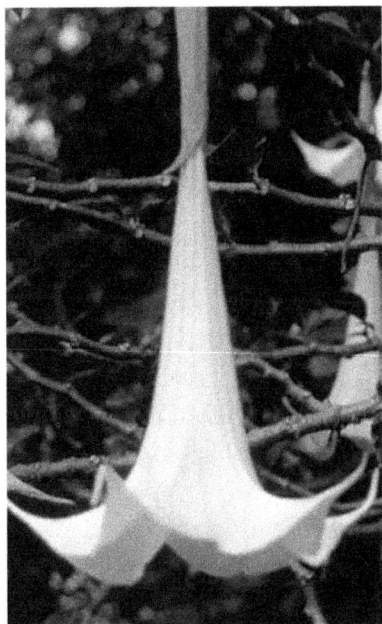

A ngel's Trumpet flower essence helps you 'blow your own trumpet' to *announce your arrival* at the next major phase on your spiritual journey. It calls forth all available angelic support and *spiritual guidance*. The white flowers signify raising the 'white flag of surrender' so that pain and discomfort can cease, and cleansing and letting go of the past can occur, with an acceptance of what lies ahead. *Rebirth and inner transformation* follows.

The Angel's Trumpet flower can be likened to a long, inverted *funnel* opening downwards to the Earth, ready to *shed light* or *draw one to the light*, for those who are ready for a clearer connection with higher spiritual realms.

If our attachment to Earth is waning and it

is no longer our higher spiritual purpose to remain, we may *surrender peacefully* to the 'pull' of our greater destiny which may lie beyond this Earth realm.

The Angel's Trumpet state of mind

When undergoing fearsome ordeals, consider Angel's Trumpet flower essence. Facing one's own impending death or the death of a loved one; becoming caught up in a war or natural disaster; when confronting seemingly insurmountable personal issues in a relationship or during therapy; when facing a fear 'worse than death' at your first public speaking engagement – in all these situations, Angel's Trumpet flower essence can support and protect you and enable you to follow the path of least resistance. All transitional phases in the cycle of life from birth to death are times when Angel's Trumpet can provide encouragement and support.

Benefits of taking Angel's Trumpet

Angel's Trumpet flower essence assists us to move through personal challenges with ease and grace, where the 'key word in understanding Angel's Trumpet is *surrender*' (Kaminski and Katz 1994) – freeing us to move with freedom through the process of inner transformation. Angel's Trumpet facilitates a spiritually safe passage through crises when our soul is challenged to be 'reborn' metaphorically or literally, to enable personal growth and soul evolution. During times of crisis we develop; our movement along the soul's evolutionary path quickens. Crises become times to look back on and give ourselves a well-deserved pat on the back! What doesn't kill you makes you stronger.

Possible physical imbalances

Angel's Trumpet flower essence is comforting and supportive when facing a potentially fatal illness. It is supportive during any major health scare or crisis when one faces mortality, especially for the first time. Angel's Trumpet is the flower essence of choice for anyone on the threshold, in the final stages of their illness.

Common uses

For those resisting inevitable major changes in their lives; to assist in surrender to what is inevitable; to support deeply transformative processes; to summon all your 'soul-mates' and allies; to follow the path of least resistance; to 'fly the coop' and SOAR!

Complementary &/or similar flower essences

Angelica, Angelsword, Arnica, Borage, Bottle Brush, Cherry Plum, Crowea, Echinacea, Forget-Me-Not, Garlic, Rescue Remedy, St John's Wort, Sweet Chestnut, Walnut, Waratah, YES formula

Supporting the changes

- Learn relaxation techniques that help you LET GO of muscular tension in the body. Focus especially on releasing those areas where you are 'holding on.' Seek help if needed.
- Explore philosophies that appeal to you which incorporate an understanding that there is 'life beyond death' and have the transience of all things at the heart of their perspective.
- Read about people who have come back from the brink and have become stronger, wiser, more 'alive' and philosophical as a result.
- Let it go, look forward, and let yourself go.

Angelsword

Lobelia gibbosa   (Blue / Aus)

Positive state

Action driven by 'inner guidance'
Strength and courage of conviction

Negative state

'Interference with true spiritual connection to higher self' (Ian White)
Confused intention

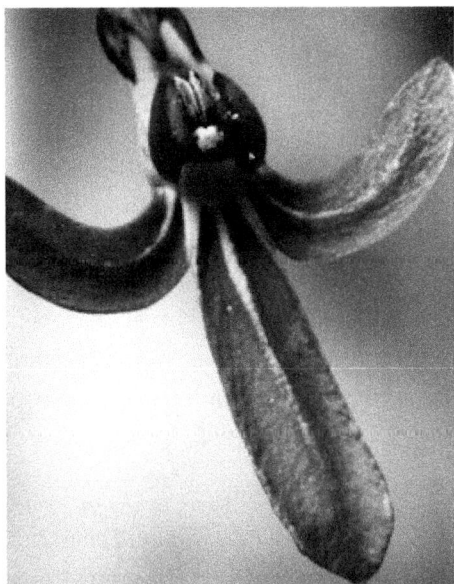

Angelsword helps you arm yourself with the *'sword of an angel'* so that you may more easily move through the *emotional and spiritual challenges* that you face. Each little flower symbolises a sword coming down from the heavens and piercing the earth with spiritual truth.

The flower essence enables people to *cut through* chaos and outside influences with piercing insight from the higher Self. They can now *'cut to the chase'* in communicating their *true intent*. The blue of the flower reminds us of its strong link to the throat chakra, the 'network connection' that enables *constructive communication* with the world.

The Angelsword personality

Sometimes we are faced with challenges that involve confrontation, whether this occurs while expressing opinions socially or at work or broaching a sensitive subject with a family member. It could be that you feel the need to stand up for an ideal or important principle at work or in the community but you fear an opposing response. Angelsword people suffer performance anxiety and wonder whether they can trust their conviction and rise to the occasion. Riddled with self-doubt, they are vulnerable to being deflected from their original intent.

Benefits of taking Angelsword

Angelsword helps you follow your true path in the face of adversity and life challenges. It helps you stay true and reach your goal even when the tide seems to be against you. Angelsword will not push you to behave in a more confrontational manner, but it can help you to be clear and resolute in your intention to resolve an issue for the eventual benefit of all. It helps you to be better understood and respected as someone who is genuine and who has an altruistic purpose, rather than being perceived as merely 'pushing your own barrow.'

I remember a client who felt strongly about environmental issues but had never taken any practical action in support of her beliefs. A sensitive environmental issue developed literally close to home for her. She decided to take a stand and take part in an organised, peaceful protest at the proposed site. She was nervous, apprehensive, embarrassed and 'just plain scared,' wondering if she could actually go through with it. She took Angelsword flower essence to help her be sure and clear about her intentions as well as to maintain the courage of her convictions. She later rang to say how much she felt it had helped her in her 'mission.'

Possible physical imbalances

Energy blockages in the throat centre can potentially lead to throat ailments of all sorts, and to thyroid issues and congestion of the lymphatic system.

Common uses

Confused in life direction; too easily swayed by outside influences; to connect with your higher Self and to spirit; for clarity of intention; for the courage of your convictions; to ground your ideals in practical action; to communicate and be loyal to your truth

Complementary &/or similar flower essences

Angelica, Angelsword, Arnica, Borage, Bottlebrush, Cherry Plum, Echinacea, Forget-Me-Not, Garlic, Mountain Pride, Mullein, Rescue Remedy, Saint John's Wort, Sweet Chestnut, Walnut, Waratah

Supporting the changes

- Seek counsel from close friends and loved ones who you know will give you HONEST feedback and counsel.
- Do your homework before embarking on any project.
- Learn to meditate to help achieve clarity.
- Acknowledge your true intent.
- Then go for it!

Apricot

Prunus armeniaca   (White / FES-res)

Positive state

Personal insight into cravings
Life is sweetened with emotional nourishment

Negative state

Strong cravings, especially for sugar/sweets
A lack of 'sweetness and lightness' in life

Apricot's sweetness gives us some indication of its relationship with sugar metabolism in the body and the part that *sweetness* plays in our lives. Apricot flower essence generally helps *raise awareness* of our emotional side and how much or little we nourish it. The *orange* of the fruit signifies its relationship to the *sacral* chakra and the quality of our intimate relationships. How much are we being *emotionally nourished* by them? Are we doing all the emotional nourishing and getting little in return? Maybe we don't allow others to add *sweetness and joy* to our lives – we just soldier on and give ourselves a reward later in the form of a sugar hit so that our moods fluctuate with each 'sugar high' (and low).

The denial of self-need and comfort is common among those for whom Apricot flower essence is useful. I once knew a seven-year-old child who had Type I diabetes. Every day she would inject herself with insulin, was diligent with her diet and regularly checked her blood sugar like a responsible 'adult'. She never complained or threw a tantrum (as other children felt free to do) and was respected highly for the way she went about her life without complaint. This is all admirable – but costly on an emotional level!

When we need apricot flower essence, we may have no idea or understanding of *how to go about getting our needs met* in everyday life. We become unable to satisfy certain emotional needs and so we reach for other forms of self-gratification to compensate for what we deny ourselves. Sugar and sweets often provide the quick fix. Apricot flower essence can help us get greater insight, mental clarity and *understanding* of the mental and emotional issues that trigger our impulsive behaviours.

The Apricot personality

Cravings, intolerances and allergies relating to certain foods are a part of everyday life for many people. For the Apricot person, there is often an unbalanced dietary response to sugar. They may crave sweets in different forms and invariably suffer mood swings after eating them. This reaction often indicates an emotional block or pain that the person seeks distraction from in eating sweet foods. Like many of my natural therapist colleagues, I have found that when a client eliminates foods to which they have an intolerance or allergy but does not also address underlying emotional issues and stress factors, they usually develop intolerances and allergies to other foods. Emotional issues can also manifest themselves in those who can benefit from Apricot flower essence in the form of excessively fluctuating blood sugar levels.

Benefits of taking Apricot

Apricot flower essence can help to process the emotional blocks or patterns that have been responsible for transference of disturbance to the physical body, for instance in the form of cravings. Repressed emotions can be allowed to surface and from a better vantage point in the mind they can be more easily negotiated. Mood swings become moderated and manageable. More sweetness and joy can flow naturally back into your life.

Possible physical imbalances

Regularly succumbing to cravings for sugar and sweet foods usually results in weight gain. Weight loss may be an indirect benefit of taking Apricot flower essence, as cravings for sugar and other carbohydrates diminish and overall diet improves. Blood sugar fluctuations, a common cause of sugar cravings, become less of an issue.

Common uses

For insight into why you crave sugar; for support and personal insight while working with eating disorders; in support of weight loss programs; for better awareness of your emotional needs; to help you find more 'sweetness' and joy in your life

Complementary &/or similar flower essences

Agrimony, Black Eyed Susan, Chamomile, Chestnut Bud, Coffee, Fuchsia, Golden Ear Drops, Iris, Lemon, Manzanita, Mariposa Lily, Morning Glory, Orange, Tansy, Zinnia

Supporting the changes

- Personal growth courses, personal counselling or psychotherapy are all supportive ways of getting to know and understand yourself better.
- Obtain personal dietary advice and include a good proportion of protein and complex carbohydrates in your diet.
- Reflect on what gives you the most pleasure and joy in life and do more of it. Try to cultivate more things that you can enjoy and look forward to every day.

Arnica

Arnica mollis   (Yellow-orange / FES)

Positive state

Healing of past and deep-seated trauma
Managing and recovering from shock/trauma

Negative state

Restriction of the vital force's full healing influence
Impediment to recovery

Arnica prefers to grow at high altitudes. It is a native of the European Alps and thrives at elevations of 1000 to 3000 metres. This preference for the *'higher ground'* is a signature of the plant's influence on the *'higher Self'* in human beings. During accidents or violent, shocking and painful experiences the higher or more subtle aspects of the human anatomy can *disassociate* from the physical body – in particular the emotional and/or etheric body can become dislocated from the physical body. In the short term this can act like a medical anaesthetic, helping us to cope and survive without feeling the full impact and pain of an extremely *traumatic experience*. Arnica flower essence can help us once again *engage the higher Self* so that the subtle levels of our being can settle back into a more stable and harmonious relationship, functioning in unison and allowing the *healing process* to progress efficiently. Arnica, in infinitesimally small doses, is to this day the standard homoeopathic remedy for trauma and shock occasioned by painful injury.

The *yellow-orange* colour of the sunflower-like blooms reflects its healing influence on the *solar plexus* (yellow) and *sacral* (orange) chakras. These energy centres take the brunt of any major *emotional (solar plexus) and physical (sacral) shock*, affecting the integrity of the emotional and etheric bodies respectively.

The Arnica personality

Consider taking Arnica flower essence as first aid after any type of trauma or shock to the system. Arnica in flower essence and homeopathic form is an essential addition to the medicine cabinet in the family home. But Arnica flower essence really comes into its own when a person is suffering from deep-seated emotional pain as a result of a past traumatic experience. Some people suffer apparently inexplicable or psychosomatic illnesses until they become aware in hindsight or during counselling that these illnesses are a direct consequence of unresolved past trauma.

Benefits of taking Arnica

Arnica positively influences our natural and vital healing forces to facilitate an efficient and more rapid recovery from emotional trauma and injury. For instance, always consider Arnica flower essence after surgery, whether minor or major. It is beneficial on a short-term first-aid basis but its true strength lies in its ability to help us recover from deep-rooted emotional trauma. Arnica can be a calming and comforting companion while undergoing professional counselling or psychotherapy, when we 'relive or re-experience the emotional trauma which accompanied the original experience' (Kaminski and Katz, 1994).

For professionals who work in the field of trauma, I have found that Arnica can provide an emotional tonic and soul support. Medical or paramedical staff involved in critical care can benefit greatly from using Arnica flower essence. People in this situation are vulnerable to losing their natural resistance to illness because of solar plexus imbalance when they are constantly exposed to, and responding to, the pain of others. Arnica flower essence can enhance natural resilience in the face of a traumatic environment. In the same way, those involved in the aftermath of natural disasters and recovery efforts can benefit from the healing and strengthening effect of Arnica.

It should be noted that the Bach Flower Remedy, Star of Bethlehem, (a component of Rescue Remedy) also has a special role in this area. The strengthening of our emotional and physical bodies and healing of deep-seated 'scars' allows our true spirit to shine through.

Possible physical imbalances

Psychosomatic or otherwise inexplicable illnesses may become manifest after a traumatic experience. Arnica is the first remedy to be considered after any traumatic physical injury.

Also, workers in the field of trauma who become unwell as a result of their work, including those suffering from burnout, will benefit from taking Arnica as a flower essence.

Common uses

After or during any shock/trauma; during counselling or psychotherapy; when reliving emotional trauma; to heal deep-seated shock or trauma from any time in the past – PTSD; to assist more efficient and rapid recovery from surgery and anaesthetic; for workers in the 'field of trauma'

Complementary &/or similar flower essences

Aloe Vera, Black Eyed Susan, Chaparral, Crowea, Dogwood, Echinacea, Fringed Violet, Garlic, Hibiscus, Love-Lies-Bleeding, Nectarine, Red Clover, Rescue Remedy, St John's Wort, Self-Heal, Star of Bethlehem, YES formula, Yerba Santa, Waratah

Supporting the changes

- Personal counselling and/or psychotherapy for recent and past trauma
- Natural healing methods and remedies to assist in recovery, especially in physical trauma
- Take extra care and be aware that just being around traumatised people has an impact on your subtle being.

Aspen

Populus tremula   (Reddish-brown / Bach)

Positive state

Secure and inwardly protected
A 'ring' of confidence

Negative state

Nameless dread
Psychically 'thin-skinned'

The leaves of the Aspen tree *tremble in anticipation* of a breath of wind on even the stillest day (Barnard, 1988), and in the same way, the Aspen personality is the first to be affected by any change in the atmosphere, living in *constant apprehension*. Julian Barnard also describes in a video on his website (healingherbs.co.uk) how the tree has a shadowy greyness, a ghostly quality to it. The patterning on the bark is 'like some runic inscription, a message from the unknown.' The bark of the tree has been used therapeutically for centuries to treat bowel complaints of a nervous origin.

Aspen people often feel as though they have been born with a *'thin skin,'* and the tree's skin or bark acts as an excellent *protective buffer* as it is thick and succulent.

The Aspen personality

Aspen flower essence is for those of us who suffer from an ever-present feeling of vulnerability or nameless dread – *fear that is of an unknown origin*. The world can feel like one huge haunted house – there is a constant sense of impending danger that has no rational basis. Waking up in the morning and contemplating the day, leaving the house for work, driving the car, greeting work-mates, coming home to an empty house – all these things may be filled with a sense of dread and apprehension.

Aspen may also be appropriate for temporary but nonetheless acute states of mind such as nightmares in either children or adults. Fearfulness resulting from the use of mind-altering drugs or just from watching a scary movie responds well to Aspen. Those days when we have an uneasy sense that something is going to happen – we know not what – are very characteristic of the negative Aspen state.

Benefits of taking Aspen

Aspen can help us to develop a thicker skin without losing the sensitivity of our nature. It helps us to comfortably bring our unconscious fears into the light of consciousness so that they no longer act as obstacles to a full and enjoyable life.

Possible physical imbalances

In the negative Aspen state, we can experience all the physical consequences of fear: shaking, goose bumps, nervous bowel complaints and even circulatory changes such as a rapid heartbeat and palpitations. Also, those of us who are constantly in a stress-induced 'fight or flight' state will become subject to kidney and adrenal fatigue.

Common uses

For fears of unknown origin; for psychic insecurity; for night terrors; for agitated (not so much anticipatory) anxiety; to bring enlightenment to unconscious fears; to develop a more secure sense of personal boundaries

Complementary &/or similar flower essences

Angelica, Angel's Trumpet, Canyon Dudleya, Corn, Dill, Echinacea, Fringed Violet, Garlic, Golden Yarrow, Indian Pink, Mimulus, Mountain Pennyroyal, Mugwort, Oregon Grape, Red Clover, Rescue Remedy, Rock Rose, St John's Wort, Violet, all the Yarrows, YES formula

Supporting the changes

- Meditation techniques, and especially visualisation of white light, can be used to strengthen your sense of inner strength and outer protection. In this way one's reserves of nervous energy are not so easily depleted.
- Avoid mind-altering drugs – even caffeine, alcohol and sugar – and other experiences that leave you negatively impressed – scary films, social situations marked with hysteria etc.
- Find or create your own special refuge – a meditation room, chapel or any place of sanctuary where you feel safe and secure. Go there in body or in spirit whenever you need to.

Baby Blue Eyes

Nemophila menziesii   (Light blue / FES)

Positive state

'No-one's fool' but open-minded
Safe and trusting in the goodness of others

Negative state

Premature loss of innocence
'It's a jungle out there – you can't trust anyone.'

Baby Blue Eyes flower essence helps people *'open their eyes'* to rediscover the qualities of trust and belief in the world. Look into the eyes of a child (perhaps your own) who has complete faith and trust in you. You will witness pure, un-ADULT-erated innocence and love. It is crystal clear that there is no greater responsibility than what you as an ADULT have been entrusted with.

Flower essence practitioner Rosana Viera, writing on the FES website (https://www.flowersociety.org/baby_blue_eyes.htm), noticed that there was a strong Piscean tone present in the astrological birth charts of many people who benefit from using Baby Blue eyes flower essence. 'The vulnerability and sensitivity of such individuals, due to their highly compassionate "water" nature, seems in the first phase of life to attract tough, disappointing, and traumatic circumstances. These situations can cast into *doubt his or her faith*, destroying trust in relationships and the larger world.' The profound healing effect of Baby Blue Eyes flower essence cannot be underestimated. Vieira credits it with the capacity to heal 'the *Father Archetype in the Soul* ... especially beneficial for those who experience the father wound through their vulnerability and sensitivity.' Baby Blue Eyes helps those who have not received adequate *emotional support and protection* through early *childhood* (Kaminski and Katz 1994). A healthy relationship with the father or a positive father figure is often absent.

It is interesting to note that as a therapist I have found that it invariably takes some time to gain the trust of those who can benefit from using Baby Blue Eyes – so it is uncommon for me to prescribe this essence at the first consultation. *Defensive layers of cynicism, mistrust and emotional guarding* often need to be shed like the layers of an onion (with the help of other flower essences) before the vulnerability of the Baby Blue Eyes nature becomes apparent. Then, as Rosana so eloquently describes it, 'this beautiful, blue-eyed flower seems to move straight to the individual's hardened personality, softening and healing the soul's conflict.'

The Baby Blue Eyes personality

Baby Blue Eyes flower essence is for those who, deep down, feel distrustful and defensive. There may be perfectly good reasons for this – it is not wise to be naive about other people, but to be hard and wary under all circumstances can limit and alienate us.

When trust is an issue it relates strongly to the nature of our early experiences in life. If we feel nurtured and safe in our formative years, we carry this sense of security with us throughout the rest of our life. It can protect us against becoming too cynical and 'hard,' as can occur if we lose our innocence too early – for example as a result of abuse at the hands of those entrusted with our care.

A classic example would be the child of a violent alcoholic parent. This child learns very early that their world is not safe and that they must never drop their guard. Over a period of time Baby Blue Eyes flower essence can help people in these circumstances to reclaim the simple trust they lost years ago. In their relationships they begin to feel safe enough to let go and display their vulnerability and so experience the joy of intimacy.

Benefits of taking Baby Blue Eyes

Baby Blue Eyes can restore a childlike innocence and trust so that we feel 'welcome' in the world rather than experiencing it as an alien or hostile environment that always has to be contested and questioned. This basic level of confidence in our environment means that we no longer need the protection of a tough exterior, and can allow ourselves to feel supported and loved by others rather than used, competed with and manipulated.

I once worked with a client whose father had died while her mother was pregnant with her. She, although unborn, FELT this loss deeply at this most formative time. According to friends and family, her mother was understandably devastated by this event but was very stoical, seemingly coping extremely well and never requesting any support. My client's difficulty was that she seemed unable to entrust anyone at her work or at home with any responsibility. She took on everything, just soldiering on with no support. It was beginning to take its toll in her relationships and was also having an effect on her physical health. She felt unsupported and emotionally isolated. As she said with a chuckle, she had gone from being 'the rock of the family to being a lonely island.' After taking Baby Blue Eyes over a couple of months she became 'a little more trusting of her husband and more open-minded' (her own words). She was more relaxed with her family, becoming less irrationally fearful and over-protective of her children and able to delegate more responsible child care roles to her husband. And of course her relationship with her husband was able to blossom again; after many years of difficulty they began to enjoy more warmth and intimacy together.

Possible physical imbalances

One can only go for so long in the negative Baby Blue Eyes state before physical health becomes an issue. Remaining stoic while carrying the burden of painful emotional trauma, especially from childhood, leads to harboured resentment that eventually undermines physical health, so that serious disease becomes a possibility.

Common uses

To restore and 'keep the faith'; to be less of a cynic; for those deprived of paternal support and protection; to sense the good nature in people; to learn to trust again

Complementary &/or similar flower essences

Angelica, Angel's Trumpet, Cherry Plum, Chrysanthemum, Dogwood, Flannel Flower, Gentian, Golden Ear Drops, Golden Yarrow, Harvest Brodiaea, Hibbertia, Hibiscus, Mallow, Mariposa Lily, Nasturtium, Nectarine, Nicotiana, Quince, Star Thistle, Sunflower, Water Violet, Yellow Star Tulip, Zinnia

Supporting the changes

- Consider having therapy. Emotional Focus Therapy (EFT) may be especially helpful.
- Try to concentrate on the good traits in people around you.
- Join a group working for an altruistic cause that you feel passionate about.
- Play in a sporting team that contains both sexes such as social netball, volleyball, mixed doubles tennis etc.
- Re-discover your inner child and have some fun!

Basil

Ocimum basilicum   (White / FES)

Positive state

Sex as a sacred and integral part of expressing love
'Integration of sexuality and spirituality' (FES)

Negative state

Secretive sexual behaviour and/or marital stress around sexual activity
Polarisation of sexuality and spirituality

Basil is well known as a culinary herb, where it features in many traditional cuisines and is favoured in tomato salads, sauces and stews. It blends well and enhances food flavours and culinary delight – permeating food with its strong character and spirit. The flower essence, too, enables permeation of *spiritual light* into areas of our life that are in the dark or form our shadow side – especially in relation to *sexuality*. The small flowers at the end of the branches are *white*, a colour that reminds us of spiritual *purification* and protection when used as a flower essence.

In herbal folklore, Basil has a strong reputation for both evil and good effects (and modern pharmacology supports the latter). As a flower essence it has the capacity to transform the polarised predicament some people experience when their *sexuality and spirituality are divided*. Basil flower essence promotes the *integration* of these aspects, making it possible to live sexuality in a spiritual way – making love in the *Light*.

The Basil personality

Basil flower essence can help those who feel unable to integrate their sexual and spiritual lives. This can include those who compulsively seek sexual activity outside a relationship, especially in the form of detached, impersonal encounters, and those who are strongly attracted to degrading and dehumanising pornography (Kaminski and Katz 1994). It can be helpful for those who feel that sex is secret, wrong or dirty and impure in comparison to some standard of spiritual purity they wish to achieve. In all these instances the soul feels great tension between the polarities of spiritual purity and physical sexuality. We suppress, deny or repress our sexual side, while on the other hand pursuing altruistic and spiritual goals in life. But this distancing and alienation of sexual desire can force it underground, bringing further guilt as it takes the form of clandestine, illicit or even illegal sexual activities.

Benefits of taking Basil

Basil helps to integrate sexuality with spirituality. Media images often separate the two, promoting sex without intimacy, sex to sell consumer products etc. The enforced celibacy of many religious practices provides further evidence of tension that occurs when spiritual purity and physical sexuality are experienced as polar opposites. In these traditions, it is believed that if a soul is spiritually evolved or in touch with divine grace, there should be no need to express love through sex. Basil flower essence signifies the integration of sexuality and spirituality into a sacred whole (Kaminski and Katz, 1994), and the remedy allows sexual acts to take their rightful place as part of our expression of spiritual communion.

Possible physical imbalances

Many people who respond well to Basil also experience a greater sense of mental clarity and better circulation to the extremities, becoming much more 'present' in mind and body. Basil and Rosemary work well together in this situation, just as they do in cooking (and as essential oils).

Common uses

For more sexual openness in your relationship; to be more comfortable in your sexuality (and in your body); to break an addiction to sex and/or pornography; for vagueness and 'out of body' discarnate states (in conjunction with Rosemary flower essence); to embrace your sexuality and your body; to make love rather than just have sex

Complementary &/or similar flower essences

Billy Goat Plum, Californian Pitcher Plant, Crab Apple, Dogwood, Easter Lily, Fairy Lantern, Flannel Flower, Hibiscus, Lotus, Manzanita, Pink Monkeyflower, Queen Anne's Lace, Rosemary, Sticky Monkeyflower

Supporting the changes

- Explore spiritual beliefs and philosophies that perceive sexuality as part of full, natural human expression.
- Consider seeking professional counselling if you feel your sexual behaviour has become too secretive or stress-producing in your relationships.
- Discuss your sex life with your partner.
- Make love!

Beech

Fagus sylvatica   (Red / Bach)

Positive state

Tolerant and unaffected by others' idiosyncrasies
Seeing the best in people

Negative state

Rigidly intolerant
Hypercritical of others (and self)

For many people, Beech represents the *perfect image* of a tree – refined and beautiful, with a lovely, balanced shape and in their European forest homelands, reaching up to forty metres in height.

Barnard (1988) provides a beautiful description of the tree as having 'smooth bark with a hard-grained and knot-free wood which can be polished to a superb finish; the young leaves covered with soft hair and minutely pleated, the purest pale translucent green, are a miracle of precision and fineness.' However, Beech trees are actually shallow rooted and *vulnerable* to being felled by storm winds once they are exposed by woodland clearance. In Beech woods, other shrubs and trees are *not tolerated* – a dense canopy and thick layer of fallen leaves *prevents* their growth. The *critical* human mind, too, is capable of reacting in a way that blocks the growth of others in order to protect itself from becoming aware of its own *underlying sensitivities, weaknesses and imperfections*, thus remaining in ignorant bliss.

The Beech personality

Beech people are often enslaved by their reactions to others who are different from them. Their intolerance of different views, behaviours, beliefs and attitudes eats away at them until they are too exhausted to care. This is the only time they get respite from their relentless over-concern about the 'incorrect' views and behaviours of others. Consider Beech when you find yourself screaming (just out of earshot) at the offender or at someone on the television screen, 'Can't you see? How can you think like that?' or 'What's wrong with these people?' How easily the fragile sense of self with its brittle mindset can be shattered by surrounding influences.

We might be in need of Beech flower essence when we see little that is good or beautiful around us. Our hypercritical nature drives away our friends and the diversity in human nature is something that confounds and annoys us rather than evoking wonder and curiosity. Even others' trivial habits or mannerisms can upset us out of all proportion to their seriousness.

The author William Hazlitt once observed that 'antipathies are always suspicious, and betray a secret affinity.' When people make us furious or earn our disapproval we should ask, 'Why am I having such a strong reaction?' And if we are honest with ourselves we will usually be able to recognise some aspect of their attitude in ourselves.

Benefits of taking Beech

As a flower essence Beech can help develop a protective buffer against feelings of invasion by different ways of being, allowing us to really appreciate, from a comfortable personal distance, the variety of styles that exist in the world. By developing better-defined personal boundaries, we are able to come to a better definition of our own truths. This makes us less judgemental of others – we no longer need to form our own protection racket! Our capacity to accept and welcome the differences that make each of us unique is increased. Variety is the spice of life.

Possible physical imbalances

Oversensitivity and over-reactivity can frequently manifest as oversensitivity to the physical environment in the form of food intolerances, allergies and skin reactions.

Common uses

For the irritability that goes with intolerance; for judgemental perfectionists; for those who are easily 'sucked in' and provoked in a negative environment; to enable one to see others' positive aspects more clearly; to be able to positively affirm more easily

Complementary &/or similar flower essences

Calendula, Chamomile, Crab Apple, Filaree, Fringed Violet, Holly, Hound's Tongue, Impatiens, Indian Pink, Iris, Mountain Pennyroyal, Quaking Grass, Quince, Snapdragon, Vine, Walnut, Willow, Yarrow

Supporting the changes

- Meditation and visualisation techniques are very useful in helping us to feel more protected and secure and develop a sense of unity and oneness at a deep level.
- Identifying and avoiding foods and other substances for which we have intolerances will mean quicker progress towards health and wellbeing. Meanwhile, Beech helps eliminate our predisposition on the subtle, emotional level at which the intolerance arises.
- Regular cleansing diets are of great value because of the tendency to become 'toxic' on all levels.
- Study the law of harmlessness – *form follows function, follows thought.*

Billy Goat Plum

Planchonia careya (White / Aus)

Positive state

At ease with physicality and our sexual being
Loving acceptance of our body (Ian White)

Negative state

Self-loathing or disgust with our body (for example a skin ailment)
Uncomfortable with physical intimacy

Billy Goat Plum's *attractive*, heavily scented flowers are large, *fleshy and moistly receptive*, with long green calyx lobes and either white or *yellow* petals (White, 2008). Numerous long stamens project from a red-orange base – *passionate projections*

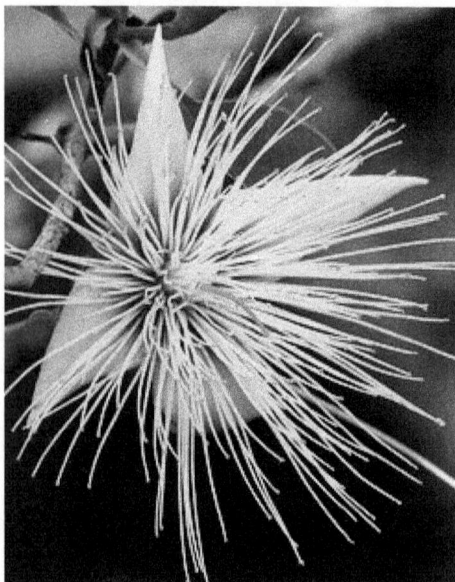

– becoming pure white toward the tips. Overall, the flower offers a *beautiful and unashamed* display of the *sexual* organs of the plant.

The *lower three chakras* are represented by the flowers' *red, orange* and *yellow* colouring. The spiritualising influence of the *crown* chakra is represented by the purity of the colour *white*. Overall, the plant's appearance symbolises an integration of the physical body with the mind and spirit and indicates the capacity of the essence to help us experience a loving appreciation of the body as a *'temple of the spirit.'*

The Billy Goat Plum personality

This flower essence relates to the spiritualisation of sexuality and a capacity to embrace the body as a temple of the spirit. Self-loathing relating to the body and its basic functions is an experience practitioners also associate with Crab Apple flower essence. In the negative Billy Goat Plum state, there may also be mental detachment from the physical body, which may be regarded as 'low,' impure and lacking spirituality (as is also the case in situations requiring Manzanita flower essence). In this state, even mentally dwelling on those aspects of the body that relate to sexual activity can prevent us from surrendering to feelings of pleasure during intimacy.

THE **ESSENTIAL** FLOWER ESSENCE BOOK

Strong feelings of disgust or repulsion accompanying physical ailments are also strongly indicative of a need for Billy Goat Plum essence. These feelings are often present in those whose physical ailments, such as skin problems, are open to view by others. Ian White (1999), founder of Australian Bush Flower Essences, informs us that First Nations people commonly used a preparation made from the inner bark of the plant as a treatment for skin problems.

Benefits of taking Billy Goat Plum

Billy Goat Plum can assist us to develop a greater acceptance of our physical body – to feel at ease and comfortable in it at all times. We can better appreciate our body as something to nurture and tune so that it can carry out its role as the precious conveyer of our spirit through life.

Possible physical imbalances

The indications for Billy Goat Plum are found more in our reactions to physical health problems than in the nature of the problems themselves, especially where there are feelings of repulsion, uncleanness and/or disgust. Billy Goat Plum may also support 'detox' and/or liver cleansing programs if there is a 'toxic feeling' element.

Common uses

For those feeling repulsed by a skin condition; for those feeling 'unclean' around sexual activity; if disgusted by some bodily functions; to help relax and enjoy your sensuality and sexuality; to love your body!

Complementary &/or similar flower essences

Arnica, Basil, California Pitcher Plant, Chrysanthemum, Crab Apple, Easter Lily, Echinacea, Flannel Flower, Hibiscus, Mallow, Manzanita, Pretty Face, Sticky Monkeyflower

Supporting the changes

- Make use of gentle and conservative cleansing diets or programs to improve how you feel about your body. Hydrotherapy or regular bathing in water blended with essential oils may also help.
- Regular, non-competitive physical exercise such as walking or swimming will improve your fitness and relationship with your body.
- Shiatsu and yoga may assist in achieving a better awareness and appreciation of your beautiful body.
- Creative visualisation can help broaden your mind. Wearing more flamboyant colours can help broaden your appeal!

Blackberry

Rubus ursinus   (Yellow/black centre / FES)

Positive state

Purposeful and decisive action
Resilient, tenacious and 'fully grounded on Earth'

Negative state

Procrastination – 'where do I start?'
'Inability to translate goals and ideals into concrete action'(FES)

Blackberry bushes' *growth* is extremely difficult to control as all gardeners know! The plant is very *resilient, tenacious and persistent*. The flower essence can confer this quality when we find it difficult to sustain the effort and focus needed to achieve certain objectives in our lives. It helps us develop persistence, *patience* and the *discipline* required to achieve any worthwhile *goal*. Just as we must wait for the fruit to ripen to full sweetness, we must persist and endure difficulties so that we may ultimately taste the *'sweetness of victory.'*

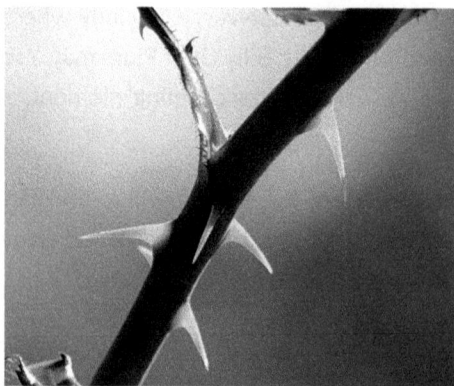

Thorns protect the plant as it grows and it persists even when cut back. Some say the only way to stop these plants regrowing is to dig out the strong root system. This strong, Earth-bound quality is also conveyed by Blackberry flower essence, which can help ground us so that we remain *focused* on the essential *groundwork* we need to do. We can then successfully *pave the way for realisation* of some of the things we have so wished for in our lives.

Protective thorns enable the plant to run rampant and this quality has been symbolically useful for humans too.

The ability to persevere, fending off all who might interfere so as to experience the sweet fruit of *persistence and patience*, symbolises a lesson the plant wishes to convey to us.

The Blackberry personality

As if stuck in brambles, Blackberry people in the negative state are trapped in the world of ideas. They may have grand plans and a clear perspective but they don't seem able to accomplish anything or put their ideas into action. They may be lazy or unmotivated, emotionally blocked or just hopelessly disorganised or distracted. Often their ideas are so grand that they feel overwhelmed and think achieving them is a remote and impossible dream. They compile a list of things to do and never do them or make New Year's resolutions that are sure to be abandoned.

Benefits of taking Blackberry

Blackberry helps you harness your will and initiative so that you can focus and achieve your goals. It helps you to organise and rationalise steps on the way to methodical achievement.

I once gave Blackberry flower essence to a friend who was feeling overwhelmed by work and other family responsibilities. He felt he was making no headway towards finishing projects at a time when his wife was due to have their second child, only eighteen months after their first. A few days after his wife had arrived home with their baby, she decided to spend a few days with her mother in the country. My friend genuinely wished to go with her and their baby but after discussion, they decided that it would be best if he stayed at home and caught up with his work. They both made a list of things to be completed during the break and at this time he began taking Blackberry flower essence.

When his wife returned home she innocently posed the question, 'How many things on the list did you get done, darling?' To which he replied sheepishly, 'Ummm, none, darling.' When pressed about what he had been doing, he explained that he had been tidying, reorganising and prioritising. He didn't yet have much to show for it but had done all the necessary groundwork for things to run smoothly and productively from now on (and they did), even allowing him plenty of quality time with his little baby. Blackberry flower essence helped him to focus on basics that needed to be done before anything else could be achieved.

Possible physical imbalances

Often Blackberry flower essence can be used to help people who are finding it difficult to establish ground rules they can follow in order to achieve a healthier diet and lifestyle. (Please also consider Tansy in this situation.)

Common uses

To ground your ideas in reality; to recognise the groundwork that needs to be done; to be 'there for the long haul' if necessary; to make it happen!; to help manifest and realise aspirations (with Cayenne essence)

Complementary &/or similar flower essences

Californian Poppy, Cayenne, (Blackberry + Cayenne is known as the 'Manifestation formula'), Clematis, Coffee, Deerbrush, Forget-Me-Not, Foxglove, Hornbeam, Indian Paintbrush, Iris, Macrocarpa, Madia, Morning Glory, Onion,

Pomegranate, Rabbitbrush, Red Grevillea, Red Lily, Shasta Daisy, Silver Princess, Tansy, Wild Oat, Wild Rose

Supporting the changes

- Regularly engage in grounding activities – working with the earth in some form (gardening or pottery for instance) and physical exercise such as bushwalking or bike-riding. If you meditate, do so in moderation.
- Balance your mental activities with physical activities.
- Set realistic goals and then focus on living and working in the moment!

Black Eyed Susan

Rudbeckia hirta   (Yellow/black centre / FES)

Positive state

Self-awareness through 'penetrating insight' (FES)
Opening of doors to our full potential

Negative state

Repressed and mentally 'edited' feelings
'Festering' emotion – 'emotional boils'

Black Eyed Susan's flower *confronts* you with its *black* central zone projecting outward (at you!) from the striking contrast of its *yellow* surrounds. You can try but you can't avoid it! Black Eyed Susan is a *powerful catalyst* to help us *confront* certain aspects of our *personality* which may have been too uncomfortable to face until now. In colour therapy, yellow is associated with the *intellect* and in those who can benefit from Black Eyed Susan essence, it is the intellect that *edits and represses*, what a person has adjudged to be his/her 'darker' emotions – *the shadow side* signified by the flower's black centre.

The Black Eyed Susan personality

In the negative state, the Black Eyed Susan person is disconnected from parts of their personality. For whatever reason – painful past experiences or suppressed anger for example – they manage to keep these dark and often painful aspects of themselves in check and 'under wraps.' They may briefly become conscious of strong feelings during a sudden, out of character, outburst. The analogy of a festering boil under the skin is often used when talking about Black Eyed Susan. Things may have been metaphorically 'getting under a person's skin' for some time until they finally erupt emotionally.

I remember a client who had been suffering from the skin condition psoriasis since his late teens. He had run his own business for two decades and had witnessed how, when under stress, his psoriasis would consistently flare up. He controlled the condition to some degree with steroid cream but it never went away entirely and he was unhappy about being dependent on the cream. I prescribed Black Eyed Susan flower essence along with some other natural remedies and dietary and lifestyle advice (especially relating to stress management). After taking the flower essence for a month he returned to inform me that he was dealing much better with the stresses of business but found that he was preoccupied by painful memories such as a difficult divorce and other unresolved family issues that he hadn't thought of for years. He commented, 'For a while there I would have preferred my stress back. In some ways it's easier to deal with than the crap I've been thinking about lately!' Fortunately, he came to his own wise conclusion and stated it in his own way: 'I suppose it's better out than in, but!' My client stuck with it and over a number of months his psoriasis improved to the point where he no longer needed steroid cream to control it. It would flare only occasionally (and not as badly as before) but he would use this as an indication that 'things were getting to him.' He would then reflect on the meaning behind it and do something constructive about it. And then he would have long periods when his psoriasis was fine. Although it was difficult at times for him to confront some emotional issues, he had learnt to appreciate the real benefits of doing so, not only for his peace of mind and wellbeing but also for his physical health. And of course his personal life was much richer for it.

(Please note that this case was not included to imply that Black Eyed Susan is the best flower essence for all psoriasis sufferers. Correct prescription always depends on choosing the flower essence(s) most appropriate for the individual at a particular time, no matter what the physical problem.)

Benefits of taking Black Eyed Susan

Black Eyed Susan helps you shed a conscious light on those aspects of Self that have remained in the dark. We all know that once you turn the light on, shadows and vague outlines are no longer so spooky, uncomfortable and mysterious as they seemed in the dark. Kaminski and Katz (1994) speak of how Black Eyed Susan 'helps the soul to integrate and transform unclaimed parts of the psyche.' A new confidence and self-assurance comes with new understanding of things that had become your demons through lack of awareness. You now know and understand yourself and others better and so become a much more enlightened being!

It takes a huge amount of energy to keep parts of our psyche repressed. Great resources of energy become available when you are no longer using energy this way, giving you a sense of vitality you may not have felt for years.

Possible physical imbalances

Many skin conditions having a marked inflammatory aspect respond well to

Black Eyed Susan. But as always for best results, be sure the flower essence matches the personality closely.

Common uses

To improve insight and perception; for support while undergoing psychotherapy; to understand what's metaphorically getting 'under your skin'; for those embarking on self-discovery; to become a more integrated person; to access your full potential

Complementary &/or similar flower essences

Agrimony, Angelsword, Arnica, Baby Blue Eyes, Black Cohosh, Californian Pitcher Plant, Chaparral, Cherry Plum, Chrysanthemum, Dogwood, Echinacea, Evening Primrose, Fuchsia, Golden Ear Drops, Milkweed, Mugwort, Pink Monkeyflower, Purple Monkeyflower, Queen Ann's Lace, St John's Wort, Star of Bethlehem, Star Tulip, Sweet Chestnut, Waratah, Yerba Santa

Supporting the changes

- Study the Jungian concept of the Shadow – that part of the unconscious that holds everything we consciously choose *not* to do or be.
- Ask a trusted friend for some feedback about yourself and the way you are.
- Pause from time to time throughout the day and ask yourself 'How am I feeling right now?'
- Stop looking solely outside yourself and look inside!

Bleeding Heart

Dicentra formosa   (Pink / FES)

Positive state

'Breathing space' in relationships
'Emotional freedom' (FES) and enJOYment

Negative state

Possessive and 'needy'
Extreme attachment

Bleeding Heart displays an obvious signature in its flower colour and shape which is like a *pink heart*. Pink is the secondary colour associated with the *heart chakra* and relates to emotional (heart) *attachment* and the *'conditional'* aspects of love. The flower essence *harmonises* affairs of the heart, especially extreme attachments

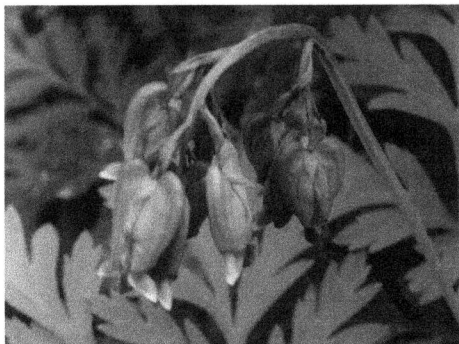

to others. The behaviour of those in the negative Bleeding Heart state is underpinned by fear of having their heart broken. Their love becomes conditional because of *fear of loss* and this fear can easily become a self-fulfilling prophecy. (When you look closely, you can often see a slight opening down the length of the heart-shaped flowers, suggesting a *broken heart*.) The overall impression of the plant when the blooming 'hearts' hang heavily downwards is precisely that of *down-heartedness*.

The flower essence's positive influence on the *heart chakra* allows a person to feel greater harmony and a sense of peace while their *loving energy* is enhanced. There is heightened ability to feel and receive *JOY*.

The Bleeding Heart personality

This flower essence is for those who fall in love too easily. They are the serial monogamists who become embroiled in one co-dependent relationship after another. Their friends and lovers begin to feel smothered and 'to feel the need for distance' (Kaminski and Katz 1994), and as they run for cover, Bleeding Heart clings to them for dear life. Once again they hear the words that have haunted them, 'I feel smothered. I need space. I need to get away for a while!' The Bleeding Heart parent may hear it expressed slightly differently by their 20-something child: 'You've got to let go, mum!'

Benefits of taking Bleeding Heart

When we are grieving over a friendship or other relationship that has finished or disappointed us (Kaminski and Katz 1994), Bleeding Heart should be considered so that both parties may feel free to love again. It can also help you to feel secure enough to give emotional freedom and personal space in new relationships. This enables you both to live, love and grow together but at the same time maintain your independence. Bleeding Heart establishes harmony in relationships, enabling an even and balanced exchange of love and support.

A number of natural therapists have also found that the Bleeding Heart flower essence is useful in assisting those in the performing arts, especially musicians. In the words of some of my clients, it helped them 'put more heart and soul' into performances, heightening their passion and their audiences' pleasure.

Possible physical imbalances

Further experience and research is required. I would recommend that it should focus on the physical organs and systems influenced by the heart chakra – the heart and circulation and the thymus gland and natural immunity.

Common uses

For emotional co-dependency; for excessive emotional 'neediness'; to help you let go emotionally; to provide personal space in relationships; to feel more emotionally secure in a relationship; to unconditionally love and be loved; to feel the joy!

Complementary &/or similar flower essences

Beech, Boab, Borage, Bottle Brush, Chicory, Foxglove, Hibbertia, Nicotiana, Pink Yarrow, Quaking Grass, Quince, Red Grevillea, Shooting Star, Sweet Pea, Sturt Desert Pea, Tall Yellow Top, Walnut, Wild Rose (Californian Wild Rose)

Supporting the changes

- Consider professional support and counselling to improve relationships.
- Cultivate passions in your life outside of personal relationships such as music, writing or some other creative outlet.
- Learn to love unconditionally. Enjoy!

Boab

Adansonia gibbosa   (Creamy white / Aus)

Positive state

'Living your own life' to your full potential
Strength and wisdom from family legacy

Negative state

'Enmeshment in negative family patterns' (Ian White)
Stuck in a stagnant dynamic with family and friends

Boab is a squat tree that grows in the tropical northwest of Australia and can live for *hundreds of years and many generations*. It is instantly recognisable by its *swollen trunk* which can be *broader than it is high* and which aids survival in a hot dry climate as it acts a *reservoir* for water over long periods of time. The *water element* is symbolic of emotion and the unconscious, and the Boab person often carries *deep-seated, ancestral emotional 'memories'* that have been *passed* on over many generations. They have been *stored* in the collective and *ancestral psyche* and lie at the root of many familial beliefs and prejudices, negative emotions and attitudes. Large, creamy white, fragrant flowers appear on the Boab tree over summer, *bound tightly* in a panicle until long after they have withered. The Boab person often needs to learn to *break free* and metaphorically 'spread their wings and *fly the coop*'!

The Boab personality

Boab people often come to recognise their parents' negative traits and fear their emergence in themselves. It could be Mum's domineering personality, grandmother's meddling, Dad's stubbornness or the unsettling feeling that we have failed to give our children space to grow, just as our parents failed to give it to us. Boab relates to the sense that 'the sins of the fathers are visited upon their children'. We feel trapped in perpetuating the mistakes and negative patterns of the past within our own families (White, 2008) and also with others to whom we may not be related but are in constant contact.

Benefits of taking Boab

The old and enduring Boab tree can bring us the wisdom of past experience and the capacity to avoid repeating old mistakes. Changing redundant behaviour patterns, especially those learned from parents, is easier said than done but Boab flower essence can help you to recognise hereditary traits that are negatively affecting your relationships or general quality of life, and be a catalyst for change. Let Boab help you to move on, be true to yourself and relinquish ingrained negative patterns.

Possible physical imbalances

The mind-body relationship is recognised as an important link in overall health. (Carl Jung described the body and mind as being two sides of the same coin.) Our emotional nature has a big influence on physical health – you only have to look at the effect of stress for confirmation of this fact. We can all recognise our parents' personality traits in ourselves – it is only logical that if Boab can influence these emotional traits it can also have a positive influence on our genetically transmitted susceptibility to certain physical health problems.

Common uses

To help survive family!; for those too easily influenced by others (especially family); to disregard what the 'Joneses' think; to follow your heart; to break free; to shine beyond everyone else's expectations; to help heal and remove negative ancestral karma

Complementary &/or similar flower essences

Almond, Bottle Brush, Chrysanthemum, Elm, Forget-Me-Not, Golden Rod, Larkspur, Lavender, Morning Glory, Mountain Pennyroyal, Mullein, Pine, Pink Yarrow, Purple Monkeyflower, Red Grevillia, Sage, Sagebrush, Saguaro, Self-Heal, Sunflower, Tansy, Walnut, Yarrow, YES formula

Supporting the changes

- Use meditation and creative visualisation to surround yourself with a shield of white light, especially in uncomfortable social or family situations.
- Consider counselling around the issue of 'surviving your family.'
- Enjoy, love and respect your family members for what they are, not what you want them to be.
- Live YOUR life!

Borage

Borago officinalis   (Blue / FES)

Positive state

'When the going gets tough, the tough get going!'
'Buoyant courage and optimism' (FES) in the face of challenge

Negative state

Succumbing to the pessimistic ('glass half empty') view
Becoming discouraged/resigned when facing personal challenges

Borage is a common annual wayside plant that was introduced to Australia from Europe and grows up to sixty centimetres in height. It is covered in soft prickly hairs and its *bright blue, star-shaped* flowers appear in drooping clusters during the warmer months. It has been valued throughout history for its ability to promote *cheerfulness and courage* and the flowers were candied as a *tonic*. Kaminski and Katz (1994) inform us that 'the "Borago" plant was originally called "Corago" referring to a state of courage associated with it ... the word *courage* [is] intimately related to the heart (*cor* is Latin for heart).' Also, the young flowers are generally pink or magenta coloured – the heart centre connection – and turn blue as they get older.

Borage is used as a salad green and the high quantities of gamma-linolenic acid in its seeds has made it more effective than Evening Primrose oil as a supplement for hormonal balance. There is also evidence that gamma-linolenic acid is beneficial to *heart* health and function, although in some cases of advanced heart disease there is a question as to whether it may be too stimulating for safe use. No such problem exists with using Borage flower essence and the plant's herbal properties add further support for the flower essence's positive influence on *heart energy*.

This essence's *uplifting* and energy-enhancing effect on the *heart chakra* helps bring about greater *bonding* in relationships so that difficult circumstances can be faced with courage. As the song says, 'He ain't heavy – he's my brother.' Borage flower essence can also be given to animals living together in confined spaces to create a better bond between them.

The Borage state of mind

When faced with apparently insurmountable obstacles, we often feel mentally burdened. The load can seem too heavy and we lose our sense of joy and humour. Borage flower essence can lift our spirits so that we can tackle problems and challenges in a much more light-hearted, energetic and direct way.

Benefits of taking Borage

Laughter and humour are now recognised as being therapeutic for many problems. We've all felt better after a good 'belly laugh.' Clowns in hospitals, laughing workshops and humour therapy can have profoundly positive effects on health and wellbeing, especially through their effects on the immune system. Borage can be a catalyst in this process of lightening up and learning to look on the bright side of life.

The loss of a loved one and the thought of life without them; keeping spirits up while nursing a loved one with a serious or terminal illness; upcoming exams, increasing work pressures and an expanding family are all challenges that Borage can help us through.

Possible physical imbalances

Borage's strong connection with the heart centre implies its positive influence on the thymus gland which is associated with the heart – and our natural immunity. Good cheer and a positive frame of mind strengthens immunity against the potentially negative and stressful effects of life's challenges. Put simply, Borage can play a strong role in maintaining natural immunity on all levels.

Common uses

For disheartened and discouraged humans and animals; while anticipating or experiencing challenging periods; for 'keeping the faith' and having a 'glass half full' view; to be UP for the challenge; to help maintain good cheer; for a therapeutic GUT-LAUGH!

Complementary &/or similar flower essences

Angelica, Angelsword, Crowea, Echinacea, Elm, Forget-Me-Not, Foxglove, Garlic, Gentian, Gorse, Harvest Brodiaea, Hornbeam, Hound's Tongue, Iris, Larkspur, Love-Lies-Bleeding, Macrocarpa, Mountain Pride, Penstemon, Scotch Broom, Self-Heal, Sturt Desert Pea, Waratah, Wild Rose, Willow, Yerba Santa, Zinnia

Supporting the changes

- Use creative visualisation to help sustain a positive outlook.

- Support your immune system with a healthy diet and lifestyle, and always consider consulting a natural therapist for professional advice.
- Surround yourself with positive people who make you laugh – engage in laughter therapy.
- Keep your own sense of humour by not taking yourself (or life) too seriously. 'You gotta laugh!'

Bottlebrush

Callistemon linearis   (Red / Aus)

Positive state

Unaffected by the past – adaptable and open to change
Confident, independent and prepared for whatever comes

Negative state

Not coping and unable to adapt to life changes (Ian White)
Early relationship attachment issues, later dependencies

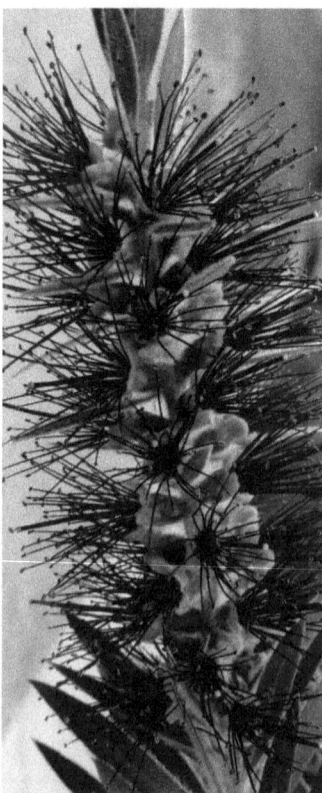

Bottlebrush's red flowers are densely packed in terminal, cylindrical spikes and actually resemble a kitchen *bottlebrush* in size and shape. This plant signature is one clue to the flower essence's effect of *sweeping away and cleansing the past* so that it cannot contaminate our experience of the present. Ian White (2008) informs us that a *'new growth* of silky shoots begins in the apex of the flower spike and in the following year a new spike will form at the growing tip.' No lateral movement here – just growth in one *direction* with no deviation off course!

The rich *red* flower signifies its relationship with the *base chakra*, enhancing a strong *presence* on Earth. It reminds us that we need to *cooperate* and encourage each other to develop (evolve) at an individual level for the sake of all humankind. A *common purpose* instils cooperation between individuals so that we can face our challenges with *acceptance and commitment*.

The Bottlebrush state of mind

We all go through various rites of passage which may daunt or challenge us – growth, starting school, adolescence, getting a job, marriage, pregnancy and birth, divorce, moving house and so on. If doubt and apprehension weigh us down, we have less chance of making these transitions safely and smoothly and this is where Bottlebrush flower essence can help.

When we lack confidence in our ability to cope with what is ahead, especially when our past hasn't fully prepared us, Bottlebrush is the flower essence to use. It is ideal for a mother who, during her first pregnancy, may be thinking, 'Oh my God! I haven't even been able to look after myself up until now, let alone a baby.' Or for the person starting a new job and thinking, 'Nothing I've ever done before has prepared me for this!' It can help us remain calm and committed, displaying poise while we negotiate important transitions.

Benefits of taking Bottlebrush

Just as the kitchen bottlebrush is used to cleanse and sweep the insides of bottles and glasses, Bottlebrush flower essence is used to metaphysically cleanse and sweep away unwanted remnants of the past (White 2008), which can easily contaminate and undermine our experience of the present and the future. In letting go of a less desirable past, we immediately let in a more desirable present and allow for a more desirable future.

Bottlebrush supports us in times of significant change by releasing us from the past and propelling us forward through life's tunnels of transition – the first of which we experience in the birth canal. And when past difficult or traumatic experiences, especially around birth and early infancy, have impacted negatively on the mother-child bond, Bottlebrush flower essence can help to heal that bond at any age.

Possible physical imbalances

Bottlebrush flower essence enhances cleansing on all levels and so augments 'detox' programs or cleansing diets. It is a catalyst for waste elimination on many levels.

Always consider this flower essence to assist in physical and emotional issues during pregnancy/labour/birth and early mother/child bonding. A common purpose instils cooperation between mother and child to enable them to face challenges with confidence.

Common uses

To assist an individual when going through life change or transition; for use during pregnancy, birth and early mother/child bonding; to help individuals stay committed to an altruistic team purpose; to adapt and cope with change and new challenges.

Complementary &/or similar flower essences

Angel's Trumpet, Angelica, Boab, Borage, Cayenne, Chrysanthemum, Elm, Forget-Me-Not, Honeysuckle, Lady's Slipper, Larch, Mariposa Lily, Paw Paw, Red Grevillea, Quaking Grass, Sagebrush, Self-Heal, Silver Princess, Tansy, Walnut, Wild Potato Bush

Supporting the changes

- Consider cleansing and elimination diets and professionally supervised fasting in conjunction with Bottlebrush flower essence.
- Investigate therapeutic and lymph-drainage massage, hydrotherapy and bathing.
- Meditate and, if already meditating, change your mantra.
- Change your tune – download a new one!

Buttercup

Ranunculus occidentalis   (Yellow / FES)

Positive state

'Radiant inner light, unattached to outer recognition or fame'(FES)
Sense of place in the greater scheme of things

Negative state

Doubting or de-valuing your worth in the world
Unable to recognise and appreciate your unique contribution

Buttercup's *brilliant, golden-yellow* flower *shines* out for all to see and appreciate. Yellow relates to the *solar plexus chakra* and just like the *sun* it symbolises, it can help us to shine brightly and confidently 'out there.' The flower essence helps us *appreciate ourselves* and our *unique contribution – our personal gift* to the world. Buttercup encourages us to accept and feel good about ourselves 'warts and all.' (The juice of the plant is traditionally used to remove warts and the homeopathic form (Ranunculus) is used to treat other embarrassing skin problems such as Herpes.) The flower essence allows our *inner beauty* to radiate. Buttercup *thrives* and grows happily in wild places often far from civilisation.

Buttercup flower essence helps us appreciate and *value* our life without any concern about whether we are noticed by peers or receive kudos in the world. If you come across this flower in some out-of the-way place you will be impressed by its *light-full-ness*, prolific growth and beauty.

The Buttercup state of mind

Whenever you come to doubt your worth in the world, consider using Buttercup flower essence. When we first start in our chosen career and wonder what we have to offer that isn't already being done better by someone else, or worry that others will laugh at our ideas or appearance, Buttercup can help us appreciate and value ourselves and be unconcerned about kudos or fame (Kaminski and Katz 1994).

Benefits of taking Buttercup

Buttercup flower essence helps us appreciate our importance and worth, the unique offering we each make to the world. Whether we are changing our baby's nappy at 3.00 am with unconditional love and without resentment or giving a Presidential address to the nation, the importance to the world's collective consciousness is the same! All life on Earth is connected, and the influence we have on each other may be overt and obvious or covert, acting on subtle levels though by no means of less importance. Buttercup allows us to get a sense of our essential role in the overall scheme of things, no matter how small or big our part may appear to be on the surface.

Possible physical imbalances

In practice, when skin problems have undermined a client's self-confidence, Buttercup flower essence often helps. (Billy Goat Plum can also be useful for skin conditions, but the feeling is one of shame, in my experience.)

Common uses

To help you share what you have to offer; to put real value on yourself and what you do; to give a clear sense of meaning in your life; to appreciate yourself like a fine wine; to unpretentiously 'shine' in life!

Complementary &/or similar flower essences

Angelica, Billy Goat Plum, Californian Poppy, Canyon Dudleya, Cerato, Cosmos, Crab Apple, Elm, Fawn Lily, Forget-Me-Not, Goldenrod, Kangaroo Paw, Lady's Slipper, Larch, Mimulus, Pomegranate, Pretty Face, Sage, Self-Heal, Shooting Star, Sunflower, Sweet Pea, Tall Yellow Top, Violet, Wild Oat

Supporting the changes

- Self-assertion, self-esteem or personal development courses facilitated by sensitive people would be very useful.
- Study creatures and plants more closely, large and small, and develop an understanding of their interdependence – their extreme importance to each other's survival. This might help you to be more appreciative of your niche and

importance in life.

- When choosing your vocation or direction in life, simply ask yourself – not others – 'Does this feel right for me?'

Calendula

Calendula officinalis   (Orange / FES)

Positive state

'Healing warmth and receptivity' (FES) in speaking and listening
Healing communication in relationships

Negative state

'Thin skinned' – easily taking offense
Cold communication – easily offending others

The fleshy and *succulent feel* of the Calendula flower reminds us of its traditional use in herbal medicine to heal injuries and inflammation of the body's internal and external membranes. In its flower essence form, Calendula heals *communication* between people so that the invisible or dynamic 'membranes' between us become *comfortable buffers* that accommodate balanced and *sensitive* exchange. The *orange* of the flower signifies its influence on the *sacral chakra* and the *intimate* way we *relate* to ourselves and others. The orange of the flower also reflects *warmth*, welcome and healing *hospitality* – a good explanation for why it is so often positioned at the entrance of gardens and houses to *greet* the visitor. Calendula flower essence enables good will and good intent to be transparent within *interpersonal communications*.

The Calendula personality

Calendula flower essence's strong affinity for the sacral chakra relates to this energy centre's tendency to store up and reflect experiences from the first seven years of life. Emotional hurt experienced in these formative years, especially from cruel words used casually, can often leave us with unresolved emotional scars. As we grow older, we may become self-protective and guarded in an attempt to avoid reactivating these painful emotional memories. But in the process of disassociating from these aspects of our psyche, we find it increasingly difficult to associate empathically with these aspects in others. In the heat of the moment we may say things that are insensitive or lack compassion, resulting in someone's feelings being hurt. Or we may be overly sensitive to what someone else has said to us. Like the gentle, soothing and healing balm of Calendula herbal ointment, the flower essence can help to heal old hurts that remain raw in our minds.

Benefits of taking Calendula

While Tiger Lily helps us trust in the potential for a win/win situation in relationships, Calendula helps us trust we won't be hurt, so that we feel free to display more warmth and openness. By promoting receptivity to our own feelings, it increases receptivity to the feelings of others. If we can develop our capacity for inner listening, intuitive understanding of where others are coming from naturally follows. We can more effectively experience 'accurate receiving' in order to understand another's perspective and engage in mutually rewarding interaction.

Calendula can help facilitate warm and sensitive contact between couples, client and therapist and those in any close personal or professional relationship.

Possible physical imbalances

Physical trauma often accompanies emotional trauma (and vice versa). This is especially so in trauma as a result of conflict between young siblings and/or other children. To help the healing process, Calendula flower essence should always be considered.

Common uses

To promote healing communication between couples in conflict; to heal old wounds resulting from verbal abuse; for warmth in communication; for a better 'bedside manner'; to facilitate 'active listening'; for conflict resolution; for those in the hospitality industry!

Complementary &/or similar flower essences

Arnica, Beech, Billy Goat Plum, Deerbrush, Dogwood, Echinacea, Flannel Flower, Hibbertia, Hibiscus, Holly, Larch, Lavender, Mallow, Oregon Grape, Quince, Shooting Star, Star Thistle, Star Tulip, Sticky Monkeyflower, Tiger Lily, Trumpet Vine, Vine, Yellow Star Tulip, Snapdragon, Zinnia

Supporting the changes

- Learn the art of active listening as part of improving your communication and counselling skills.
- Resist the urge to fix, prescribe or give advice. Just practise really listening to the other person, and try to sense the feelings being conveyed. Truly be there for the other person.
- Spend more time with people you have learned to really trust.
- Be kind to yourself!

Californian Pitcher Plant

Darlingtonia californica   (Green & purple / FES)

Positive state

Passionate and present
'Earthy vitality' (FES)

Negative state

Disassociated from raw, instinctual emotion
Lacking vitality, pallid

Californian Pitcher Plant is a *carnivorous*, insect-eating plant that is very much in touch with its 'meat eating,' masculine side. The flower essence is helpful for people who have insufficient protein or iron in their diet, or for those who just need to assimilate protein better. While the ideals of those who do not eat animal flesh or animal products may be admirable in principle, I have also observed that there are some, although in the minority, whose physical health might improve if they occasionally ate a little meat, or at least considered taking Californian Pitcher Plant flower essence to help the *assimilation* of protein and minerals such as iron from the many excellent vegetable sources that are available.

The Californian Pitcher Plant personality

People who benefit most from this flower essence are those with an idealistic and spiritual nature who cannot efficiently access the basic, raw energy for living. Their higher Self cannot connect completely with the grounding and energising qualities of the lower chakras, the seat of instinctual desires and reactions. The flower essence helps us establish a better relationship with the physical plane of existence so that we can really embrace BEING HERE and passionately engage in life!

Benefits of taking Californian Pitcher Plant

The flower essence helps us to accept basic aspects of ourselves that we may have self-judged as unacceptable – what Carl Jung would call our Shadow side. If we have denied our raw, untapped passion and vitality, Californian Pitcher Plant can help us to use this life-force energy creatively, guiding us to transform suppressed anger and frustration into strong personal presence and decisiveness. By gaining access to our primal, innate energies, we can turn our passions and desires into refined fuel for energy and creativity.

Possible physical imbalances

Poor digestion and assimilation, especially of protein, is common among those who respond well to Californian Pitcher Plant. Poor assimilation often results in lethargy and sometimes anaemic conditions.

Common uses

To come to terms with your 'shadow side'; for repressed anger; to help a person get in touch with their masculine side; to assist digestion of protein and complex foods; for energy and vitality; to tune in to your passionate desires

Complementary &/or similar flower essences

Black Eyed Susan, Blackberry, Cayenne, Cherry Plum, Clematis, Corn, Flannel Flower, Forget-Me-Not, Fuchsia, Hibiscus, Lotus, Madia, Manzanita, Morning Glory, Red Lily, Rosemary, Scarlet Monkeyflower (and all the Monkeyflower essences), Shooting Star, Snapdragon, Tall Yellow Top, Tansy, Wild Rose

Supporting the changes

- Jungian psychotherapy may help you integrate and bring into consciousness previously denied strong emotions (and passion) for use in creative pursuits.
- Regular vigorous exercise (with proper preparation) will help to get the blood flowing.
- Engage in any type of grounding activity, especially work with earth.
- Eat more root vegetables and legumes. It may be worth considering eating a little red meat occasionally.
- Get down and dirty and swear a bit!

Californian Poppy

Eschscholzia californica   (Golden orange / FES)

Positive state

Heartfelt understanding, inner knowing (FES)
Discernment in life choices

Negative state

Seeking outside oneself for illumination, especially through escapism or addiction (FES)
'Restless seekers' or those for whom 'the grass is always greener on the other side of the fence'

Californian Poppy's solitary, saucer-shaped, *deep-orange* flowers convey the universal allure of the *cup of gold or holy grail*.

Native Americans used Californian Poppy as a herbal remedy to alleviate the pain of toothache, which can often be a physical manifestation of an inner struggle to find and 'sink our teeth into' our true life's work.

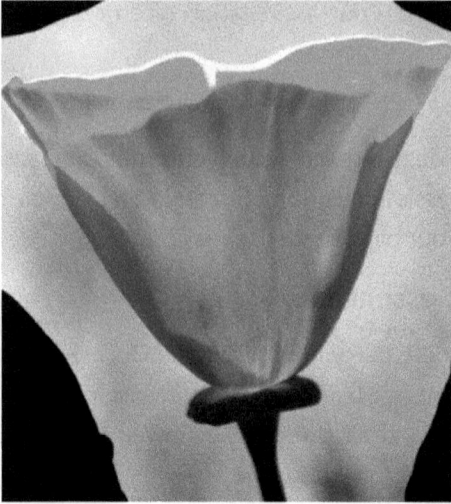

It is said that before modern industrial and residential development, the poppy-covered hills of California would shine so brightly that sailors far out at sea used them as beacons to guide their course. I have often used this flower essence to ignite my own (and others') 'heart light' and help me to *direct my course in life*. The Californian Poppy is also California's State Flower. California owes its early rapid population growth to a gold rush to which people flocked in the belief that they would find their 'pot of gold' and live happily ever after. In a different kind of Californian gold rush, Hollywood has also attracted many a desperate soul in search of stardom and the realisation of dreams. 'The saying *"all that glitters is not gold"* is an apt one to describe the lesson of the Californian Poppy' (Kaminski and Katz 1994).

In the 1960s and 70s many engaged in a misguided quest for rapid *enlightenment* and the *'ultimate high'* through drugs, which were seen as an opportunity to fast-forward personal growth and 'personal evolution.' While this age-old aspiration was and is admirable, this particular path to it was misguided. This was especially evident in the widespread use of psychedelic drugs, as many humanistic psychology and personal growth books written at the time testify. (It is interesting to see renewed mainstream interest today in the use of mind-altering drugs for the treatment of depression.) However, it soon became clear that enlightenment was not to be found in drugs for the simple reason that they have their primary effect on the mental level rather than in the heart and are not *grounded* in practical reality. Californian Poppy enables balanced distribution of our intelligent life force into all levels of our being, notably our heart.

As people began to recognise this, many started to seek *heart consciousness* through practices such as meditation. (Transcendental Meditation ™ is just one form of meditation that was presented in a way that appealed to many Westerners and is still practised widely.) The well documented journey of the Beatles through drug experimentation and Eastern spirituality epitomised the times for many people. A need for psychic and *spiritual balance* is a major indication for the use of Californian Poppy flower essence, especially in *restless seekers* who are cerebral or 'heady.'

The Californian Poppy personality

Restless seekers who may benefit from this flower essence spend their time in the expectation of complete fulfilment once their nirvana is found. However, their quest is endless as they find that wherever they are, the grass seems greener on the other side of the fence. As Carl Jung put it, 'Who looks outside, dreams; who looks inside, wakes.'

In this high-tech, speedy and hyper-stimulating world, it is very easy to be distracted and seduced. We can end up seeking outside ourselves for inspiration and false forms of higher consciousness, especially through escapism or addiction. Like a moth that is drawn to a light, we can easily become disorientated, exposed and vulnerable to predators and find ourselves burned or trapped by that which attracts us. Most of the different forms of media tend to play into this in order to get your attention.

Californian Poppy flower essence is for the 'restless seeker' in us all – 'workshop junkie' 'guru chaser,' 'fame seeker,' 'fleeting fad follower,' 'retail therapy' addict, 'perfect partner pursuer' or seeker of the 'ultimate high' through natural or chemical means. Californian Poppy helps bring the outer journey into balance with a greater awareness of the inner journey. The need for psychic and spiritual balance is a major indication for the flower essence. It helps maintain inner balance during personal growth and psychic awakening.

Benefits of taking Californian Poppy

When you chop and change constantly, never really getting to where you want, let Californian Poppy help you find the way back home to your heart. Rediscover the guru within because the best answers lie at the heart of your being, not outside you.

Many clients for whom I prescribe Californian Poppy begin to feel calmer, more discerning in their decision-making and generally more content with the way their lives are unfolding.

Possible physical imbalances

The inner calm that Californian Poppy brings is reflected in its use as a herbal relaxant, bringing restful sleep to those who have trouble stilling themselves.

Common uses

For the restless seeker; for workshop junkies; to learn that 'all that glitters is not gold'; when 'the grass is always greener'; for vocational guidance; to help make discerning life choices; to follow the heart rather than the head towards inner peace; for deep contentment

Complementary &/or similar flower essences

Agrimony, Angelsword, Blackberry, Buttercup, Canyon Dudleya, Cerato, Chrysanthemum, Dill, Forget-Me-Not, Hibbertia, Lotus, Pomegranate, Pretty Face, Sunflower, Tall Yellow Top, Wild Oat

Supporting the changes

- Study the concept of glamour from a theosophical perspective and ask yourself why it is so attractive to you.
- Many 'restless seekers' have found some peace of mind in the philosophies and teachings of Buddhism.
- Engage in solitary and grounding activities such as gardening or walking.
- Meditate in moderation in order to develop a more contemplative and reflective approach to life.
- Learn to follow your gut instincts. Does it really feel right?

Californian Wild Rose
(see Wild Rose)

Calla Lily
Zantedescia aethiopica   (White-yellow / FES)

Positive state
Comfortable with your sexual identity
Dynamic balance in relationships or friendships

Negative state
Imbalance between masculine and feminine qualities
Confusion about sexual identity/gender (FES)

Calla Lily's signature is immediately evident in the structure of the flower, which distinctly displays *male and female sex organs.*

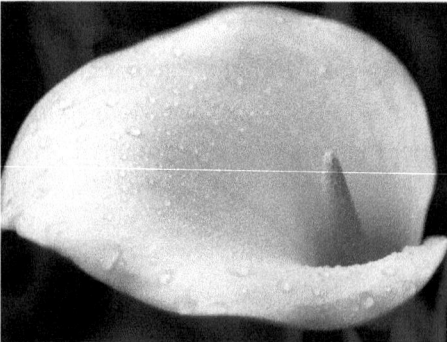

The physiological male-female division is unique to Earthly existence, unlike the balanced, androgynous state of existence in the spiritual realm. Sometimes on an emotional and spiritual level there may be *resistance to a male or female role* while on a purely physical level, sexual characteristics are determined by *hormonal changes.* (I have found in my practice as a therapist that this resistance can also manifest on a physical level in the form of hormonal imbalance and associated symptoms.) The Calla Lily flower expresses sexual duality in perfect balance and the flower essence is used to help people reach their own *balance* in expressing their sexuality and *masculine/ feminine qualities.*

The Calla Lily state of mind

It is not uncommon to find ourselves playing a subservient role in some relationships and a dominant one in others. Sometimes roles within a relationship go from one extreme to the other and it is hard to find that happy medium in which we feel on equal and fair terms with each other. Our interpersonal relationships will become more harmonious once our internal masculine-feminine relationship reaches a harmonious balance.

Calla Lily flower essence has been helpful for many of my clients during significant life-stage transitions. In prepubescence, for example, we prepare on a physical and spiritual level to make a conclusive statement to the world about our gender identity by developing secondary sexual characteristics. However, there may be some ambivalence about this process, and this may bring about discontent, emotional problems and issues, especially in relationships. Calla Lily can help us gain confidence and 'clarity about our sexual identity' (Kaminski and Katz 1994) at this crucial time.

Calla Lily is also useful at midlife and/or menopause when a person inevitably revisits and revises their sexual and gender identity.

Benefits of taking Calla Lily

Calla Lily encourages balance and 'equal opportunity' in your sexual and intimate relationships and in all interactions with others. It helps you attain clarity about your sexual identity and self-acceptance in your role in relationships. Calla Lily helps to enable honest and comfortable expression of sexuality.

Possible physical imbalances

Calla Lily can be very supportive and balancing during those periods when spiritual and emotional change and development is quickening and manifesting on a physical level through dramatic hormonal change. Prepubescence and midlife/ menopause for both men and women are naturally such times, but it is not necessarily confined to these times at an individual level.

Common uses

Dramatic oscillation between subservience/dominance in relationships; ambivalence or confusion around sexual identity; for prepubescence and early puberty; clear acceptance of sexual identity; balanced expression of masculine/ feminine qualities; equality in relationships; during menopause and midlife

Complementary &/or similar flower essences

Alpine Lily, Billy Goat Plum, Crab Apple, Easter Lily, Fairy Lantern, Hibiscus, Lady's Slipper, Manzanita, Orange, Pomegranate, Queen Anne's Lace, Quince, Sagebrush, Scleranthus, She Oak, Snapdragon, Sticky Monkeyflower, Sunflower, Tansy, Tiger Lily

Supporting the changes

- Study the masculine, the feminine and androgyny in Jungian psychology.
- Personal growth and assertiveness courses may be helpful.
- Read inspirational stories about individuals who have survived and prospered despite being subject to discrimination because of their gender or sexual preferences.
- Be yourself!

Canyon Dudleya
Dudleya cymosa   (Orange / FES)

Positive state
Grounded/balanced life perspective
Spiritual insight arising from everyday life

Negative state
Drawn to 'distorted psychic experiences' (FES)
Too easily 'sucked in' by charisma or 'sensationalism'

Canyon Dudleya's *orange-red* flower has an open structure which resembles that of a sea anemone as it waits to *engulf and consume* its prey. Those in the negative Canyon Dudleya state are all too ready to be *lured by sensationalism*, whether in the media or in approaches to healing and spiritualty, but they are not drawn to anything 'ordinary.' They have a *fascination* that borders on *addiction* to 'trauma-dramas' and *psychic experiences*. The Canyon Dudleya plant 'lives on the edge,' attaching itself to sun-baked ledges in river canyons and mountain hillsides.

The flower's *orange-red* colour relates to the *lower chakras (the base chakra and sacral chakra)* and the essence helps to ground us in a more 'earthly reality' which in turn allows us to act with more *discernment* and make better choices in life.

The Canyon Dudleya personality

The person in need of this flower essence can be too easily 'sucked in' by others and drawn into 'sensationalised' experiences, especially on a psychic level. There is a craving for dramatic psychic-emotional experiences. The colour orange *sacral chakra* sometimes reflects a fascination with glamour and easy distraction (see Californian Poppy) but because in Canyon Dudleya it is integrated with red *base chakra*, there is a further dimension related to personal survival and the possibility of being consumed by a cause, belief or intense experience. At its most extreme, this can take the form of psychic domination and brainwashing of the kind practised in some cults. In everyday circumstances, it can take the form of hysterical surrender to an experience or to a cause or system of worship.

When the lower chakras are properly enriched and balanced, the higher chakras become securely rooted in Earthly reality and are protected from being too easily influenced or taken over.

Benefits of taking Canyon Dudleya

Canyon Dudleya helps to secure and create boundaries for those with a vulnerable or suggestible mind. It can assist in earthing the wandering psyche of the mental 'space cadet.' When necessary, it can also help contain an inflated psychic life within the realms of everyday reality. Some people interested in alternative healing look for intense psychic and emotional experiences through rebirthing, past-life regression or healing crises. It is as through dramatic catharsis is experienced as a direct reflection of the effectiveness of the cure and of the healer's competence and charisma. The inaccuracy of this position is attested by many disillusioned clients and burnt-out healers. Genuine spiritual or personal growth is usually gradual and quiet and the 'growth spurts' that do occur may even go unnoticed at the time, to be recognised only in retrospect. When the qualities of a remedy relate profoundly to a client's life situation, healing often begins with the insights that arise during quiet self-reflection. Only over time does the depth of internal change express itself outwardly.

Canyon Dudleya can lead to psychic wisdom by bringing depth of understanding to over-the-top spiritual experiences. Kaminski and Katz (1994) speak of how Canyon Dudleya teaches us discernment by guiding the soul 'towards more balanced spiritual opening and contained emotional presence.'

Possible physical imbalances

Vulnerability at a psychic-emotional level is often accompanied by a lowering of overall immunity. This inevitably leads to physical vulnerability and adrenal fatigue and energy depletion.

Common uses

For those easily 'sucked in' by charismatic 'guru' figures; psychic drama queens (or kings); for distorted psychic experiences; for 'healing crisis' junkies; for those always seeking the sensationalist and/or psychic 'WOW' factor; for loss of Self and consequent psychic vulnerability; for grounding and directing energy; for discernment and healthy spiritual growth; to experience a peaceful and balanced reality

Complementary &/or similar flower essences

Aloe Vera, Angelica, Angelsword, Arnica, Californian Poppy, Chamomile, Chaparral, Corn, Dill, Echinacea, Garlic, Fringed Violet, Hibbertia, Indian Pink, Lavender, Mountain Pennyroyal, Mugwort, Queen Anne's Lace, Red Clover, Star of Bethlehem, St John's Wort, Sunflower, Walnut, all the Yarrows, YES formula

Supporting the changes

- Any grounding activity will be beneficial – physical exercise, especially walking, gardening, pottery – anything that brings you into close contact and interaction with the earth.
- Use creative visualisation to surround yourself with white light whenever you sense a need for protection.
- Cultivate friendships with people you regard as very down-to-earth and the 'genuine article.'
- Always remember the Buddhist saying: 'Before enlightenment, chop wood and carry water; after enlightenment, chop wood and carry water.'

Cayenne

Capsicum annuum   (White / FES)

Positive state

Invigorated and able to enjoy the 'spice of life'!
Energy 'for change and transformation' (FES)

Negative state

Stagnating, stuck and sluggish
Unable to gather forces to move forward (FES)

People often associate Cayenne with the cuisines of Asia. However the chilli plant is actually native to South America and didn't get to India until the early sixteenth century. Numerous cultivars of this shrubby, tropical plant with varying degrees of *pungency* have since been developed all over the world. Native Americans used chilli to treat pain and illness, including fevers and sore throats. Chilli peppers *stimulate* the salivary glands and were believed to cleanse the whole digestive tract. We have all experienced the way chilli can really 'stir up' things in the gut region!

The physical *heating effect* of cayenne pepper is an important aspect of the plant's signature. Cayenne flower essence *speeds up* action (*heats*) on a spiritual level. The energetic 'heating' effect gently stirs the *heart centre*, so that our deepest desires and spiritual aspirations become more defined and the energy for their manifestation can be used in a more deliberate and focused manner. In this way, Cayenne assists in *removing blockages on a soul level* so that people can perceive, understand and remove the outer obstacles that arise as a result of these blockages.

The Cayenne state of mind

Those in need of Cayenne feel generally 'stuck.' They may see themselves as being in a rut of repetitive or monotonous behaviour governed by routine and habit, and mentally they are tired of the same old thought patterns and desires. They find it difficult to motivate themselves to move out of their stagnation because they are 'caught in a pattern of procrastination and resistance' (Kaminski and Katz 1994). Although they may be able to identify the problem, they feel lethargic and disinclined to engage in activity.

Benefits of taking Cayenne

Cayenne, and chilli in general, is often used to strengthen and bring out the flavour in food. As a flower essence, Cayenne is used to strengthen and bring out the flavour in life. When your life seems monotonous and repetitive, and you get the sense that you are 'going nowhere,' you might consider adding Cayenne to spice things up.

Cayenne is the ideal catalyst when you need to move on in life. It can also add a stimulating element to a flower essence mix, enhancing your overall receptivity to the other essences. The combination of Cayenne and Blackberry is a good example. Often referred to as the Manifestation formula, this combination is used to help bring into existence important things we may feel are missing from our lives. It is also useful when we need extra motivation.

Cayenne flower essence enables proper pre-performance 'warm up,' stirring your physical energy and mental clarity to help you pursue your vision of what you want from life.

Possible physical imbalances

Physical lethargy and indolence accompanies the negative Cayenne state of mind. Most people experience a new sense of physical vitality after taking the flower essence, the proverbial 'rocket under you'!

Common uses

To help overcome ingrained habits; when you are stuck in 'idle'; to 'put a rocket under you'; to catalyse quick change; for energy to mobilise action

Complementary &/or similar flower essences

Blackberry, Californian Pitcher Plant, Coffee, Hornbeam, Iris, Macrocarpa, Madia, Morning Glory, Nasturtium, Olive, Onion, Peppermint, Rosemary, Silver Princess, Tansy, Waratah, Wild Oat, Wild Potato Bush, (Californian) Wild Rose

NB: Blackberry + Cayenne = Manifestation formula

Supporting the changes

- Any physical and grounding activity will be beneficial – especially physical exercise such as gardening.
- Work on developing a clear vision of what you want in (or from) life. Practise creative visualisation.
- Make a plan!

Centaury

Centaurium erythraea   (Pink / Bach)

Positive state

Service in mutually beneficial relationships
Co-operation without loss of personal power

Negative state

Servile, neglecting one's own needs
Prone to developing co-dependent relationships

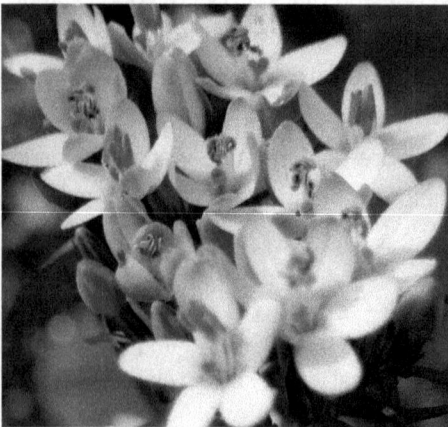

Centaury is an annual wild flower found in dry, grassy places throughout Europe and many other parts of the world. It 'grows strongly where many other flowers cannot *find a footing*' (Barnard 1988). It is little wonder that the flower essence can teach us to *'stand our ground'* when necessary. Each pale *pink* flower opens in warm sunshine and closes towards evening, displaying *purposeful*

clarity in a gesture of *heartfelt cooperation* with the greater forces of nature. The flowers are also held in clusters. Such growth implies that the plant possesses healing qualities that relate to the social dimension – 'humility, inclusiveness or the absorption of the individual identity in the larger collective' (FES). Dr Bach made his flower essence from these clusters, seeing them as a symbol of *cooperation* in the service of love *amongst equals*.

Hippocrates related how Centaury was used by Chiron the centaur, the founder of medicine in Greek mythology, to heal the wound inflicted on him by Hercules. Chiron is sometimes referred to as the *'wounded healer'* – a good description of the way many natural therapists heal themselves through healing others. A life of *service* is implied by this plant's name.

The Centaury personality

The Centaury flower has a small yellow centre surrounded by pink petals. It is as though the pink – the colour associated with the heart chakra – draws the Centaury person to the needs and affairs of others like a magnet. Unfortunately, this can occur at the expense of a Centaury person's own inner needs – a denial represented by the confined yellow centre (the colour associated with the solar plexus chakra), which governs the energy of personal power and assertion. Centaury people can be completely at the beck and call of others, so focused on external needs that they lose contact with their own.

When you are overly helpful to others, you risk being a hindrance. Not being in touch with your own needs makes it easy to fall into the trap of automatically responding to the requests of those around – family, friends, clients – who then don't fulfil their own responsibilities. Both parties lose in the end because neither learns to be truly independent – a co-dependent vicious cycle easily develops.

In certain stereotypical relationships, those over-served by the Centaury person may include: mummy's boy, daddy's girl, he who 'marries his mum' (a wife who takes over from where his mother left off) and the patient who rings their accommodating health practitioner every day. Those who can benefit from taking Centaury include parents who do everything for their children without giving them the opportunity to learn from their own mistakes and Centaury employees who always oblige, accommodating every workmate's demand. In these situations unhealthy, dependency-based relationships can develop.

Those on the receiving end of over-care often come to resent their dependence and feel stifled and restricted in their growth towards self-sufficiency. In healthy relationships, we are able to create enough space to empower each person to grow as a capable individual. This is the true art of service – to create a mutually beneficial exchange that facilitates personal growth for all involved.

Benefits of taking Centaury

The Centaury plant can easily be overlooked and accidentally stepped on. This characteristic in the Centaury person earns them the unkind nickname of 'doormat.' Up close, however, the flower is admired for its delicate beauty of form and colour. Centaury flower essence can help us raise and maintain our awareness of this beauty within, allowing the needs and dreams of our inner child to remain in our awareness, keeping us in contact with our joy and vitality.

Possible physical imbalances

Digestive complaints are common in those who benefit from taking Centaury flower essence. All areas of the gut are vulnerable, related as they are to the solar plexus, where our feeling-reaction to life resides. It is often only as a result of physical illness that people in the negative Centaury state will give themselves a reprieve from service to those dependent on them.

Common uses

For the 'yes-person' or doormat mentality; for those who allow themselves to be routinely exploited by others; for those who lose the Self in servitude; for the 'wounded healer'; to help contact the inner child and its needs; to help understand what your own needs are and learn how to meet them yourself; to heal co-dependency; to joyfully act in service amongst equals

Complementary &/or similar flower essences

Bleeding Heart, Buttercup, Calla Lily, Cosmos, Echinacea, Fawn Lily, Elm, Garlic, Indian Pink, Lady's Slipper, Larkspur, Mariposa Lily, Mountain Pride, Mullein, Pine, Pink Yarrow, Pomegranate, Red Grevillea, Scleranthus, Tansy, Violet, Walnut

Supporting the changes

- Take time to discover what you really desire for yourself.
- Before you say 'yes', ask yourself, 'Is this going to benefit both of us?'
- Make time for yourself on a regular basis, and in particular, allow for some enjoyment and 'playtime.'
- It is OK to throw a little tantrum sometimes!

Cerato

Ceratostigma wilimottianum   (Blue / Bach)

Positive state

In tune with inner guidance
Self-assured and autonomous

Negative state

Distrust of own judgement – self-doubt
Conditioned by advice from (many) others

Dr Bach first noticed Cerato in a garden in Norfolk, England. The shrub was relatively unknown in the area and he was unaware of its Himalayan *origins*. The thirty-seven other Bach remedies are gathered from the wild, so Cerato is a puzzling exception – and also, significantly, a remedy for *uncertainty*! The Tibetan connection is also significant. When a Tibetan student monk asks a question of his lama, the teacher immediately turns the question back to the student. The student must find *an answer within* if they are to achieve satisfaction and lasting insight. An *internalisation* of intention is facilitated by the lama so that students are forced to seek and find their *own truth*.

The Cerato state of mind

When we are in the negative Cerato state, we feel uncertain and seek answers from others. (This Cerato process of seeking answers is more overt than in the Scleranthus state, where there is a tendency to internalise indecision.) When we are in need of Cerato we actively seek the advice of family and friends, health practitioners and so on.

Self-doubt can rock the foundations of our life. With no lasting faith in the fundamental structure of our world-view, we constantly seek guidance from external sources to gain meaning and structure. The analogy of a child with a colouring-in book is useful – in the negative Cerato state we are good at colouring our lives to the last detail but we desperately seek someone else to provide the outline. The final effect is never truly our own and we feel as if we are only a proxy, filling in someone else's vision. As Dr Bach said in his *Collected Writings*, in the negative Cerato state we 'concentrate too much on the details of life, and miss the main principles: convention and small things count above main issues.'

Some element of self-doubt is constructive, as it leaves us open to change and growth, but an excess can leave us unable to recognise what change is appropriate for us. Stuck in destructive habits or a mindset of uncertainty, we can become doctor-shoppers, always in search of the advice we want to hear. Paradoxically, this apparent search for the new may simply be another form of sticking with 'the devil you know,' seeking advice that will give permission to stay the same. We may even take advice we know is wrong because we are unable to hear the inner voice that can tell us what is right. We do not trust our own judgement enough to recognise the right advice or direction, even when it is in front of us.

Benefits of taking Cerato

Cerato helps release us from the habit of seeking external authority, freeing us to contact the wise Self that is waiting to guide and direct our lives from within. With this comes refreshed enthusiasm for life and an eagerness to learn.

Possible physical imbalances

Cerato has a special influence on the throat centre which in turn strongly influences the body's lymphatic 'rubbish disposal' system. A lack of discernment on a mental and emotional level can manifest as a similar problem in the lymphatic system, which becomes cluttered with waste, leading to congestion, immune system weakness and proneness to infection.

Common uses

For self-doubt; for the chronic advice-seeker (who rarely takes the advice they are given!); for the doctor-shopper who moves from one therapist to another (waiting for the diagnosis they want to hear!); for the character actor unsure of their own identity; to help develop your intuition; for the Gemini type who needs a holiday from their normal surroundings; to discover your own truth; for a new and fresh view of life; to help create a life that reflects one's truth

Complementary &/or similar flower essences

Angelsword, Angelica, Californian Poppy, Cayenne, Chrysanthemum, Deerbrush, Dill, Filaree, Forget-Me-Not, Foxglove, Goldenrod, Iris, Lotus, Mullein, Onion, Paw Paw, Pretty Face, Rabbitbrush, Red Lily, Sagebrush, Saguaro, Scleranthus, Self-Heal, Shasta Daisy, Silver Princess, Star Tulip, Sweet Pea, Sunflower, Wild Oat

Supporting the changes

- Take on a position of responsibility where you run the show – chair a committee or captain a team for example.
- Put yourself in a situation where you will be called upon for guidance you know you are competent to give.
- Take a holiday or change your circumstances to gain a fresh perspective.
- Change the theme of your life!

THE **ESSENTIAL** FLOWER ESSENCE BOOK

Chamomile

Matricaria recutita   (White/yellow centre / FES)

Positive state

'Emotional balance' (FES)
Serene and even disposition

Negative state

Emotionally welling up
Moody and easily irritated (FES)

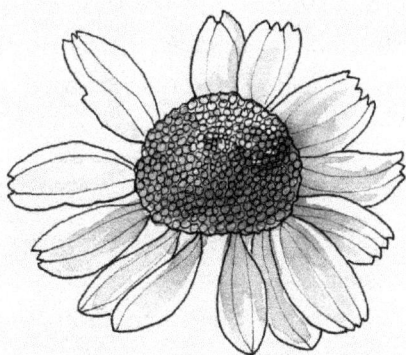

Chamomile (both the Roman and German species) is used herbally and as a flower essence to help achieve a sunny, *even disposition*. From ancient times it has been used to enhance deeper relaxation and meditative practices. The *golden-yellow* and *white* flowers, the plant's chemistry and its geometric patterns point to its usefulness in facilitating meditative practices aimed at gaining *inner peace*. Chamomile's beneficial effect on the entire *nervous system* has also been corroborated by scientific studies.

Another signature can be seen in the small white flowers with yellow centres which mimic the structure of the glands of the stomach lining. The yellow heart of the flower, which appears to protrude from the surrounding petals, also symbolises the *solar plexus* and *'gut feelings,'* reminding us of the *'emotional swellings'* that can occur, especially in children, which often result in *stomach upsets.*

The Chamomile state of mind

Both the flower essence and homeopathic forms of Chamomile have an anti-inflammatory effect on the emotions. The remedy helps when you are 'emotionally inflamed,' especially when you perceive what others say as provocative or inflammatory.

In Europe, Chamomile is probably best known for its beneficial effects on digestive disturbances because it is calming (anti-spasmodic) and stimulates the appetite. The 'swollen belly' signature of the flower in its relationship to the solar plexus is enlightening in this respect. Chamomile can help us settle and better negotiate emotional upheavals which are at the root of many digestive upsets.

Benefits of taking Chamomile

Chamomile can help us win the 'battle of the emotional bulge.' Chamomile may be of benefit for mood swings characterised by anger and irritability, and for emotional unevenness and restlessness. When we are easily irritated and respond in an emotionally reactive way, a mutually hostile relationship is created with those nearby. Chamomile flower essence is very useful to promote co-operation and calm thinking in people who work together.

When we are stressed to the point where we feel 'beside ourselves,' the emotional body is in fact 'beside' us – dislocated – and therefore seems to be out of our control. Chamomile helps the mental body rein in the emotional body, so that strong feelings can be examined with more objectivity. There is increased emotional stability and this creates calm in the region of the stomach and the solar plexus. Always consider Chamomile for children's ailments when the characteristic irritable emotional upsurge is present. Chamomile also helps dispel nervous tension, insomnia and nightmares.

Possible physical imbalances

Chamomile flower essence has a beneficial effect on the central nervous system and its development in much the same way as Vitamin B. Chamomile in its herbal and homeopathic forms has traditionally been used in acute ailments in children, from colic and stomach upsets to teething symptoms and nervous irritability. A calming and ameliorating effect on irritability, pain and inflammation is a common theme.

Common uses

For the child who is 'beside him/herself'; as an emotional 'anti-inflammatory'; to ease emotional tension & irritability; to lessen the tendency to angry outbursts; to learn to be more objective; to assist meditative practices; to help attain an emotionally even disposition

Complementary &/or similar flower essences

Black Eyed Susan, Calendula, Californian Poppy, Canyon Dudleya, Corn, Crowea, Dandelion, Dill, Filaree, Fuchsia, Impatiens, Indian Pink, Lavender, Lotus, Mugwort, Purple Monkeyflower, Quaking Grass, Red Clover, Scarlet Monkeyflower, Shasta Daisy, Snapdragon, Tiger Lily, Vervain

Supporting the changes

- Investigate relaxation and meditative techniques such as yoga and tai chi as ways of de-stressing and 'grounding' yourself, leaving you calm and emotionally balanced.
- Eat foods that are rich in the Vitamin B group, drink nervine-type herbal teas and

avoid mood-altering substances such as sugar, coffee and alcohol. Get sufficient sleep, which means having some sleep before midnight and sticking to a regular sleep pattern.

- Calm down!

Chaparral

Larrea tridentata   (Yellow / FES)

Positive state

Deep self-perception (FES)
At ease within, de-stressed

Negative state

Psychic, emotional & physical toxicity – 'Guts in a knot!'
Long-standing stress, disturbed (dream) sleep

Chaparral, like most desert-living plants, has the ability to *endure* harsh environmental conditions – drought, temperature extremes, fire, pestilence and pollution – for long periods. These plants can access what they need to *survive* despite the barrenness and lack of fertility in their environment. For this reason Chaparral can assist those who have experienced difficult or *stressful times*, especially for extended periods. A good example is someone who lives in a rural area in drought where the risk of bushfire is high. The stress of living with the constant threat of fire over summer, let alone living through a wildfire, leaves people severely *traumatised over time.* In my practice I once worked with a client who had endured a long, hot summer in an area where her home had been under constant threat of fire. Her sleep was restless, with *disturbed dreams* and she felt exhausted; her body was tense and she experienced cramps and tension headaches. She explained that her digestion was 'all over the place' and she had 'put on weight that won't budge.' She had suffered from shingles two years previously and had seemed to have totally recovered until recently, when she started to have some 'uncomfortable, niggling sensations' in the areas of her face and scalp that had been previously affected. After taking Chaparral flower essence she was feeling far less stressed, and many of the associated symptoms improved significantly.

Just as the Chaparral plant survives soaring extremes of temperature and remains relatively unscathed, iits flower essence enables us to recover and minimise the effects of ongoing trauma and external stressors. Chaparral herb is known as an *adaptogen* – that is, it increases resistance to a broad spectrum of physical, chemical and biological stressors. Adaptogens have a normalising effect, counteracting or preventing disturbances brought about by stress.

The *yellow* of the flowers signifies the plant's connection with the *solar plexus chakra*. Chaparral flower essence helps ease the 'stressed' solar plexus, allowing a reassuring spiritualisation of the intellect. *Worrying, 'guts in a knot,' tormented thinking and disturbed dreams are dispelled as a result of the cleansing of the mental body*. A fresh and better-organised way of thinking results in mental clarity and *quiet*.

The Chaparral state of mind

When we feel psychically toxic and traumatised, burdened or worn out as a result of being subjected to 'chaotic experiences ... actual violence or disturbing images in the media' (Kaminski and Katz 1994) Chaparral flower essence helps cleanse, protect and preserve the psyche. When the mind is clouded and cluttered, lacking clarity as a result of the impact of past experiences and trauma, Chaparral can help cleanse a heavily burdened mind. Our dream life acts as an important channel for psychic cleansing both on a day-to-day and long-term basis. Dreaming provides the opportunity to cleanse residual 'astral-emotional debris' resulting from stressful experiences in our daily lives. Chaparral can help us achieve better, more restful sleep when our dreams have become disturbed and restless.

Benefits of taking Chaparral

Chaparral's ability to help protect from burnout and the intensities of modern life is vividly symbolised by its ability to conserve energy by using it slowly; Chaparral inhibits its own oxidation and burns with a very slow flame. There is a plant in Imperial County, California, which has been carbon dated at over 13,000 years old! The preservative action of the herb has been further displayed in the area of free radical research, where it has been shown to contain compounds with strong anti-oxidant qualities that protect the liver and lungs from free radical damage. The herb is a true adaptogen and the flower essence helps us to adapt with ease to life and all that it throws at us!

Possible physical imbalances

An accumulation of mental, emotional and psychic 'toxicity' will, over time, find an outlet through the physical body. For Chaparral people in the negative state, this toxicity is most often expressed as problems in the digestive system, particularly the liver. The liver responds to how we feel, being especially affected by feelings of anger and frustration according to Traditional Chinese Medicine, whether consciously felt or suppressed, and whether it occurs in the present or past – it is as though the liver retains our emotional memory (not always consciously in sync with our brain's cognitive recognition) of past experiences and events. A good response to appropriately chosen Chaparral flower essences therefore includes a positive influence on the liver and digestive system. Plants with yellow flowers (relating to the solar plexus) have traditionally been used as herbal medicines for their beneficial effect on the liver and digestion.

Common uses

After long-term stress; when feeling burnt out; when your 'gut is in a knot' from stress; for disturbing dreams when under stress; as part of a (supervised) detoxification program (including drug detox); to clarify your 'gut' sense of things; to aid regression therapy (and recall of significant past experience); to help you adapt; to rediscover the quiet within.

Complementary &/or similar flower essences

Aloe Vera, Agrimony, Arnica, Black Eyed Susan, Borage, Dandelion, Dill, Dogwood, Echinacea, Golden Ear Drops, Indian Pink, Love-Lies-Bleeding, Morning Glory, Mugwort, Nasturtium, Nectarine, Nicotiana, Olive, Penstemon, Sagebrush, St John's Wort, Star of Bethlehem, Star Tulip, Sturt Desert Pea, all the Yarrows, YES formula

Supporting the changes

- Professional counselling/psychotherapy (Emotional Focus Therapy) for past trauma may be very useful in some situations.
- Natural liver cleansing and elimination diets may be appropriate. Seek advice about a gentle approach to diet from a qualified natural therapist.
- Take up up relaxation exercises such as yoga, tai chi and/or meditation as part of healthy lifestyle changes.

Cherry Plum

Prunus cerasifera   (White or pale Pink / Bach)

Positive state

Spiritual surrender/trust
Calm and poise under stress

Negative state

Fear of losing control
Pushed-too-far feeling; 'at wit's end!'

Cherry Plum's flowers are mainly white, signifying a white flag of unconditional *surrender* to God, the universe and/or the Great Plan, allowing us to *'go with the flow'* rather than guard against anticipated events which may or may not happen. This surrender is akin to those moments just prior to a performance, examination or other test when, realising that there is nothing more you can do to prepare, you put your *trust* in your inner resolve and say, 'I can do it.' And usually you do it well. You *survive* the performance – and you're not only still alive, but more alive than before this close encounter with your darkest, *innermost fears*.

Barnard (1988) reminds us how Cherry Plum flowers 'appear towards the end of winter,' so we can *take heart* (note the few pale pink flowers) knowing that the light and warmth of spring is on the way and winter storms and bitter cold will soon ease. Cherry Plum flower essence helps us find *'the calm amid and after the storm'*!

The Cherry Plum state of mind

Most of us like to maintain a sense of control in our lives and we take practical steps to insure ourselves and our families against difficult times and threatening circumstances. We invest money, often at the expense of our present quality of life, in order to assure our independence upon retirement, when we believe that peace of mind will be guaranteed by the nest egg we have put aside. However, no matter how much we try, we cannot control all of life's variables. Freedom from worry and anxiety depends largely on our trust in fate.

Fears of losing control can inhibit the experience and appreciation of life for ourselves and those around us. We may withdraw emotionally into a guarded existence or, in particularly stressful times, we may be terrified that we will do something unthinkable. Normally relegated to our Shadow side, vivid fears arise that we will lose our sanity or harm ourselves or others. Of course these emotional urges and mental images rarely become reality but they cause great pain and anxiety. When feeling desperate, out of control and fearful of doing something destructive to ourselves or others, always consider Cherry Plum (or Rescue Remedy which contains this 'emergency' essence) and seek professional help immediately.

Benefits of taking Cherry Plum

Cherry Plum helps us have faith in our higher Self, so that we can surrender to inner guidance and meet life with poise and calm. In letting go of our concerns around our mortality, we take a better grip on life and living.

Possible physical imbalances

The condition of our stomach says a lot about our receptivity to life-experience – how 'at-ease' we are about meeting the next moment in time. Accordingly, stomach problems are common for those in the negative Cherry Plum state. Muscle tension and 'guarding' can also be a sign of resistance or fear of what's coming up next in our lives.

Common uses

For fears about doing something desperate; for fear of losing your mind; for fears about what you might do if pushed too far; for fear and denial of our Shadow side; to support trust in the Self; to surrender to what is out of your control; to help keep a 'cool head' in difficult situations; to help 'get a grip'

Complementary &/or similar flower essences

Agrimony, Almond, Angel's Trumpet, Aspen, Black Eyed Susan, Chamomile, Crowea, Garlic, Glassy Hyacinth, Indian Pink, Lady's Slipper, Mimulus, Nectarine, Olive, Pear, Scarlet Monkeyflower (and all Monkeyflowers), St John's Wort, Star of Bethlehem, Sweet Chestnut, Waratah

Supporting the changes

- Investigate the Jungian concept of the Shadow – that part of the unconscious that holds everything we consciously choose not to do or be.
- Practise relaxation techniques or activities that enable you to let go. Become familiar with how it feels.
- Just for once, allow someone else to drive the car, run the finances or initiate love-making.
- Trust!

Chestnut Bud

Aesculus hippocastanum   (Green / Bach)

Positive state

Learning/growing from experience
Full awareness, insight

Negative state

Not learning from life experience
Repeating old mistakes, lack of hindsight

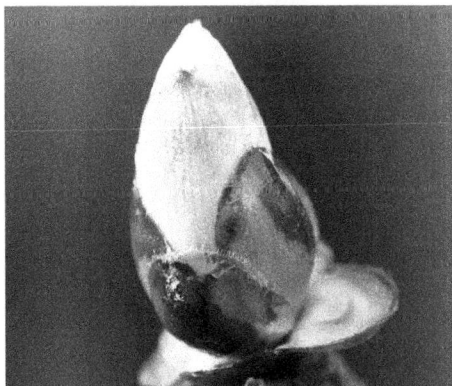

Chestnut Bud, from the majestic Horse Chestnut tree, bursts forth in the spring *awakening* of Nature. A bud represents both immaturity and also new beginnings and great *potential for growth*, learning and development. The tree's equine association (the name *hippocastanum* derives from the Greek word for horse) is due to the peculiar horseshoe-shaped scars left on the smaller branches by the previous years' leaf stems. This aspect of the plant signature represents scars left by life experiences but also the *lessons learnt*, etched in our memory for future reference. The *green* colour of the bud can represent the greenness of immaturity, inexperience and naivety. It also signifies an openness of *heart* to new experience and the *wisdom* gained from it.

The Chestnut Bud personality

Chestnut Bud is suitable for anybody who continually falls back into old, self-defeating habits – the child at school who makes the same mistakes over and over so that learning is impeded; the worker who doesn't recognise a recurring problem and repeats the same errors of judgement; people who repeatedly fall back into addictive, self-destructive habits relating to food, drugs, sleep patterns and so on, without seeming to gain any insight.

Benefits of taking Chestnut Bud

Chestnut Bud helps to raise our awareness of the warning signs that point to a recurrence of destructive patterns, allowing us a better overview of life as we contact our inner wise teacher and receptive student for guidance. It can help us maintain concentration, clarity and focus, allowing us to see our goals more clearly, as well as how to reach them more easily. Most of all, Chestnut Bud helps us gain wisdom from life experiences.

Possible physical imbalances

In those who can benefit from Chestnut Bud flower essence, there is often 'selective memory' and a lack of awareness when it comes to choices relating to food and lifestyle. Habitual unhealthy choices can result in food sensitivities and intolerances and even addictions, which all take their toll on bodily health and vitality.

Common uses

For the slow learner of life's lessons; for those who don't seem to learn from their mistakes; for self-awareness; to help contact the 'inner guide' (Centaury is for the 'inner child'); to get the best out of a learning experience; for a 'budding' situation; to 'wise up'

Complementary &/or similar flower essences

Black Eyed Susan, Blackberry, Boab, Bottlebrush, Californian Poppy, Chrysanthemum, Clematis, Dill, Fairy Lantern, Filaree, Forget-Me-Not, Gentian, Iris, Kangaroo Paw, Lotus, Madia, Mullein, Paw Paw, Red Grevillea, Sage, Sagebrush, Saguaro, Self-Heal, Shasta Daisy, Star Tulip, Tansy, Walnut

Supporting the changes

- Try to be more accountable to yourself for your progress in learning from experience. Make a daily chart of how well you're doing. Be honest with yourself – show how often you really ate chocolate this week, or how often you left the side gate open and accidentally let the dog out!
- Create learning systems that will allow you to check your progress and observe yourself and your patterns of behaviour.
- 'Listen up.'

Chicory

Cichorium intybus (Blue / Bach)

Positive state

Recognised and appreciated
Unconditional giving and receiving

Negative state

What about me?
Conditional love and attention

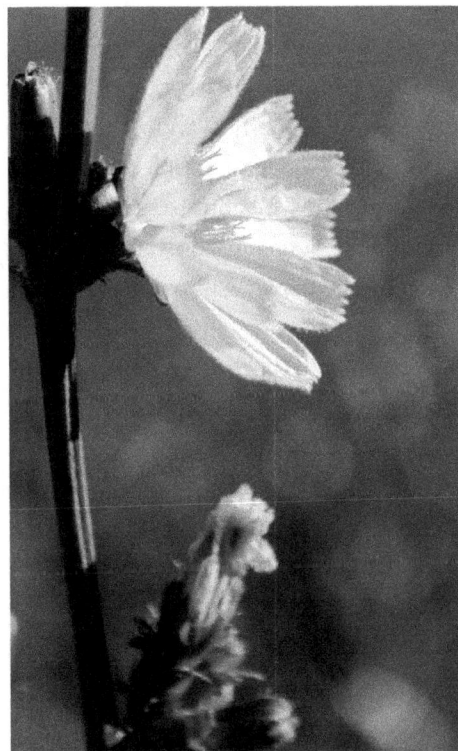

Chicory is a perennial herb that grows wild in fields, hedges and roadsides in Europe and has been introduced to Australia. It has been used in herbal medicine since ancient times and the dried, roasted and ground root is often blended with coffee or used as a caffeine-free coffee substitute. Chicory's *sky-blue* flowers can be totally relied upon to open and close at the same times each day, unconditionally responding to and serving nature.

Chicory flower essence's quality of *unconditional love* reminds us of the mythology of Mother Earth (Gaia) and the Jungian concept of the feminine or *archetypal mother*. The pure blue colour of Chicory flowers also reminded Dr Bach of the blue of Mary, the mother of

Jesus, and *pure spiritual love* – 'a wellspring of love found in the mother whether in the family or in the world' (Barnard 1988).

Another important plant signature is that the flower buds form in clusters and open one after another in succession. Each flower lasts only a day, opening at sunrise and closing after midday but each bud always gets its time to blossom and be radiant. Each gets its 'day in the sun' and then unconditionally gives way to another flower the next day.

The Chicory personality

Chicory people have a lot of love and help to give – 'as Bach put it, we "long to open both our arms and bless all around"' (Barnard 1988) – but often feel unappreciated. Sometimes this makes them sulk and put conditions on their love and offerings, even manipulating situations in order to get the recognition, attention and appreciation they feel is their 'due'.

In the negative Chicory state we often feel that our voice is not heard and we lose trust in life's ability to meet our emotional needs. 'No one looks out for me! Look at all I've done for you and this is how you repay me!' are typical Chicory complaints. When we feel like this we may scheme and go to great lengths to change the situation. Unfortunately, we often do this in unproductive ways, resorting to clingy and manipulative behaviour that only decreases our chances of getting what we want.

If we don't trust that our needs will be met, our love can become conditional – we count it as a sort of currency. We may have a sense of missing out on our fair share, when fear has stopped us responding to opportunities and others have snapped them up. Sibling rivalry is another example of a negative Chicory pattern. With the arrival of a new baby, the older child desperately sets out to re-establish a sense of his or her place and importance in the family dynamic, constantly seeking the attention they believe has been taken away by the baby. 'What about me?' is a common refrain.

Whenever illness arises (especially in children) and there is a feeling of being powerless and not receiving enough attention and support, always consider Chicory to assist recovery.

Benefits of taking Chicory

Chicory helps us effectively communicate our needs to those around us, and then trust that those needs will be met. Chicory helps us trust in life's abundance and increases our ability to perceive its flow in our lives, enabling us to act and love unconditionally.

Possible physical imbalances

Any illness that arises when we feel powerless or feel we are not receiving the attention and support we deserve will respond well to Chicory. It is useful for physical illnesses in children, especially in situations, for example, where it is a big inconvenience on a workday for one of two working parents to stay at home with them. Through illness, the child may be unconsciously saying, 'What about me, Mum and Dad!! Stop for a second and let's BE together.'

Common uses

For sibling rivalry; for the relentlessly attention-seeking child or adult; for the 'sulker'; for feelings of being unappreciated and powerless; for fear of missing out, feeling 'What about me?'; to help you mother, not smother!; to operate with unconditional love; to tap into universal emotional abundance; to trust that you will get what you need in life

Complementary &/or similar flower essences

Almond, Bleeding Heart, Buttercup, Chrysanthemum, Cosmos, Deer Brush, Dogwood, Larkspur, Mariposa Lily, Quaking Grass, Quince, Star Thistle, Tiger Lily, Trillium, Willow

Supporting the changes

- Learn effective communication and self-assertiveness so that you can use overt rather than covert ways to get what you want.
- Learn to criticise constructively, especially in relation to those close to you.
- Try to engage in activities that are self-nurturing. For example, seek the company of people who appreciate you and follow interests that truly delight and nourish you.
- Learn to give and receive gifts or compliments for no other reason than the joy of it.

Chrysanthemum
Chrysanthemum morifolium   (Red-brown / FES)

Positive state
Philosophical and less materialistic focus
Grounded in one's own spiritual identity

Negative state
Facing one's mortality and the inadequacy of materialism
'Losing my religion'; mid-life crisis (FES)

Chrysanthemum's earth-coloured flower conveys its intimate relationship with *material existence* on Earth. The flower essence is helpful in *grounding* our higher spiritual nature in the realities of a materialistic world – not just confining one's higher *spiritual identity* to church on Sunday for instance. The *red-brown* colour of the flower also relates to the energy of the *base chakra* (grounding) and *sacral chakra*, which can provide unique 'colour' to individual expression within a group *belief system* such as an organised religion. The flower essence is particularly helpful, for example, to help us expand upon or *transcend* traditional religious beliefs from childhood which have now become too rigid, inhibiting or shallow for us.

The Chrysanthemum personality

If you are tired of just chasing the almighty dollar and being totally devoted to material concerns, and have become receptive to deeper, more personally meaningful experiences, your new-found wisdom may draw you to this flower essence. The appearance of brown in the aura can indicate a condition of toxicity and encumbrance and may signal the need for purification and change. When the stream of your life has become clouded by stagnant, muddy waters, it would be wise to consider Chrysanthemum flower essence. This red-brown flower has a strong connection with midlife (healing) crises and can help steer a course that enables a person to age with grace in body and heart.

As the body loses its youthful exuberance and it is no longer possible to take physical strength and vitality for granted, a more philosophical perspective becomes advantageous to wellbeing. If you are questioning your belief system or looking for a new one that respects and embraces all your life experiences and wisdom gained therefrom, consider Chrysanthemum.

Benefits of taking Chrysanthemum

This flower essence can help you connect with your higher spiritual identity and your better nature and judgement. As a health practitioner, I see people every day who are confronting their mortality because of physical incapacitation and illness. The ego fears its own demise and as a result, forms a soul-draining dependence on this life. Fear of death, whether conscious or unconscious, cannot really be alleviated by blind faith in medical science or outgrown religious doctrine. It can be eased by faith in our higher Self or soul nature that is not physically constrained and impermanent (Kaminski and Katz 1994). This need not mean a diminished commitment to life – in fact commitment can become stronger, as what is truly fulfilling and right for your life becomes clearer when a materialistic view isn't the only one available to you.

Possible physical imbalances

Chrysanthemum flower essence is often indicated for women experiencing midlife crisis. If this also accompanied by difficult physical menopausal symptoms, they will likely be helped indirectly.

Common uses

Breaking old, ingrained habits that no longer serve you; 'losing my religion' (as the REM song says); coming to terms with mortality; re-sensing your soul's immortality; for finding true spiritual identity; self-actualisation; ageing wisely and gracefully

Complementary &/or similar flower essences

Angel's Trumpet, Angelica, Angelsword, Easter Lily, Filaree, Forget-Me-Not, Hibbertia, Honeysuckle, Hound's Tongue, Iris, Lady's Slipper, Lotus, Love-Lies-Bleeding, Nicotiana, Pretty Face, Purple Monkeyflower, Quaking Grass, Queen Anne's Lace, Sage, Sagebrush, Saguaro, Silver Princess, Star Tulip, Zinnia

Supporting the changes

- Take renewed interest in your diet and lifestyle. Eat mainly 'live' foods such as fresh fruit, vegetables and nuts and consider cleansing diets. Regular physical exercise will help to get a sluggish metabolism moving. Feel better being 'out of your head' and in your body'!
- Explore different philosophical approaches to life, especially those of people you admire and respect. Read about successful, natural negotiation of menopause, midlife and other life crises.
- As the old cliché says, today is the first day of the rest of your life!

Clematis

Clematis vitalba   (White / Bach)

Positive state

Stable and 'down to earth'
Practical, alert and focused

Negative state

Vague, 'split off', not grounded in the moment
Dreamy (dis)orientation

Clematis is a creeper that hasn't any means of supporting itself and *so depends upon others* – the small trees and shrubs around it – to carry it aloft (Barnard 1988). The creamy-white, tufted flowers *lack intensity or strength* of colour and give off a very faint vanilla scent. Despite these *unremarkable* features Clematis grows very *prolifically*, successfully covering large areas and was one of the first three flower essences discovered by Dr Bach. It has a strong hold on life and on the plant on which it finds *stability*, learning 'to hold on when there is nothing in you except the will which says to you – hold on!', as Dr Bach said (Barnard 1988). Clematis is a great example of *strength in apparent frailty* and the flower essence can help us turn our perceived weaknesses into strengths.

The Clematis personality

People in the negative Clematis state have vivid and colourful thoughts that are seldom converted into action because their mental world absorbs all their energy. They constantly escape to the future from present responsibilities. It is easy for them to disappear into reading, watching films, daydreaming or planning ahead at the expense of things and people of more immediate concern. It is useful to compare Clematis with Honeysuckle: while Clematis often escapes from the present into the future, Honeysuckle escapes from the present into the past; both seek happier times.

Fantasy and daydreaming can be therapeutic in moderation and are quite normal for children, but when they are constant in adult life they can prevent us from living our full potential. Like the Clematis vine which has no means of supporting itself and relies on other plants to hold it up, we can become dependent on others for support and structure in our lives if we don't put enough energy into day-to-day practicalities. I describe some of my clients who can benefit from Clematis as 'detached but held firm' by family, partner or friends.

Benefits of taking Clematis

There are times when we find ourselves easily distracted from mundane and unattractive tasks, whether studying for an exam or an unappealing project at work. Clematis is very helpful during temporary lapses in motivation, allowing us to convert thought into action. Clematis helps ground us so that our thoughts and ideas can take tangible form on Earth. We begin to feel more comfortable in the present, and so become more productive and self-fulfilled. Optimism about life is renewed and, like the Clematis plant itself, spreads fast.

Possible physical imbalances

Consider Clematis for the effects of concussion and shock (always seek medical advice as well) and for the after-effects of drug abuse (especially marijuana), jetlag or anaesthetics, when disorientation results from a dislocation or distortion of our multidimensional anatomy.

Common uses

For the unrealistic dreamer or mental 'space cadet'; for mind-body dislocation; for inability to concentrate or focus; for procrastination; to help commit to 'being here'; for 'grounding' in the present; to become fully conscious; to 'wake up' to yourself!

Complementary &/or similar flower essences

Arnica, Blackberry, Californian Pitcher Plant, Cayenne, Corn, Echinacea, Fairy Lantern, Honeysuckle, Lotus, Madia, Manzanita, Morning Glory, Mugwort, Nicotiana, Peppermint, Red Lily, Rosemary, Shooting Star, Star Tulip, Sundew, Tall Yellow Top, Tansy, Wild Rose, YES formula

Supporting the changes

- Engage in as many grounding activities as possible, such as working with earth in some form (gardening or pottery, for instance). Physical exercise such as bike-riding or bushwalking will get the blood flowing through your veins, making you aware of your body and giving you a sense that it belongs to you.
- Create some routines in your life. They will help you develop a sense of responsibility and self-reliance, making you more accountable to yourself and others and keeping you mentally in tune with the present.
- Avoid spending too much time in meditation or other passive, mental activities.
- WAKE UP!

Coffee
Coffea arabica   (White / FES-res)

Positive state
Enthused and focused
Mental acumen and decisiveness

Negative state
Lethargic and lack of mental clarity
Mentally slow and lacklustre

Coffee's white, scented flowers grow in clusters for only a few days in spring – their blooming is *short and sharp* like the quick, *stimulating effect* we expect from a cup of coffee or other caffeine 'hit'. *White* relates to the *crown chakra*, which *inspires* and sheds *'light'* on the subject – you! Flower clusters relate to *working together* in relationship, which is a characteristic of *heart chakra* consciousness. These aspects stimulate the mental and emotional bodies simultaneously, so that head and heart work together, giving us the ability to make quick and *insightful decisions*.

We use coffee to sustain us and allow us to access energy for moving towards a desired result or vision we have for the immediate and long term future. However, over time, over-consumption of coffee causes the visionary aspirations of the mental body to develop but leaves us lagging in our ability to bring our plans to fruition.

Coffee addicts are often visionaries who see how life could be in the future and are determined to function that way now, without having developed the necessary physical capacity (Cunningham and Ramer 1988). In other words, they get 'aHEAD of themselves' and risk the burnout associated with serious adrenal and physical fatigue from an overstimulated sympathetic nervous system.

The Coffee state of mind

Consider the effects you seek from your next cup of coffee and you will understand the positive state to which Coffee flower essence naturally leads you. Striving to boost productivity and alertness, we often drink coffee as a tool to alter the body's natural rhythms, cranking ourselves up and bypassing necessary quiet times in both physical and mental rhythms. This can create a problem of caffeine-dependence and eventually, a real possibility of burnout and/or other health issues.

Benefits of taking Coffee

Coffee flower essence raises the vibration of caffeine to the equivalent of a homeopathic frequency and in this way nullifies its negative physical effects and potential addictiveness. This action assists in lessening our dependence so that we may more comfortably and effectively cut back or eliminate our coffee intake. Most importantly, Coffee flower essence can help us consciously reconnect with natural body rhythms, so that we can become more effective and productive by using natural energy peaks and then resting and recovering sufficiently afterwards.

Possible physical imbalances

As mentioned above, Coffee flower essence helps lessen our physical dependence on caffeine. Coffee flower essence nullifies the effects of caffeine residue and enhances its elimination from the system. Once the residue of any drug of dependence is eliminated from the body, physical cravings for it rapidly subside.

The health benefits of lessening caffeine intake to moderate amounts are well documented.

Common uses

To help give up coffee or cut back on intake; to help overcome lethargy and/or indifference; to help quicken perception; for better decision-making under pressure; to improve efficiency and become more productive; to 'switch on'!

Complementary &/or similar flower essences

Blackberry, Californian Poppy, Cayenne, Clematis, Corn, Cotton, Forget-Me-Not, Grapefruit, Hornbeam, India Paintbrush, Iris, Lemon, Macrocarpa, Madia, Morning Glory, Nasturtium, Nicotiana, Olive, Peppermint, Rosemary, Silver Princess, Sundew, Tall Yellow Top, Tansy, Wild Oat, Wild Rose

Supporting the changes

- Get back in sync with your body's natural circadian rhythms. Have adequate sleep, including at least an hour before midnight. Take short breaks throughout the day - relax during these time-outs and enjoy a bit of productive daydreaming.
- Engage in moderate exercise every day to get the blood flowing through your capillaries right to the extremities (especially your head!)
- Ask yourself, 'Do I really like my work and feel it has a fulfilling future?'

Corn

Zea mays   (Yellow-white / FES)

Positive state
Grounded and well-orientated
Well-adjusted in social interaction and urban living

Negative state
Easily disorientated and 'stressed out'
Feeling 'uprooted and scattered' by crowded city living (FES)

Corn seeds display *different colours* and this implies the plant's potential for balance in diversity – in other words, the potential to diversify or *adapt to diversity* in the environment. Corn's potential for change and adaptation to its environment is also reflected in its fairly *simple DNA structure*. Lots of mutational change has been possible through easy manipulation of the corn plant to generate new and different types of crops (non-laboratory 'genetic engineering'). The way plants and animals adapt to the ever-changing environment is through mutation, which is the basic process that drives evolution. Today, Corn essence assists individuals to adapt to increasingly crowded and 'built up' urban environments where there is great diversity, especially in terms of race, culture and behaviours. The plant's predominantly yellow colour relates it to the solar plexus chakra and the comfortable assimilation ('digestion') of what is happening in our immediate environment while remaining grounded.

The Corn state of mind

We need Corn essence when we are thrown off balance by the city's frenetic activity and diversity. Confined to crowded city life with its melting pot of peoples, cultures, colours, art forms, buildings, machines and noise we can easily become disconnected and 'scattered.' Disharmony is created by this inability to really connect, engage and ground oneself in a mutually respectful and sustaining relationship with the environment. Stressed and disorientated, 'sea change' or 'tree change' lifestyles in the wide open spaces may become increasingly attractive. Our reveries about a different way of life are usually interrupted when we are called back to the reality of urban living. Corn essence can help us to respond to the innate urge to foster the evolution of our soul's inner sanctum despite the convolution of the city's complexity and commotion. In other words, energetically we grow outwards from within in order to compensate for external pressures of city life and cope better with them. Or as Kaminski and Katz (1994) put it, 'Corn essence addresses the soul's need for spaciousness – its desire to live freely within the vast matrix of Nature and Cosmos.'

Benefits of taking Corn

Corn essence helps us balance our emotions, creating an inner calm that buffers us from what is outside. This allows us to remain grounded, well-orientated and strongly present, countering the hyperactivity and destabilising effects of urban life. We can then practise discernment, remaining receptive to what is beneficial while remaining protected against debilitating factors in our environment. Spiritually we can connect and cooperate with the finest in our surroundings, transcending what is harsh, especially in city life.

Potential physical imbalances

Always consider Corn (along with other appropriate flower essences) when the stresses of living in the 'rat race' create health issues. Digestive problems are common, as are other slow-developing and insidious illnesses that seem to be strongly psychosomatic in origin.

Over-use or daily use of some foods can create allergies or intolerances – for example potatoes, sugar (and alcohol), dairy products, wheat (and other grains, including corn) – and temporary elimination of these foods from the diet while taking flower essences, especially Corn flower essence, will help to solve the problem.

Common uses

To 'get your feet back on the ground'; to 'ground and centre' oneself; to connect and commune with your environment; for grounded presence that creates personal space (in crowded urban/city life); for better natural orientation; to become more relaxed and in harmony with one's environment

Complementary &/or similar flower essences

Aloe Vera, Angelica, Arnica, Californian Pitcher Plant, Canyon Dudleya, Cayenne, Clematis, Cosmos, Crowea, Dill, Echinacea, Garlic, Golden Rod, Golden Yarrow, Indian Pink, Lady's Slipper, Lavender, Madia, Mountain Pennyroyal, Nicotiana, Quaking Grass, Rabbitbrush, Red Clover, Red Lily, Shooting Star, Star Tulip, Sweet Pea, Walnut, all the Yarrows, YES formula

Supporting the changes

- Being able to properly ground and centre oneself is of utmost importance. All activities that further this end should be encouraged, from physical exercise and gardening through to relaxation techniques and meditation.
- Make brief 'time out' periods to contemplate what you intend to do well in the next few hours. In other words, be the director of how you want your day to pan out!
- Escape to the country sometimes, or at least to a park or garden haven.
- Create a personal refuge you can visit when you need to.

Cosmos

Cosmos bipinnatus   (Red-purple & yellow / FES)

Positive state

Speaking and living your heartfelt truth
Emotionally articulate (FES) – coherent speech

Negative state

'Overwhelmed by too many ideas' (FES)
Emotionally inarticulate – overexcited or erratic speech

Cosmos' *deep red-purple flower* immediately commands attention; you cannot help but notice. It *'speaks'* to you with clarity and colour and these extrovert qualities can help you *unravel and externalise* what you really feel inside. Some people even find the flower's colour a *'bit rich'* when confronted by its clear and uncompromising, *honest expression*. Cosmos helps the *heart chakra (passion)* and *throat chakra (communication)* to work in harmony, bringing composure in *self-expression* when speaking and *creative expression* in life generally.

The Cosmos personality

People in the negative Cosmos state find it hard to express their thoughts and feelings, which may be verbalised in a disordered or confused way. They may feel frustrated in their ability to clearly articulate opinions on certain issues that are important to them. This can significantly inhibit their ability to define who they really are, clearly sense what is their heartfelt truth and speak it. In my practice I have often prescribed Cosmos flower essence for children who feel verbally intimidated (not necessarily aggressively) and/or entranced by the language of their parent(s) and always feel stifled or unsure how to respond. Cosmos has helped them to 'find their voice.'

Benefits of taking Cosmos

With the help of this essence you can speak more from the heart, honestly expressing yourself. Your heartfelt sentiments become CLEARER TO YOU and therefore CLEARER TO OTHERS, enabling them to hear and respond. And, as with anything straight from the heart, it rarely offends and usually heals. You can live your life as you see it and agree to disagree if need be in a democratic and caring environment. Your new direction in life, following the true aspirations of your heart, becomes much clearer.

Cosmos can also help you gather your composure before public speaking or a before musical, artistic or dramatic performance so that you can eloquently express your passion and genuine feeling.

Potential physical imbalances

Cosmos helps release emotional tensions stored in the heart area, freeing them up for more ease of expression via the throat centre. This has the potential to ease physical conditions associated with the lung and throat areas that might, for instance, manifest as asthma.

Common uses

To help you say what you feel; to help ease emotional tension in the heart; to help a child who feels stifled to find their voice; for composure in (public) speaking; to improve communication skills; to help you define your passion so that you can express it clearly to the world

Complementary &/or similar flower essences

Angelsword, Bleeding Heart, Calendula, Californian Poppy, Centaury, Deer Brush, Fuchsia, Golden Rod, Indian Paintbrush, Indian Pink, Iris, Lady's Slipper, Larch, Madia, Mountain Pennyroyal, Mullein, Pink Monkeyflower, Pink Yarrow, Pomegranate, Rabbitbrush, Red Grevillia, Snapdragon, Trumpet Vine, Violet, Yerba Santa, Zinnia

Supporting the changes

- Learn some form of relaxation exercise which uses the breath, such as yoga, tai chi or meditation. Breath work is important in the release of emotional tension and stress in the heart area and can help you to gain composure. These rituals can become an integral part of your preparation for the day but especially for public speaking or other kinds of performance and for important social events.
- Take a deep breath.

Cotton

Gossypium hirsutum (White to yellow (cream) / FES-res)

Positive state

Clear headed – progressive outlook
Aware, self-assured, and discerning

Negative state

Feeling vague and 'in a mental limbo'
Mistrusts own judgement – insecure

The Cotton plant has many *fine hairs*, signifying extreme *sensitivity* to what is around. When we say, 'It made my hair stand on end' or 'It gave me goose bumps' we describe a capacity to *'cotton on'* to subtle aspects of a situation, which may be hidden from view. With the help of Cotton flower essence, a *dreary/fuzzy outlook* can become more *spiritually sensitised* and a new *mental clarity* will prevail.

The expression 'wrapping something up in cotton wool' describes Cotton's *protective* capacity. In Greek mythology, cotton plants were described as 'wool-bearing trees' or 'vegetable lambs.' 'Certain trees ... bear for their fruit fleeces surpassing those of sheep in beauty and excellence and the Asian natives clothe themselves in cloths made therefrom.' This theme of animal-like 'protective clothing' applies to the qualities of the flower essence, which provides an *insulating and protective etheric 'skin'* – the essence metaphorically 'wraps you up in cotton wool' while you undergo a *spiritual awakening* and reach a point of acute mental clarity that accompanies the emergence of a new and wiser mindset. In other words, you've finally 'cottoned on'! (Walnut flower essence, similarly, helps to create a *protected psychological space* that allows us to be free from distraction as we undergo internal changes that lead to a new mental outlook.)

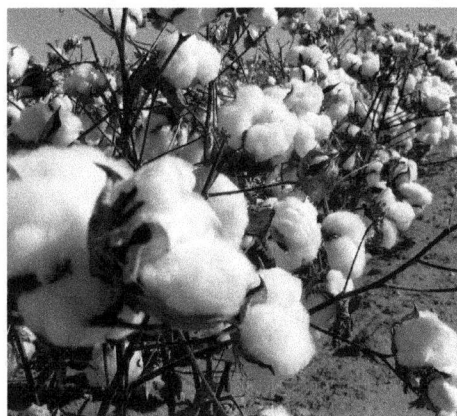

The Cotton state of mind

People who can benefit from Cotton flower essence often feel 'woolly-headed' and clouded in their thinking – as if 'the (cotton) wool has been pulled over their eyes.' They are unsure of themselves and fear that they will be taken advantage of or even 'taken over.' On a subconscious (soul) level they are opening up to a new level of being but on a conscious level they feel uneasy, with an unexplained sense of being vulnerable. It's a bit like shedding an old skin and feeling raw and over-exposed during the process of metamorphosing into a new form.

When people complete personal development courses or go through a major experience that challenges their previous belief system, for a short period they may feel 'out of it,' in a kind of limbo in their thinking. And then a fresh, new and invigorated perspective and philosophy of life begins to emerge.

Benefits of taking Cotton

Cotton flower essence strengthens and energises the aura, allowing you to feel more secure and protected and less susceptible to unwanted outside influences. You can carry on your normal everyday activities with more mental clarity, heightened awareness and sensitivity, without feeling as vulnerable as you did before. Your mental faculties are exalted and your mind becomes more attuned to your higher Self, like a radio tuned to a clearer signal.

Potential physical imbalances

In my practice as a therapist I have found that many people who are in need of Cotton flower essence suffer from 'congestion' in the head – whether in the form of sinus congestion, tendency to headache, light-headedness or mental vagueness.

Common uses

For mental clarity; to protect you ('wrap you up in cotton wool') when feeling vulnerable; to 'clear the head'; to safely and securely heighten your psychic awareness and sensitivity; to welcome a new and progressive outlook on life

Complementary &/or similar flower essences

Angel's Trumpet, Angelica, Angelsword, Baby Blue Eyes, Canyon Dudleya, Chaparral, Chrysanthemum, Clematis, Deer Brush, Garlic, Forget-Me-Not, Fringed Violet, Honeysuckle, Hound's Tongue, Lady's Slipper, Lavender, Lotus, Madia, Morning Glory, Mountain Pennyroyal, Mugwort, Nicotiana, Peppermint, Purple Monkeyflower, Queen Anne's Lace, Rabbitbrush, Red Clover, Red Lily, Rosemary, St John's Wort, Star Tulip, Sundew, Violet, Walnut, all the Yarrows, YES formula

Supporting the changes

- Develop dynamic methods of self-protection such as visualising white light around you, other forms of meditation or performing protective rituals.
- Retreat to your special 'safe haven' on a regular basis, metaphorically 'wrapping yourself up in cotton wool' for short spells.
- Get some fresh air!!

Crab Apple

Malus sylvestris   (White tinged with pink / Bach)

Positive state

Broad-minded
Self-love, aware of the beauty in all around

Negative state

Finicky, nit-picky and 'crabby'
Feeling toxic (yucky!), unclean or ashamed

Crab Apple's flowers are *white*, reflecting the potential *purifying* qualities of the essence, with a tinge of *pink*, signifying an affinity with the *heart chakra* and the cleansing of *toxic feelings and thoughts*. While the flowers are sweet the fruit is sharp and sour *(bitter-sweet!)*, reminding us of the positive and negative states addressed by the flower essence. The fruit's sour taste is also suggestive of the flower essence's *astringent*, toning and cleansing qualities. This flower essence offers us another good example of how action on the metaphysical level can influence the physical level, particularly in relation to the purification processes in the body.

Crab Apple is the wild apple that domestic varieties were originally bred from. The ancient belief that 'apples confer *eternal youth*' has found its way into the contemporary psyche in the form of the saying 'An apple a day keeps the doctor away' – the idea that apples have a therapeutic, cleansing effect which is life-prolonging. Our quest for longer life brings us into consciousness of mortality and our obligation to the immortal/eternal Self, an awareness that *puts small problems into proper perspective.*

The Crab Apple personality

A feeling of contamination or of being unclean is a primary indication for the use of Crab Apple flower essence – something doesn't feel right or, as a child would put it, 'I feel yucky.' A typical human response to internal disquiet is to externalise the problem, separating it from the psyche as a way of dealing with it. This externalising process may take the form of a focus on one part of the body, becoming obsessed with a perceived imperfection and losing perspective about what is really important. In the negative Crab Apple state, we get caught up in annoying details, becoming disconnected from the big picture. Or we may become pedantic, wasting time on trivia to the point where the magic of full experience is lost. We may lose appreciation of the exquisite pleasure of love-making by focusing on body parts and details of the physical act. A small skin blemish, a birthmark or slight body odour may destroy our capacity to see our own beauty or that of others. We project all our shame and self-condemnation onto these minor idiosyncrasies, focussing on them out of all proportion.

When you feel 'toxic' or 'unclean' to the point of shame or feel repulsed or disgusted by your own and others' physical attributes, consider using Crab Apple flower essence.

Benefits of taking Crab Apple

Crab Apple is a cleanser at all levels, bringing a feeling of purity and freedom of spirit, so that we are able to sense more clearly the glow of inner beauty in ourselves and others. You will be better able to accept and see beyond your own imperfections, niggling fears and physical blemishes and feel free of shame about your appearance and behaviour. You will go with the flow, enjoying the moment without any inhibiting self-consciousness.

Possible physical imbalances

Crab Apple will support any detox/cleansing diet or treatment if a sense of uncleanness (or toxicity) is part of the presenting problem. It is often useful during brief periods of feeling yucky/toxic, guilty or ashamed after a period of overeating, or when similar feelings arise acutely before and during menstruation.

Common uses

For those who feel contaminated (or 'yucky') in mind or body; for a sense of shame; for those obsessed about impure thoughts and unclean bodies; to be less pedantic; to be less prudish; to be more broad-minded; to help put our (body) parts, our problems and lives in perspective

Complementary &/or similar flower essences

Basil, Billy Goat Plum, Black Eyed Susan, Bottlebrush, Chaparral, Chrysanthemum, Crowea, Easter Lily, Filaree, Flannel Flower, Hibiscus, Hound's Tongue, Impatiens, Lemon, Manzanita, Pine, Pretty Face, Rabbitbrush, Shasta Daisy, Sticky Monkeyflower, Wild Potato Bush

Crowea

Crowea saligna (Magenta-pink / Aus)

Positive state

Calm and centred
Open and worry-free mind

Negative state

A sense that something is 'not quite right' (Ian White)
Niggling worries and agitated anxiety

Crowea is a small shrub common to the coastal sandstone ridges of New South Wales and southern Queensland. Its *magenta-pink* flower has a *pronounced centre* due to long appendages on the stamen tips. Ian White, developer of this Australian Bush Flower Essence, describes its usefulness in helping to *'centre and balance'* a person prior to treatment. The flower's distinctive *magenta-pink* centre relates to its strong affinity to the *heart chakra* or *heart of our being*. People in meditation aspire to *heart centre consciousness* – a profoundly aware and accepting but completely relaxed state of mind.

All flower essences with an affinity to the heart chakra, and especially Crowea, have a significant centring and balancing influence on the physical/etheric, emotional and mental subtle bodies whose energies contribute to the personality.

The Crowea state of mind

Crowea is a flower essence to consider when you just don't feel right in yourself. Perhaps you are worried, even though there is nothing in particular to worry about, or you're so wound up you worry even if you have nothing to worry about! You may feel as though there is something you haven't checked or locked or attended to, but there isn't!

Crowea can help calm the mind when it is cluttered by incidentals – little concerns and worries that are simply not very important. People can find themselves in this state when they have been worried about business or family matters for a long period of time and, even when the worst is over, the state of worry persists. It also helps people who find it difficult to switch off from work concerns in the evenings or on weekends.

Benefits of taking Crowea

Crowea helps us feel balanced, calm and centred, which results in a sense of vitality and energy. It is a good remedy for worry and stress.

At one time I was travelling an hour and a half from where I lived to the clinic where I worked from Monday to Thursday. On Thursday afternoons I would leave the clinic and not return until the following Monday. The distance I lived from the clinic, as well as the time I spent away from it, added to my worry each Thursday afternoon. As I was leaving, I always felt that there was something I had left unfinished or a door I had failed to lock or someone I had not contacted. This uneasy feeling would stay with me well into the weekend, despite the fact that everything was under control at the clinic. I decided to take Crowea for a couple of weeks and within the first week I noted some subtle but welcome changes to my state of mind. I was generally more relaxed mentally, worrying less and in time I was able to leave the clinic each week with less apprehension. As my mind became less cluttered, I felt more assured that I had attended to all important matters as needed.

Possible physical imbalances

An agitated and/or worried mind leads to tension in the body. Crowea flower essence will always support the practice of relaxation techniques, body balancing or stress-reducing activities. People who constantly worry about what may or may not happen next often develop stomach problems ranging from over-acid conditions to ulcers. Crowea flower essence can help us to 'greet and digest' each moment calmly, allaying the anticipatory anxiety that leads to digestive problems.

Common uses

To stop worrying and be mentally more at peace; to 'ground and centre' oneself before (or after) important events; to prepare for performing and public speaking; to facilitate meditation; to be more receptive to other more specific flower essences or therapies

Complementary &/or similar flower essences

Californian Poppy, Chamomile, Clematis, Corn, Cosmos, Crab Apple, Dandelion, Dill, Echinacea, Garlic, Filaree, Indian Pink, Lavender, Lotus, Nicotiana, Paw Paw, Red Clover, Red Lily, Shasta Daisy, Star of Bethlehem, Star Tulip, White Chestnut, Zinnia

Supporting the changes

- Learn meditation and/or other mental relaxation techniques.
- Any regular physical activity will help bring balance back to mental activity. Gardening, going for walks and even housework can have this effect.
- Yoga, tai chi and other physical disciplines are also relaxing and mentally calming.
- Get balance back into your lifestyle!

Dandelion

Taraxacum officinale (Yellow / FES)

Positive state

At ease; energy flowing freely
Relaxed, with a feeling that 'time is on your side'

Negative state

Physically and mentally uptight
'Over-striving' (FES); time-driven

Dandelion flowers are *yellow*, which is the colour that relates to intellect and the *mental body. Release of tension* associated with mental strain and over-striving is symbolised by the gesture of the plant's fluffy white seed-head releasing its seeds – a gentle metaphor for the *'tossing to the wind' of ingrained ideas and thought patterns.*

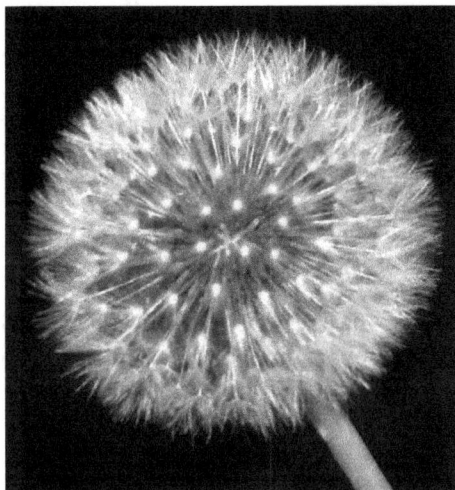

A strong aspect of the Dandelion plant's signature lies in its natural cycle. The yellow bloom, rich in mineral elements, represents the mental body. The nebulous and fragmenting white seedhead, at the mercy of the weather, represents the emotional body. And finally the dispersing seedlings which eventually fall to the ground represent the etheric/physical body. Through the *natural transformation of thought forms* of the mental body, *new and calmer mental patterns* flow to the physical body. (As Carl Jung states, 'the body and mind are just two sides of the same coin.') We are also reminded again of the saying that *'form follows function, follows thought'* – where the form of the physical body follows the function of the emotional body, which follows the thoughts of the mental body.

The Dandelion personality

In the negative Dandelion state, people strive to achieve a goal but then find it difficult to let go and simply allow what they want to happen. A tense, stress-driven mind causes a tense body and vice versa. Dandelion can assist in breaking this vicious cycle by helping to release tension in the mental body.

It is a suitable remedy for people who have an overwhelming zest for life (FES) and find it difficult to restrain themselves from going full speed to their destination, often driven by an inner sense of urgency. Dandelion can help high-achieving go-getters, hard-driven, overzealous, compulsive movers and shakers and those who continually overcommit themselves. It helps them take time out to 'experience more contained moments of reflective activity' (Kaminski and Katz 1994), so that they can relax, recover, consolidate and avoid physical and mental burnout.

Benefits of taking Dandelion

Dandelion flower essence can help you achieve a level of relaxation that eases the inner agitation which causes outward tension. If you're uptight and highly strung, with a 'motor' that keeps running even when you're stationary, Dandelion can help you wind down. Dandelion will help 'ground' and calm you so that you can better appreciate the present moment.

Possible physical imbalances

If your body's musculature is tense, energies don't flow easily and organ systems are prone to toxic build-up in their tissues. Dandelion can help you relax and allow a proper release and flow of energy. It is ideal in conjunction with massage and relaxation techniques and for use in sport/exercise recovery regimes. Release of nervous tension in the body will always aid liver function and it is not surprising that Dandelion has been traditionally accepted as a one of the first herbs to consider for treating the liver.

Common uses

To assist in deeper relaxation; to enhance therapeutic and relaxation massage; to aid recovery from strenuous exercise; to help the 'try-hard' person to let go; to help you wind down; to help the overly 'high achiever' achieve balance in life

Complementary &/or similar flower essences

Arnica, Bottlebrush, Californian Poppy, Chamomile, Cherry Plum, Corn, Crowea, Cosmos, Dill, Dogwood, Filaree, Fuchsia, Hibbertia, Impatiens, Indian Pink, Lavender, Nectarine, Nicotiana, Paw Paw, Shasta Daisy, Snapdragon, Vervain, White Chestnut, Yerba Santa, Zinnia

Supporting the changes

- Learn meditation and/or other mental and physical relaxation techniques.
- Any regular, preferably non-competitive, physical activity/exercise will help bring balance back to mental activity. Gardening and going for walks will have this effect.
- Yoga, tai chi and other physical activities where the breathing is a focus will also

assist in achieving a more relaxed and calm mental state.

- 'Chill out!'

Deerbrush

Ceanothus integerrimus   (White / FES)

Positive state

Purity of intention, 'clarity of purpose' (FES)
Clear and direct communication

Negative state

Giving 'mixed messages'
'Beating around the bush' in communication

Deerbrush's flowers are *white*, the colour associated with purity, and in this case the flower essence helps us live and act with greater *purity of intention*. The *soft* and *fluffy flowers* are like the padding of a pillow. People who can benefit from taking Deerbrush often *'pad'* what they are saying in order to *'soften the blow'* but unfortunately this merely confuses the listener, as does the fact that individual flowers may be *disguised* amongst the bunch. The little flowers are white, with *a dome-like shape at the end of the stalk* similar to Dill, and reminiscent of the *pineal gland*, which is governed by the *crown chakra*. The crown chakra is often described as our most direct channel to the *higher (spiritual) Self* which enables us to act with purest intention according to our highest good.

The Deerbrush personality

The person who can benefit from taking Deerbrush flower essence is often prone to self-deception in relation to their motives and intentions when communicating with others. They may allow themselves to remain unaware that they have an ulterior motive and that what they are saying or doing is not consistent with what they genuinely feel. When this is the case, people close to them feel that they have been deceived when true intentions become clear. On the other hand, sometimes a person's intentions are in fact quite noble and the problem is that over-politeness causes them to be indirect for fear of offending. In either case, indirectness is the problem and those on the receiving end may be exasperated by what seems like an inability to 'talk straight.'

Many years ago I participated in a course devoted to personal growth. During the course we were given a simple but profound model to help us measure where we were in relation to our personal issues and development. The model proposed the following stages of development: At the start we are unconsciously unskilled at living out aspects of our potential, then through self-reflection we gain further self-understanding and become consciously unskilled. By taking personal responsibility and acting on this greater self-awareness we become consciously skilled, until finally after more work, we start to live our true potential, becoming unconsciously skilled. In the negative state, the Deerbrush person struggles to synchronise conscious intention with skilled action. Kaminski and Katz (1996) state that the personality needs to self-observe and maintain inner scrutiny 'in order to align inner motive with outer deed.' Deerbrush essence can help us on the path to living consistently in an unconsciously skilled manner.

Benefits of taking Deerbrush

Deerbrush helps us to be more pure in our intention, clear in our communication and direct in our action. We become consistently conscious of our motives and are able to be clear about them with others. Being more honest and open allows us to display our inner truth and this earns us respect for acting with integrity. Our sincerity is appreciated, making those in our presence all the more receptive to the grace we bestow on them.

Possible physical imbalances

Many people who have benefited from Deerbrush have also suffered from ailments associated with 'congestion' in the head, including headaches and sinus conditions. As Traditional Chinese Medicine (TCM) informs us, sinus congestion often indicates that 'the heart is trying to get into the head' and headaches often indicate that the 'head is aching to go the way of the heart.' Both these sayings describe a person struggling to respond directly to the pure intent of the heart.

Common uses

To stop 'beating around the bush'; to learn to be more direct in communication; to help 'walk the talk'; for sincerity and good intent; to help you and others understand what you really mean and intend!

Complementary &/or similar flower essences

Agrimony, Angelsword, Black Eyed Susan, Blackberry, Boab, Calendula, Californian Pitcher Plant, Corn, Cosmos, Goldenrod, Lady's Slipper, Madia, Mullein, Quince, Red Grevillea, Red Lily, Rosemary, Queen Anne's Lace, Snapdragon, Tansy, Violet

Supporting the changes

- Consider doing some personal (psycho-)analysis.
- Practise methods that help you become better attuned to your inner Self. Meditation, contemplation, regular 'time out' to gather your thoughts, or any

process that helps you achieve more clarity of purpose in your daily life will be useful.

- Say what you mean!

Dill

Anethum graveolens   (Yellow / FES)

Positive state

Mutually beneficial environmental exchange
Calmly 'digesting' life, purposeful

Negative state

Hyper-reactive to what's around
'Overwhelmed due to over-stimulation' (FES); abuzz

Dill's aromatic seeds have been used for centuries to treat a wide variety of digestive ailments. In its more subtle form as a flower essence, this healing ability helps us better *'digest' and process life experience*, assimilating what we need from the environment and discarding what we don't. Clients in my practice often comment on how 'busy' the flower bunches look, as if there is too much excitement, too much going on.

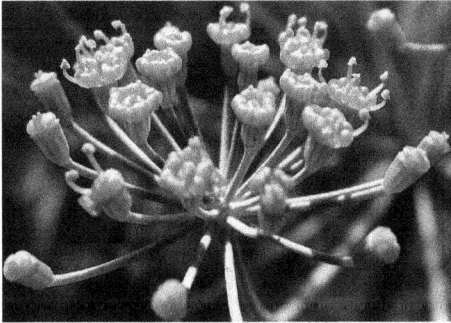

Dill has been a traditional colic remedy for babies, going by the name of 'gripe water' and can also promote the flow of mother's milk. This further emphasises how it may assist us to *calm down* and be more receptive to *assimilating* the soul food available in our immediate environment.

The name 'Dill' is derived from the Old Norse word *dilla* which means *'to lull.'* Another strong aspect of the plant's signature is the *dome-like arrangement of flowers on a stalk*. This flower form is symbolic of the *human pineal gland*. The pineal gland has been acknowledged as playing an important role in the body's hormonal processes, in particular those that influence circadian (24-hour) rhythms. The reception of light via the optic nerve is a critical factor in balanced functioning of the pineal gland. Lack of sleep or disturbed sleep as a result of shift work or jetlag have an effect on the amount and timing of light reception and so upset the body's 24-hour biorhythms. Any person who travels rapidly between time zones will be all too familiar with these effects.

Dill flower essence has a beneficial effect on the *crown chakra* which conditions the pineal gland and can help those who are constantly on the move to *adjust to new surroundings*. The crown chakra receives spiritual light – *shedding light on the subject* (you) – just as the pineal gland functions through the regulated reception of natural light. As we learn more about the pineal gland and its significance for health and wellbeing, many more opportunities for the use of Dill flower essence will arise.

The Dill plant grows by itself and has a very distinctive and recognisable odour. This gesture of *individuality and standalone independence* signifies the ability of the essence to help us maintain our focus and intention, allowing us to express what is inside, *despite what is happening on the outside!*

The Dill state of mind

Consider Dill flower essence when you feel that you are in the fast lane, with life and its experiences flashing by. You may have become overstimulated and overwhelmed by the amount of activity around you. In the city environment, many things compete for attention and it is hard to discern what we need to take in and what we can ignore. We may become overloaded and unable to effectively regulate incoming stimuli. This results in 'psychic indigestion' (Kaminski and Katz 1996), and as a result our nervous system is pushed to the brink. We suffer from psychic 'colic' or become desensitised, our senses temporarily numbed into submission. In these situations, only a holiday in a remote, simple and soothing environment or a dose of Dill flower essence can help.

Benefits of taking Dill

Dill flower essence helps us establish a calmer and more mutually beneficial relationship with our environment. A better balance (and relationship) is achieved between our emotional and etheric bodies – our feelings and sensations. This allows us to be more objective and helps us to discriminate between mere sensationalism and those sensorial impressions that can be of real benefit to us.

Dill flower essence helps us to take a more intelligent perspective on our predicament in life and sheds light on the subject — you! Then you can stand back, calmly 'digest' and assimilate what you need for soul nourishment and sustenance from your environment and respond in kind. You become like a renewable energy source, illuminating your environment just as the smile of a happy and contented (colic-free!) baby does.

Possible physical imbalances

Stress-related nervous problems such as an inability to unwind physically, disturbed sleep patterns, nervous fatigue and nervous digestive complaints are very possible when people become 'strung-out' in the negative Dill state of mind. Always consider Dill when travelling, to assist with time and spatial adjustment and to help ameliorate jetlag and maintain good sleep patterns (also consider Morning Glory.)

Common uses

To get out of life's fast lane and slow down; for when overstimulated by what's around; to help adjust to new surroundings after travel; when life is going through you 'like a dose of salts'; to help calm your 'digestion' of life experience; to spiritually enrich and be spiritually enriched by your environment

Complementary &/or similar flower essences

Aloe Vera, Arnica, Blackberry, Californian Poppy, Canyon Dudleya, Cayenne, Chamomile, Chaparral, Corn, Crowea, Dandelion, Echinacea, Filaree, Fringed Violet, Golden Yarrow, Indian Pink, Lavender, Madia, Morning Glory, Paw Paw, Rabbitbrush, Red Lily, Shasta Daisy, Walnut, YES formula

Supporting the changes

- The ability to properly ground and centre oneself is of utmost importance. All activities that further this end, from physical exercise and gardening through to relaxation techniques and meditation should be encouraged.
- Yoga, tai chi and other physical activities where breath is a focus will also assist in achieving a more relaxed, mentally clear and calm state.
- Learn to balance, shield and protect your auric field, especially your solar plexus, from unwanted impressions and influences. Creative visualisation of white light, for example, can be very useful.
- Develop your own safe 'haven of contemplation' to retreat to when you need.

Dogwood

Cornus nuttallii   (Creamy-white / FES)

Positive state

'Grace-filled movement' (FES) and coordination
Emotional and physical resilience/flexibility

Negative state

'Scarred' physical/etheric body (psychosomatic conditions)
'Awkward' (FES); 'uncomfortable in your body'

Dogwood's tiny yellow flowers form a central cluster surrounded by four showy, notched, creamy-white bracts that look like *thick and succulent* petals. The predominantly white bract – its succulent look and protection and support of the flower cluster – conveys the capacity of Dogwood flower essence to foster human

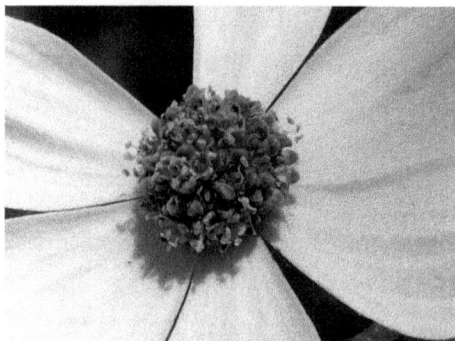

qualities of *self-protection* and the ability to *physically absorb or buffer* the impact of emotional shock and trauma. Native Americans used an extract of Dogwood bark to relieve sore and aching muscles.

Hopi Indians held that the use of tough, gnarled wood was important in the treatment of cramps and convulsions and part of Dogwood's signature is that it is known for its *extremely hard timber*. The flower essence can help *soften* a person who has become *scarred and hardened* by unresolved emotional trauma/hurt. Dogwood flower essence helps them become *liberated from* past *emotional injury* and *'freed up'* on emotional, etheric and physical levels. In my practice, some clients who responded well to Dogwood experienced an initial very brief period of intense, often tearful, emotional release after taking the essence, followed by a lovely sense of relief and lightened mood. It is interesting to note that in springtime the *bursting forth* of the blooming Dogwood trees was a signal to the Native Americans that it was time to plant corn, symbolising *new beginnings*, new growth and new ways of expression.

The Dogwood personality

Taken too far, our capacity for self-protection can make us overly guarded and defensive, unable to let go of the hurt we experienced in life. When we are in need of Dogwood flower essence, much emotional hurt has been absorbed and the memories remain firmly entrenched in our psyche, especially at the etheric and physical levels. 'Once bitten, twice shy,' is a very appropriate saying for Dogwood people in the negative state. Like those needing Willow flower essence, we may experience an accumulation of emotional trauma (or one particularly traumatic experience may stand out in our mind). We cannot or will not recover. Not only does our attitude become hardened but in sympathy, our physical body may also display rigidity and lack of resilience. In response to painful or abusive life circumstances the etheric body may shrivel and retract – receding from the source of pain. As a result the physical body hardens, lacking the fluidity of movement that would be a consequence of a normal healthy and fluid etheric body (Kaminski and Katz 1996).

I have found that many people who respond well to Dogwood are painfully aware of their body in some way – muscular stiffness in response to real or anticipated pain often causes awkwardness and a lack of fluid movement. This awkwardness escalates the problem by making the person more prone to accidents. This guarded and defensive attitude also aggravates the problem on another level – when people protect themselves from life's emotional hurts, they also protect themselves from receiving the nurturing that can strengthen their spiritual and emotional nature and heal deep-seated scars. As a therapist I have found that parts of a client's body are often affected asymmetrically (for instance, one knee only) by rheumatic or arthritic pain.

Benefits of taking Dogwood

When Dogwood is appropriately chosen it can have very positive effects. It is not uncommon to experience an improvement in nagging, inexplicable joint and muscle afflictions that have been unresponsive to other treatments. Sometimes emotional release occurs in the form of apparently unprovoked tears, followed by a sense of relief. Kaminski and Katz (1996) describe how 'the individual is able to feel more gentleness and inner sanctity, as the soul regains its state of grace through harmonious communion with the life or etheric body.'

Possible physical imbalances

Dogwood may be supportive in deep tissue therapy or any intense therapeutic bodywork. It will aid and support the release of past emotional trauma that has contributed to musculoskeletal problems and will also assist in the release and resolution of emotional issues that have resulted in inflexible attitudes and/or postures or a negative and 'stiff-necked' stance.

Common uses

'Once bitten, twice shy'; to help release and resolve past emotional trauma and hurt; to help learn to trust in life again; to become more flexible and adaptable on all levels; to help the 'old you' to blossom forth once again

Complementary &/or similar flower essences

Arnica, Baby Blue Eyes, Black Eyed Susan, Chaparral, Dandelion, Echinacea, Fuchsia, Golden Ear Drops, Hibiscus, Nicotiana, Vine, Willow

Supporting the changes

- Study the law of karma and investigate the power of thoughts and attitudes in creating your reality.
- Regular stretching and limbering-up exercises have a direct effect on the physical body's flexibility and resilience and will have a positive influence on your wellbeing. Consider yoga!
- Massage may help, from subtle therapeutic touch to deep tissue body-work. Remember that the depth of therapeutic action is not necessarily proportional to the force of physical action.
- Let it go! No one is to blame.

Easter Lily

Lilium longiflorum   (White / FES)

Positive state

'Ability to integrate sexuality with spirituality' (FES)
Reconciled and at ease with one's sexuality

Negative state

Ambivalence or 'feeling that sexuality is impure' (FES)
Inner conflicts with sexuality and morality

Easter Lily's flowers are *white*, a symbol of *purity and spiritual light*. Flower essences made from white flowers foster the ability to shed light upon what psychotherapist Carl Jung would call our *Shadow side* – those aspects of our emotional and mental patterning that we are uncomfortable with or would rather not acknowledge. The greater self-understanding provided by these essences allows us to view these aspects in a wider, more spiritual and meaningful context. Like Basil, Easter Lily relates especially to the *integration of sexuality and spirituality.* White lilies have also long been associated with reproduction and child-bearing. Easter Lily essence can be of great assistance to women, especially at midlife, when procreative energies associated with sexuality are being channelled into other areas of their lives. This is a time when many unreconciled attitudes and feelings about one's sexuality can surface.

The Easter Lily personality

For Christians, Easter is a time of spiritual cleansing and transformation through Christ's death and spiritual rebirth in the Resurrection. People who may benefit from Easter Lily are often going through a cleansing process, a symbolic death of parts of their persona – often in relation to their sexuality – which allows their pure spirit to shine through. Plants of the Lily family have fleshy underground parts, usually in the form of bulbs that allow the plant to stay alive but dormant in harsh conditions. Many women, particularly of previous generations, describe themselves as performing their 'duty' for the greater part of their sexually active years, 'going through the motions' without experiencing sexual intimacy as a truly loving and spiritual exchange. I am definitely not implying that it is only their responsibility! The potential for sexual fulfilment can remain dormant, often as a result of harsh and insensitive sexual encounters, cultural traditions and societal behaviours. Easter Lily flower essence, like all essences prepared from members of the Lily family, can help people whose potential remains untapped in certain areas because of conditions of deprivation. Flower essences from the Lily family bring forth awareness that can compensate for what was lacking during harsh and painful experiences in the past. (Lily flowers often have an upright posture, resembling a cup that is receptive to the provisions of the universe.) For example, Mariposa Lily makes it possible to be more receptive to the nurturing and 'mothering' that is available from one's environment, especially if these qualities were lacking as an infant.

New attitudes to sexuality associated with Easter Lily often coincide with a general change of life. Menopause or midlife may be times when a more spiritual perspective develops in a range of areas apart from the realm of sexuality. As spirituality begins to find expression, sexuality may be seen initially as something physically crude and less than pure (see Crab Apple). Past sexual habits and behaviour may be viewed as unclean or even promiscuous and, in reaction, there may be a swing towards celibacy or prudish behaviour 'which severs the soul from the life forces of the lower body' (Kaminski and Katz 1996). Easter Lily can help to integrate sexuality and spirituality by utilising 'the psychic currents which are associated with the sexual and reproductive organs.'

Benefits of taking Easter Lily

Easter Lily flower essence helps us reconcile sexuality and spirituality and allow sexual energy to enhance personal and spiritual growth. Untapped potential can find many more avenues of expression, enhancing a more creative and fulfilling lifestyle.

Possible physical imbalances

Many women have found Easter Lily flower essence very comforting and reassuring during midlife/menopause. On an energetic level the increasing activity of the throat chakra draws up energy from the sacral chakra for use in planning and structuring creative lifestyle pursuits. This pre-empts and coincides with hormonal changes which occur at menopause involving the thyroid and ovaries, which are governed by the throat and sacral chakras respectively.

Common uses

Midlife mind, body and spirit purifier; to help cleanse the system of past (sexual) traumatic experiences; to help resolve sexual/moral tensions; to press the 'refresh' button on your personal and spiritual growth; to resurrect ALL of yourself!

Complementary &/or similar flower essences

Basil, Billy Goat Plum, Calla Lily, Chrysanthemum, Crab Apple, Hibiscus, Iris, Lady's Slipper, Manzanita, Morning Glory, Nicotiana, Pomegranate, Queen Anne's Lace, Sticky Monkeyflower, the rest of the Lily family

Supporting the changes

- Explore or expand your spiritual nature through appropriate reading and study.
- Practise meditation with visualisation exercises that flood the sacral area with orange light and the throat centre with blue healing light.
- Yoga, tai chi and pilates exercises that energise the pelvic area are very beneficial.
- Consider diets that cleanse or encourage the eliminatory organs of the body. Drink more pure water.
- Learn to love yourself more – others will follow.

Echinacea

Echinacea purpurea   (Pink-purple / FES)

Positive state

Physically and mentally 'together' – 'core integrity' (FES)
Strong sense of Self, establishing resilience

Negative state

'Feeling shattered by severe trauma or abuse' (FES)
Under threat, lack of natural defence/immunity

Echinacea, in its herbal form, is famous for its beneficial effect on the immune system. In a more subtle way, this *'natural defence'* quality is also conveyed by the flower essence. Single, long-stalked flower heads have drooping, purple-pink petals which ray out from a *proud central core* of clustered flowers that are *exposed* to the elements. (It is no coincidence that a similar gesture is displayed by the Arnica flower, which is also used to restore *inner/dynamic strength* after physical trauma.)

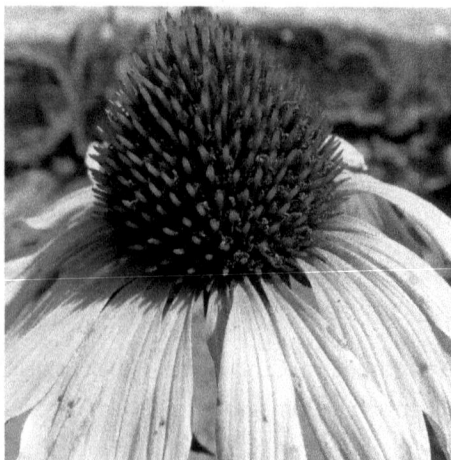

This is symbolic of the *core strengthening* quality that the flower essence conveys to the subtle elements (or inner layers) of our being. Just as the core strengthening exercises of pilates or yoga can improve overall strength and agility and protect against injury, the Echinacea herb can strengthen our natural physical immunity against germs and infection. Taking it to another level, Echinacea flower essence can strengthen the subtle body's *'core'* against destructive forces and assaults on its *essential integrity* and *spiritual identity*.

Echinacea herb is an *adaptogen* and the flower essence allows us to adapt to and welcome change in our environment.

It is very interesting to note the way in which the Echinacea plant has come to the fore in the past few decades! When we consider the increasingly harsh impact of chemical pollution, overcrowding, geopathic stress, the threat of new viruses, etc, and the not unrelated recent development of so many auto-immune diseases, Echinacea has a significant role to play in restoring the core integrity of our natural immunity to help us adapt.

Kaminski and Katz describe how 'many souls [seem] to have a functioning persona when in fact [there is] only a meagre connection to the true spiritual self [the core of our being]. This is one of the underlying reasons, at the level of the soul reality, for the vast outbreak of immune-related diseases' (1996).

The Echinacea state of mind

In the negative Echinacea state, our spirit has been traumatised by harsh life circumstances, like a 'street kid' who weathers dangers, climatic exposure and poor nutrition. In these circumstances, our natural protective life force and immunity becomes eroded, just like a cut piece of untreated wood left outdoors.

Benefits of taking Echinacea

Echinacea flower essence can help to repair a damaged aura. It can aid in the recovery of subtle integrity so that a person can develop a better sense of Self, unique and distinct but still in touch with others. A new inner strength can develop to help them discover a safe, secure and comfortable niche in life. A seventeen-year-old woman came to consult me some months after she had returned to her family after living homeless on the streets for a year. The consequences of her prolonged ordeal had only really started to emerge. She underwent emotional pain and upheaval, like coming out of an extended state of shock, and her immune system broke down, leaving her vulnerable to every infection around, so that she never fully recovered before she became ill again. She found this especially upsetting because up until then she had rarely been ill. In the months that followed, Echinacea flower essence was instrumental in helping her to recover emotionally and physically from her trauma and 'fit back in' comfortably to her new, more nurturing environment.

Possible physical imbalances

Over time, constant stress/trauma affects the more subtle life forces and will inevitably result in the manifestation of immune-related physical ailments. After extended exposure to geopathic stress and/or harsh physical, emotional and psychological environments, our etheric template for physical health becomes compromised, and there is often a delay before physical symptoms manifest.

Echinacea flower essence will be restorative of this etheric template as it acts at a causal level to prevent further physical natural health issues associated with our natural immune system.

I have found from experience (in practice and personally) that a combination of Echinacea, Arnica, Star of Bethlehem and Crowea flower essences is very useful when recovering from surgery that involves general anaesthetic.

Common uses

To aid recovery after trauma; for people who are or have been 'living on the street'; to assist in post-operative recovery; after emotional and physical abuse; to help restore a sense of dignity after 'shattering' life experiences; to help restore one's natural 'core' immunity

Complementary &/or similar flower essences

Aloe Vera, Angelica, Arnica, Baby Blue Eyes, Chaparral, Corn, Crowea, Dogwood, Fringed Violet, Garlic, Golden Ear Drops, Indian Pink, Morning Glory, Mountain Pennyroyal, Nicotiana, Red Clover, St John's Wort, Star of Bethlehem, Walnut, Waratah, all the Yarrows, YES formula

Supporting the changes

- Nurture yourself physically and emotionally – learn to take time out to metaphorically 'wrap yourself up in cotton wool.'
- Eat well, get adequate sleep and exercise regularly to maintain your immune system.
- 'Make over' your room and your living/working environment so that it makes you feel good.
- Hang out with those who love and care about you.

Elm

Ulmus procera   (Reddish-brown / Bach)

Positive state

Coping well with all your responsibilities
Confident, calm and capable

Negative state

Anxious thoughts about how much needs to be done
Feeling overwhelmed by responsibilities

Elm is a large tree that can grow up to 20–25 metres high, with a massive trunk, thick, deeply-fissured greyish bark and numerous spreading branches.

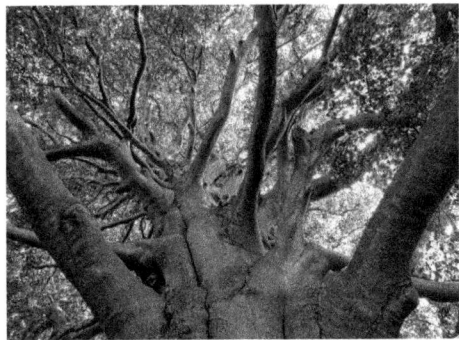

Timber from the Elm tree has been used for making furniture for centuries because of its *strength and durability*. However, as evidenced by the fineness of the twigs and subtle pattern of the branches, there is also a marked *sensitivity* which is usually accompanied by a level of *vulnerability*. Dutch Elm disease has killed many mature trees throughout the world. 'The thought that such handsome and majestic trees could be laid low by a passing fungus seems ironical but the strongest of us can be assailed by weakness' (Barnard 1988). But Elms have survived, and despite the fact that populations have become very localised, the *innate strength* of the Elm will allow it to endure.

Another important signature of the plant is the way Elm flowers appear before the leaves. This signals the potential of Elm flower essence to help those who blossom prematurely or 'peak too early' and *struggle to cope* with their rapid rise to the top of their field. The pressure of *responsibility* and *expectation* on those who achieve early or 'overnight' success in sport, business or entertainment can become *overwhelming* and lead to collapse or dysfunctional behaviour.

The Elm personality

Elm people are found on every committee, at every working bee, busy fulfilling every commitment they have made, always available to others in need, like the Rock of Gibraltar. But even the Rock of Gibraltar can wear down and crack eventually! Elm flower essence is useful for people who have the same qualities as the tree – they are strong, capable and responsible – until they suddenly become overwhelmed by what is expected of them. Elm flower essence should be considered at times when we become anxious and overwhelmed by the thought of what needs to be done. We are daunted by tasks and responsibilities which we have previously taken in our stride but which now seem as if they will bring us down. Elm people typically accumulate responsibilities to provide a secure structure for themselves and a sense of worth in their lives. When commitments and obligations build beyond a tolerable level, a personal crisis occurs and they are forced to choose between the desire to take on more work in order to maintain a sense of worth, and the need for relief from overwhelming responsibility. In the end our own needs and those of people close to us make the choice clear.

Benefits of taking Elm

Elm teaches us to acknowledge the responsibility we have to ourselves and to recognise that meeting our own needs is a God-given right. 'Only rogues give more than they've got to give' is a proverb that Elm people can benefit from. We cannot spend our lives trying to achieve the impossibly high standards set for us by authority figures or role models such as our parents. Fortunately, Elm can help restore the self-assurance that is a trademark of classic Elm people in the positive state. It does so by raising awareness of our personal integrity, value and right to a reasonable workload, relieving us of the constant urge to externally validate our existence. 'Ah, what a relief.'

Possible physical imbalances

Elm can be useful as a protection against 'burnout' and other threats to the immune system during periods of great responsibility or heavy workload.

Common uses

For anxiety associated with overwhelming responsibility; to help the 'overnight' success to cope; to help achieve a healthier and more balanced lifestyle; for weak moments in the lives of the strong (or weaker moments in the lives of the not-so-strong); for those with something to prove – often to their father; for self-assurance under pressure; to honour the inner child's needs

Complementary &/or similar flower essences

Boab, Bottlebrush, Buttercup, Cherry Plum, Corn, Cosmos, Cotton, Crowea, Dandelion, Dill, Filaree, Gentian, Indian Pink, Larch, Larkspur, Lavender, Madia, Oak, Paw Paw, Rabbitbrush, Sagebrush, Self-Heal, Shasta Daisy, Sunflower, White Chestnut, Zinnia

Supporting the changes

- Get your priorities right. Choose the things that support your own needs as well as those of your loved ones or co-workers.
- Spend more quality time with your father or a father-figure, or do some therapeutic work on issues that relate to your relationship with him.
- Put a higher value on yourself and your time.
- Remember the saying, 'Only rogues give more than they've got to give,' and look after yourself!

Fairy Lantern

Calochortus albus   (White / FES)

Positive state

Balanced body/mind/spirit development
Maturity, independence, creative expression

Negative state

Delayed or 'splintered' body/mind/spirit development
'Immaturity ... childish dependency' (FES)

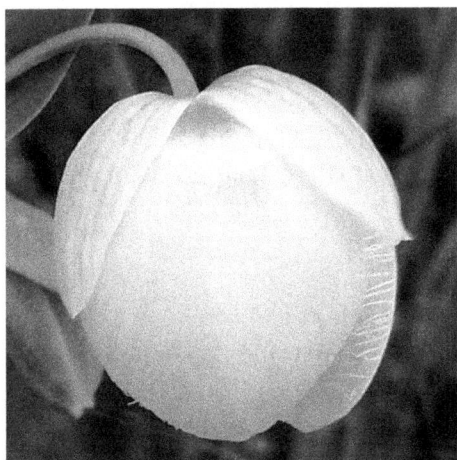

Even when Fairy Lantern is in bloom the flowers never properly open.

Fairy Lantern flower essence helps people who are reluctant to *'open up'* and *'state their case'* to the world. This can manifest as *frustrated creative expression* or more profoundly as *delayed development*, physically and emotionally. The flower's *soft and delicate* appearance symbolises the *childlike* aspect some individuals may wish to present and remain in to avoid the responsibility of changing their relationship dynamic with the world and the people close to them.

The Fairy Lantern personality

Fairy Lantern is for 'late bloomers' – for example a girl who remains on the verge of physical and emotional maturity for a prolonged period. After her peers have negotiated the transition to womanhood, she may remain immature, especially on an emotional level, clinging to inappropriately childlike behaviour. This may be also reflected in delayed physical development.

Benefits of taking Fairy Lantern

In addition to being useful during early puberty, this flower essence can be helpful during menopause, which is also a move into a new phase of womanhood. At midlife, women often face issues relating to sexuality and creative expression, during the move from procreation to a different style of creative contribution in the world.

Fairy Lantern flower essence enables us to accept the responsibilities that go with these changes more easily. The personal reward is the empowerment that comes through recognising a whole new level of creative ability and independence.

Kaminski and Katz (1996) describe how 'the soul who needs fairy lantern still clings to a childlike personality … Such a person learns that she or he will receive love only by remaining in an arrested, over-dependent childlike state.' Many years ago a young woman came to me for a consultation. Her main concern – or should I say her mother's main concern – was a delayed and irregular menstrual cycle. Although she was nineteen, she had only experienced two periods, eighteen months apart, the first of which occurred when she was fifteen. She came to the first consultation with her mother, with whom she behaved like a very young child despite the fact that she was nineteen. When talking to her, I felt that I was talking to someone in her early teens or younger. Mother and daughter dressed the same and spoke in a similar manner and the relationship was like that of a 'baby' sister with her older sibling. The young woman took Fairy Lantern flower essence over the next few months and I observed considerable changes and personal development. It helped her to reach a new level of maturity and healthy independence from her mother (who supported her daughter's personal growth) which coincided with the establishment of a regular menstrual cycle.

Possible physical imbalances

As in the case mentioned above, Fairy Lantern can often be helpful for physically 'late maturers,' especially when there is difficulty in taking on the next level of responsibility associated with maturation to adulthood. Sometimes Fairy Lantern can also be useful at menopause when past issues may re-emerge for revision.

Common uses

For late bloomers; for females with significantly delayed menarche; to help girls accept the move to womanhood; to accept and develop one's creative and positive feminine side.

Complementary &/or similar flower essences

Almond, Angelsword, Basil, Billy Goat Plum, Bottlebrush, Californian Pitcher Plant, Calla Lily, Chestnut Bud, Chrysanthemum, Easter Lily, Honeysuckle, Indian Paintbrush, Iris, Kangaroo Paw, Lotus, Manzanita, Mullein, Onion, Pomegranate, Violet, Wallflower, Walnut, Watermelon

Supporting the changes

- Consider professional counselling during puberty.
- Look to good female role models for advice and/or inspiration.
- Investigate the Jungian concept of the anima.
- Recognise the beauty in yourself and nurture it.

Filaree

Erodium cicutarium   (Violet / FES)

Positive state

Broad perception
Attention to priorities

Negative state

Overwhelmed and unable to 'see the wood for the trees'
Distracted, side-tracked by irrelevancies

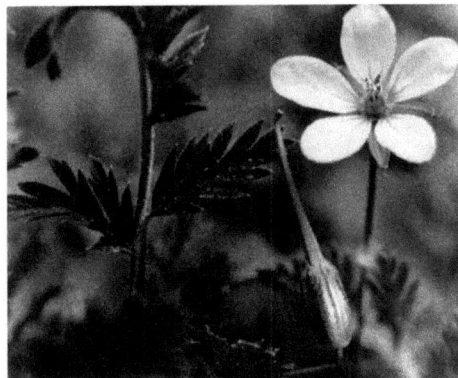

Filaree's flower bud is sharp and pointed like a teacher's cane but undergoes transformation into a beautiful, *well-rounded* flower.

This reflects the flower essence's ability to help people gain a *wider perspective* when they are constantly worried or stressed over minor details and inconsequential concerns. The *violet* colour of the flower relates to the *crown chakra*, which is the subtle *'overseer'* of our lives. Filaree can help us to see minor and inconsequential problems within a *larger context*, bringing about a *clearer perspective* on what is really important. It is particularly useful when we become *bogged down and overwhelmed* by many details, distracting us from perceiving the few most salient ones.

The Filaree personality

Many managers who have too much to oversee become stressed and caught up in petty concerns and worries, unable to discern the most important issue and remain focused on it. Filaree can help these people gain a clear and holistic perspective of the job at hand and enable them to convey it to those under their supervision.

Benefits of taking Filaree

Filaree helps us contain our energy instead of becoming side-tracked and wasting it on incidentals, leaving plenty in reserve for productive activities that get results and/or fulfil our higher purpose. Kaminski and Katz (1996) describe how it 'liberates overly suppressed psychic energy, allowing greater receptivity to spiritual inspiration and vision.' Like a general in the field summoning the troops and directing them to a common goal, we can achieve the best outcome at work or in everyday life.

Possible physical imbalances

An overwhelmingly stressful state associated with the need for Filaree can lead to all sorts of physical problems, especially the exacerbation of pre-existing ailments.

Common uses

To help one MANAGE better; for those in managerial positions (work or family); to help you 'see the wood for the trees'; to help you prioritise and focus; to improve your spatial perception; to broaden your vision but 'lower your eyes' to focus on what is necessary

Complementary &/or similar flower essences

Angelsword, Calendula, Californian Poppy, Chrysanthemum, Coffee, Cotton, Crab Apple, Crowea, Dill, Elm, Forget-Me-Not, Heather, Hound's Tongue, Madia, Nicotiana, Paw Paw, Rabbitbrush, Red Lily, Shasta Daisy, Silver Princess, White Chestnut

Supporting the changes

- Learn to manage your time and prioritise better by getting a good diary!
- Regularly take time out for short walks, meditations etc and step back a little to gain better perspective.
- Integrate more relaxing, physical exercise into your life – get out of your head and into your body!
- Broaden your view ahead and lower your eyes when necessary.

Flannel Flower

Actinotus helianthi   (White / Aus)

Positive state

Receptive – openly 'feeling your way'
At ease with physical contact and intimacy

Negative state

Dislike of being touched (Ian White); emotionally closed
Overly 'macho' or 'butch'

The entire Flannel Flower plant – flowers, buds, stems and foliage – is covered with a *soft, silky* down. Ian White, founder of Australian Bush Flower Essences, comments on the *soft, sensuous* texture and appearance of the flower. It invites

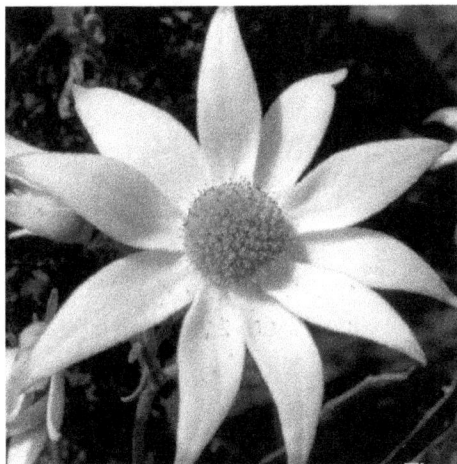

us to stroke and feel it and experience the joy of being in physical contact. The first time I saw the flower, something inside me just melted. Their white colour signifies the plant's ability to help us feel *safe* in *surrendering* to the moment.

As with Dogwood, the thick, velvety white bracts *embrace* the comparatively smaller flowers, emphasising the qualities of support, protection and *nurturing* offered by the flower essence.

The Flannel Flower personality

The protective qualities symbolised by the white flowers enhance this essence's healing effects, especially for those whose personal space has been invaded and traumatised in the past. Sexual and physical abuse, physical assault and trauma can have consequences that remain unresolved and leave us apprehensive and unable to trust others. As a result, we develop defences such as hardening or withdrawal from intimate emotional expression and physical contact. This defensiveness can be eased by using Flannel Flower essence. Even the green velvety tips of the bracts express the quality of protection and natural immunity through its association with the primary colour of the heart chakra.

Benefits of taking Flannel Flower

Flannel Flower essence helps us contact, appreciate and savour our physical and emotional sensitivity. It can help us be more open to receiving healing, therapy and pleasure through the experience of physical contact and emotional intimacy. This remedy allows us to be 'touched' in a deeper way by life.

Sometimes the ability to touch is separated from the ability to be touched. For example, some people enjoy giving a massage but find it more difficult to receive one. There are also people who enjoy touching but lack sensitivity and gentleness in their approach. When you lack confidence about knowing when, who, how and what to touch – and especially, whether or not it is appropriate to touch! – consider using Flannel Flower essence to help you respond more naturally (and genuinely) to each individual situation.

Flannel Flower can help us feel safer, more secure and less vulnerable about emotional expression. Trust is a key issue for the person in need of Flannel Flower. Developing trust improves our ability to be open and to avail ourselves of all the 'yummy' emotional experiences life has to offer.

Possible physical imbalances

Many people who respond well to Flannel Flower essence experience physical tension and 'guarding' in their bodies. The release of emotional tension through using this flower essence results in the softening of stiffness and tension held in the body. Always consider Flannel Flower essence when there are problems in sexual relations.

Common uses

To help soften 'macho' or 'butch' extremes; to feel more comfortable relating intimately; to feel safe to let go; to get a better 'feel' for situations; to surrender to the tenderness of the moment; to allow yourself to be nurtured

Complementary &/or similar flower essences

Agrimony, Arnica, Baby Blue Eyes, Billy Goat Plum, Calendula, Crab Apple, Dandelion, Dogwood, Easter Lily, Echinacea, Fringed Violet, Golden Yarrow, Hibiscus, Kangaroo Paw, Mallow, Mariposa Lily, Mimulus (and all the Monkeyflowers), Oregon Grape, Quince, Star of Bethlehem, Star Thistle, Star Tulip, Tiger Lily, YES formula, Zinnia

Supporting the changes

- Explore the many tactile therapies available and engage in those you are comfortable with.
- Professional counseling/psychotherapy, especially in relation to developing trust, may provide a catalyst for change in your intimate physical and emotional relationships.
- Relaxation or meditative techniques and practices that enable you to fully let go physically and mentally can be helpful.
- 'Let go, let in.'

Fuchsia

Fuchsia hybrida   (Red-purple / FES)

Positive state

Deep awareness / Self-understanding
Genuine (primary) emotional expression; grounded

Negative state

Psychosomatic symptoms resulting from emotional repression (FES)
'False states of emotionality' (FES); 'over the top' reactions

Fuchsia flowers face downwards towards the ground and the flower essence has the ability to *ground* people and allow them to embrace their *true feelings*.

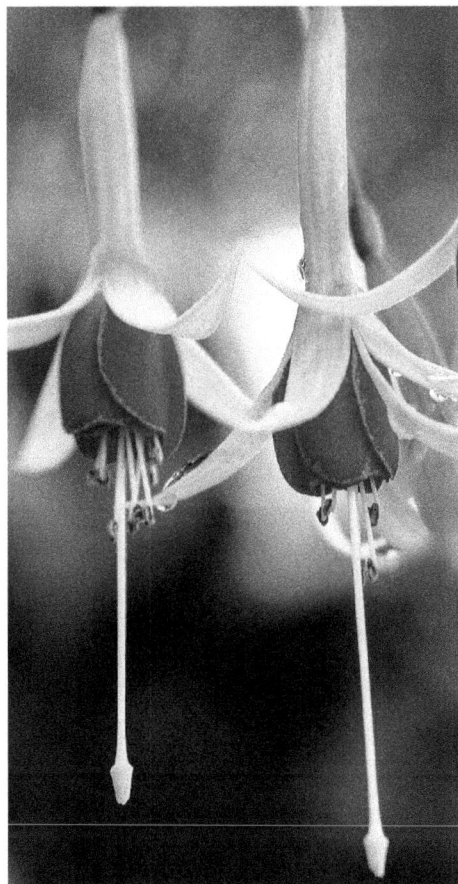

The flower's rich red-purple, *blood-earth* colour gives a clue to its usefulness in allowing us to fully experience the richness of life so that we *genuinely feel and live* in the moment and react accordingly.

The Fuchsia personality

When we are in need of Fuchsia flower essence we often miss opportunities for conscious self-expression due to repression of our true emotional responses.

However, the emotional 'charge' associated with all of life's experiences continues to accumulate until the slightest trigger can provoke an 'over the top' reaction.

This hyper-emotional release is small compensation for those times when we don't respond, as the reaction is so disproportionate to the incident that no one takes us seriously. Those around respond either by ignoring it completely or by dismissing it: 'There he goes again!' Or worse, 'Oh, she's off again, it must be that time of the month.' No one takes your reaction seriously despite the fact that there may be strong justification for it. You feel as though you are not heard and consequently become frustrated beyond reason; you retreat emotionally and the vicious cycle continues.

The most tragic aspect of this pattern is that we may deny ourselves the opportunity to explore and understand 'core emotions ... such as grief, deep-seated anger or rejection' (Kaminski and Katz 1996). These unaddressed issues continue to cause hyper-emotional outbursts but may also become associated with psychosomatic symptoms as the body processes the physical consequences of unexpressed, painful emotions.

I have found that when clients' premenstrual tension and hormonally related mood swings improve while taking Fuchsia flower essence, they also find that they are more able to speak up 'on the spur of the moment' and be heard at other times of the month as well.

Benefits of taking Fuchsia

Repression implies an unconscious process, whereas suppression of emotion is a more conscious choice. Of course, there are very good reasons why emotions, especially those of a painful or overwhelming nature, are relegated to our unconscious or Shadow side. Taking Fuchsia flower essence will not unleash painful emotions indiscriminately from the unconscious into an already vulnerable psyche. However, it can provide inner freedom to make emotional choices from a position of greater awareness.

A friend who relied heavily on daily, strenuous, physical workouts as his only means of dealing with stress came to see me after suffering an injury he knew would incapacitate him for a long time and which was part of his journey as an athlete facing the inevitable processes of ageing. After much consideration, we decided Fuchsia flower essence might be helpful. Its effect was to help him to react with greater awareness and in a more grounded and constructive manner to mental and emotional stresses as they occurred at his business and in his everyday life. His stress levels didn't build to the same degree, giving him more freedom of choice about whether he needed to work out or not. He still exercises regularly, but now he does so mainly for pleasure and with obvious health benefits, rather than out of absolute necessity.

Possible physical imbalances

Always consider using Fuchsia flower essence when there is emotional and physical tension associated with hormonal changes and imbalance. Although there are many other useful essences to consider for emotional issues associated with pre-menstrual syndrome, I have utilised Fuchsia in my practice more than any other essence for this condition.

Common uses

To become more grounded; to embrace, enjoy and express feelings as they arise; for spontaneity; for a more even disposition; for genuine and dynamic emotionality

Complementary &/or similar flower essences

Agrimony, Almond, Black Eyed Susan, Californian Pitcher Plant, Calla Lily, Canyon Dudleya, Chamomile, Cherry Plum, Corn, Cosmos, Deerbrush, Dogwood, Lotus, Scarlet Monkeyflower (and all the Monkeyflowers), Snapdragon, Willow

Supporting the changes

- Take part in grounding activities such as non-competitive physical exercise, the more vigorous forms of tai chi and yoga, gardening, bushwalking and so on. If meditation is practised, it is best done in moderation, as some people unintentionally use it as a way to keep at bay, rather than transform, deep-seated emotions.

- Study your body rhythms and learn to use them rather than be a victim of them. Try to keep your blood sugar levels stable.
- Ask yourself on a regular basis, 'How do I feel right now?'

Garlic

Allium sativum   (Violet / FES)

Positive state

Vitality, multi-level natural immunity
Confident, good humoured and 'tuned in'

Negative state

Over-susceptible to negative environments
Debilitating sense of foreboding

Garlic is said to have given *strength* to the pyramid builders, courage to Roman legionaries and fighting spirit to English gamecocks, not to mention its reputed magical protective powers against 'dark' forces in the environment. The strengthening and protective qualities of Garlic flower essence do not come from rigid shielding or denial but rather by enabling us to understand and be less fearful about the subtle dimensions in which our life is embedded. It helps us to become comfortable in all our 'skins'! Rudolf Steiner spoke of the *parallel spiritual dimension* and how we have learned to filter it out of our awareness in order to go about our daily lives. Garlic flower essence enables us to develop a *comfortable and secure 'sense,'* mainly subconsciously, of the *'other side,'* without developing fears and distracting us from our everyday business. The way in which the portion of the plant that grows above ground (including the flower) dies some time before the Garlic clove is ready to be harvested is a signature that relates to a sense of *permanence* beyond this life.

Garlic helps us to become more accepting of our physical body's mortality.

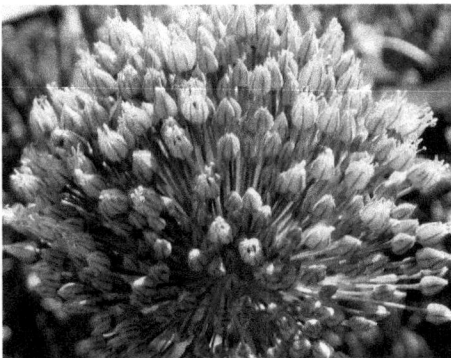

Consciously or unconsciously, death is most people's greatest fear and if this fear can be ameliorated in some way, other more minor fears will also be eased.

Another aspect of the plant's signature is the way the flowers grow at the top of a long stem in a *tightly integrated tassel* enclosed in a protective papery bract and this relates to the way Garlic flower essence protects and helps us to *get ourselves together,* integrating all aspects of our being. This greater sense of wholeness delivers us into a more *unitive consciousness* that imparts *strength and security.*

The Garlic state of mind

Garlic flower essence can be used to help calm the fears that overcome us when we feel that 'the world is our stage' and we are called upon to perform. It helps calm niggling uneasiness as we go about our everyday activities, easing 'butterflies' in the stomach which are associated with anticipatory anxiety. Think about using Garlic flower essence before public speaking or playing competitive sport, before a job interview or important meeting, commencing a new job or facing people you feel in awe of or intimidated by, socially or at work. Garlic flower essence can help allay fears of public humiliation, especially before a hostile or unsupportive audience. I have used it myself when about to give a talk on flower essences to a group of scientific 'fundamentalists'! The flower essence gives you a 'sense of wholeness which imparts strength and active resistance' (Kaminski and Katz 1996) that helps *protect the integrity of your own thoughts.* You can then more easily maintain contact with your feeling side in a predominantly intellectual and 'cerebral' atmosphere (as in the example above). How we 'keep our act together' in these circumstances is described by Kaminski and Katz (1996) as being the result of the Garlic flower essence helping to bring the astral body 'into greater harmony with the physical and etheric and the spiritual ego.'

Benefits of taking Garlic

Garlic helps us remain positive. As the famous sixteenth century English physician and herbalist Nicholas Culpeper said of the herb, 'In men oppressed by melancholy it will attenuate the melancholic humour.' Use this flower essence when you feel unusually sensitive to the world and it will help you develop a strong, protective aura. Use Garlic to protect yourself from your own and others' 'demons,' as people have done for centuries.

Many of the herbal properties of Garlic pass over to the flower essence. Some of them, such as immunity-enhancing qualities, are actually expanded upon by the flower essence to include immunity beyond the physical dimension.

Possible physical imbalances

Those who can benefit from taking Garlic flower essence are often 'prone to low vitality' (Kaminski and Katz 1996) which renders their immune system far more susceptible. The immune system of those taking this flower essence will be enhanced.

Common uses

For those who are facing death or are oppressed by a great fear of death; for anticipatory anxiety; for a sense of dread or foreboding; to remain positive when surrounded by negativity; as an adjunct to improving your natural immunity; for self-confidence when 'facing the world' every day; to feel safe in the universe!

Complementary &/or similar flower essences

Angelica, Angelsword, Angel's Trumpet, Aspen, Echinacea, Fringed Violet, Golden Yarrow (and all the Yarrows), Lotus, Mimulus, Mountain Pennyroyal, Oregon Grape, Red Clover, Rock Rose, Star Tulip, St John's Wort, Sweet Pea, Violet, Walnut, YES formula

Supporting the changes

- Exercises and practices that enhance a sense of wholeness and a feeling of being grounded are useful. Tai chi and yoga, creative visualisation, meditation in moderation, walking, gardening and pottery may be considered.
- Developing good physical and mental fitness, perhaps through martial arts or competitive sport, may help to foster inner security and self-assurance.
- Find your safe haven, Earthly temple or place of worship, whether it's a seat in your favourite café, a spot in a restful park or at home in your most comfortable chair and most tranquil room.

Gentian

Gentiana amarella   (Purple-violet / Bach)

Positive state

Ability to oversee and understand
Resilient – undeterred by setbacks

Negative state

Depressed; narrow-minded view of problems
Discouraged by setbacks

Gentian is a low-growing herb with bell-shaped, dull purple flowers that grows wild in alkaline soils and on dunes. It doesn't tolerate agricultural chemicals and has become scarce, but its struggle for survival echoes its subtle healing qualities – it can foster a sense of *positivity even after setbacks*.

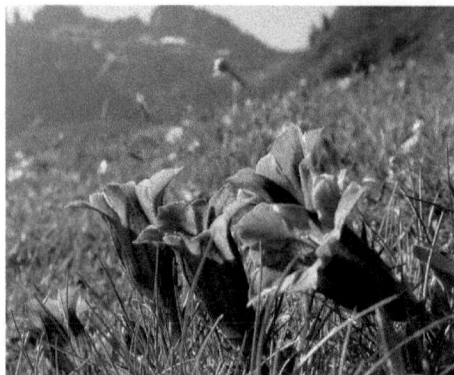

The plant seeks to establish itself on *hill top* grassland – this signature relates to how the flower essence helps us gain a *broad perspective* of the world so that we are able to sense the *bigger picture and put things in context*. The flowers' *purple/violet* colour reminds us of the *spiritual realms (crown chakra)*, *inspiring* and providing a *'view from on high.'* Gentian helps us to see our worries, obstacles and setbacks as the trivial incidentals that they really are in the wider scheme of things. Gentian *flowers late* in the season, proving that 'it is never too late' (Barnard 1988). The lesson it teaches us is *'Never say never'!*

The Gentian state of mind

Gentian helps when we have become discouraged and disheartened by setbacks in achieving our hopes and aspirations, particularly when we have worked hard. Failure to achieve a desired performance level at a chosen sport, setbacks in promotion or business projects, the failure of a personal relationship that appeared at first to have great promise, or the loss of a loved one can all leave us disillusioned, struggling to find the will to try again.

A big part of the problem is that our ideas about how life should be are often inflexible and not grounded in reality. When situations occur that do not fit neatly into our dreams, we feel disappointed and are prone to give up. In the same way, when faced with a phenomenon that doesn't fit into our world view or belief system we can too easily dismiss it. Gentian flower essence can help us when our heart wants to believe that something new is possible but our head's old ideas won't let us!

Benefits of taking Gentian

Gentian helps us to face life's challenges with courage, a light heart and a buoyant view. It broadens our perspectives and allows us to see the positive aspects of our situation. We learn to tolerate the ups and downs of life with a resilient, positive and purposeful attitude.

Possible physical imbalances

The discouragement experienced in the negative Gentian state sometimes develops into depression, especially after setbacks in recovery from physical illness.

Common uses

For discouragement after setbacks; for those who give up too easily; for depression of a known cause; to help flexibility of outlook and a broader perspective; for perseverance; to help 'keep the faith'

Complementary &/or similar flower essences

Baby Blue Eyes, Borage, Elm, Filaree, Forget-Me-Not, Gorse, Harvest Brodiaea, Hibiscus, Hound's Tongue, Iris, Love-Lies-Bleeding, Larch, Mountain Pride, Mustard, Pine, Sage, Scotch Broom, Self-Heal, Sturt Desert Pea, Sweet Chestnut, Tansy, Waratah, Willow

Supporting the changes

- Explore the Zen Buddhist philosophy which suggests that the road travelled is as important as the destination reached: 'Before enlightenment, chop wood and carry water; after enlightenment, chop wood and carry water.'
- A more philosophical and spiritual outlook will give you a better context in which to view your problems.
- Above all, have another go – nothing ventured, nothing gained!

Golden Ear Drops
Dicentra chrysantha   (Yellow / FES)

Positive state
'Releasing painful memories from the past' (FES)
Empowered by one's childhood experience

Negative state
Repressed painful memories from (early) childhood
The past undermines current experiences

The Golden Ear Drops plant comes from the same family as Bleeding Heart *(Dicentra)* and its properties also relate to affairs of the heart, especially

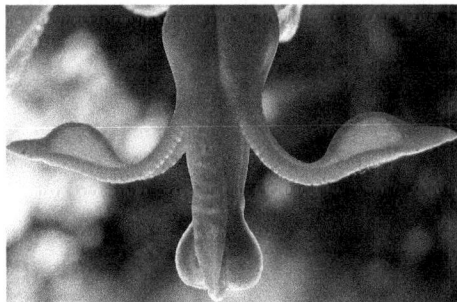

those that relate to the *past and early childhood*. The *yellow* flowers show its connection to the *solar plexus chakra* and our *feeling* nature. The shape of the flower can be likened to a *suspended teardrop*.

Painful feelings from *old hurts*, especially the negative emotional charge associated with certain *childhood experiences*, can become entrenched deep in our psyche. Golden Ear Drops flower essence can help us gain a wiser and more comfortable perspective on these *old, painful memories*, allowing us to gain *resolution*. Remember, flower essences help to reveal only what we are prepared, ready and able to understand and accept – our free will always stays intact.

The Golden Ear Drops state of mind

Some therapists refer to 'emotional amnesia' as being a necessary survival mechanism which allows us to cope with harsh or traumatic events. When physical pain becomes too intense we lose consciousness and in the same way, when emotional pain becomes too intense we sometimes block it by relegating it to the unconscious. This is especially likely to happen during childhood and at other times when we have little personal power and are vulnerable. However, these blocked-out feelings can cause emotional problems later in life resulting from emotional desensitisation or 'numbness,' and/or cause maladaptive responses to certain situations. We may not recall the 'trigger' events or experiences in a clearly conscious way but if the feelings associated with them have never been properly processed, they remain 'raw' in our psyche.

Benefits of taking Golden Ear Drops

When we have reached a stage of readiness in our personal growth or just a comfortable time in our life, 'the unconscious residue of traumatic memories ... [can] be encountered with more awareness' (Kaminski and Katz 1996). At this time, Golden Ear Drops flower essence can help us let go of painful episodes from our past. When the emotional charge associated with these experiences is freed, a load of emotional baggage we have been carrying for many years lightens and we feel liberated. Past experiences no longer weigh so heavily on the psyche and we can 'reclaim this past, so that it becomes a source of strength, wisdom and insight' now and in the future.

Possible physical imbalances

On an energetic level, the liver is the organ that holds and 'edits' emotional reactions associated with experiences. Repressed and unresolved emotionality burdens the liver and emotional toxicity can result in physical toxicity. Natural liver support may be beneficial when Golden Ear Drops flower essence has been chosen for use.

Common uses

To let go of the past; to help release painful memories from childhood; for those who can't (or weren't allowed to!) cry; to 'lighten the emotional load'; to allow the whole of you to live in the now; for enjoyment and spontaneity

Complementary &/or similar flower essences

Arnica, Baby Blue Eyes, Black Eyed Susan, Bleeding Heart, Borage, Chaparral,

Dogwood, Echinacea, Evening Primrose, Fuchsia, Hibiscus, Mariposa Lily, Star of Bethlehem, Sturt Desert Pea, Waratah, Willow, Yerba Santa

Supporting the changes

- Make yourself familiar with the qualities of Golden Ear Drops flower essence before you take it and have a practitioner, partner or friend around for support.
- Professional counselling may be useful. Emotional Focus Therapy (EFT) may be an option. Things can (and will) get better.
- Always remember, flower essences will help to reveal only what we are ready and able to understand and accept.

Goldenrod

Solidago californica   (Yellow / FES)

Positive state

'Comfortable in your skin'
'Well-developed individuality [along with] social consciousness'(FES)

Negative state

Too easily influenced by family, peers and social groups (FES)
Unable to be true to oneself and adhere to inner conviction

Goldenrod has a round, *upright* stem and a cylindrical root, which finds the depth of soil it needs to establish a *firm grip* on Earth. Its *singular, forthright and direct* habit of growth reflects the qualities the flower essence can enhance in those who use it. Kaminski and Katz (1996) describe how Goldenrod 'encourages a vertical or individual axis to counterbalance the overly broad, horizontal axis, which influences the personality too strongly.' It encourages us to be *unambiguous* and *genuine* in our intentions and the expression of our feelings, and *stops us being easily distracted from our truth by external social pressures.*

The plant's Latin name *Solidago* (from *solidus*, meaning whole) indicates its use as a wound-healing herb. The flower essence helps heal deep emotional wounds so that we can become whole and integrate all aspects of the Self, enabling our full potential as an individual to develop and remain solid.

The Goldenrod personality

Unresolved emotional wounds cause us to act in a less-than-integrated way and make us more inclined to express a false or negative persona to the world. We can get stuck in limited, antisocial behaviour which masks the authentic Self and may push people away, including our loved ones.

Those in need of Goldenrod flower essence may find themselves compromised by pressure from peer groups, family, school and social expectations. When we are too easily diverted from living in a way that is true to our inner convictions, we can become trapped in behaviours that bear little relationship to who we really are. We may become ultra-conservative and conform to rigid social conventions in a bid to gain acceptance and approval or on the other hand, in an attempt to create a unique social identity (Kaminski and Katz 1996) we engage in antisocial or obnoxious behaviour, especially during childhood and teenage years. This in turn has consequences which may prevent us from achieving the very thing we crave – social acceptance and self-respect.

Benefits of taking Goldenrod

Goldenrod helps heal old hurts and damaged egos. It helps us to feel more relaxed about ourselves and remain true to our higher Self in social situations. Our true identity can shine through in family, school, work and social arenas.

Possible physical imbalances

The tendency to be easily influenced by external (social) factors can play havoc with our attempts to live a healthy and balanced lifestyle. Goldenrod flower essence helps us to remain firm and stick to healthy goals, for example in relation to our intake of fast foods, alcohol and other substances even more detrimental to our physical health and wellbeing.

Common uses

To improve self-esteem; to become more comfortable with the Self; to restore a shattered ego; to be less susceptible to peer group pressure at any age; to help express your true individuality; to be the 'genuine article'!

Complementary &/or similar flower essences

Agrimony, Angelsword, Buttercup, Calla Lily, Chrysanthemum, Cosmos, Deerbrush, Fairy Lantern, Hibbertia, Larkspur, Mallow, Mountain Pride, Mullein, Pink Monkeyflower, Pink Yarrow, Pomegranate, Quaking Grass, Red Grevillea, Sagebrush, Saguaro, Self-Heal, Sunflower, Tall Yellow Top, Tansy, Violet, Walnut

Supporting the changes

- Courses devoted to personal growth and self-realisation can be helpful.
- Seek vocational guidance from practitioners of disciplines such as psychology and/or astrology.
- Ask yourself regularly, 'Am I acting and behaving in a manner true to myself?'

Golden Yarrow

Achillea filipendulina   (Yellow / FES)

Positive state

Mutually strengthening social relationships
Integrity of life force in dynamic social involvement (FES)

Negative state

Oversensitive and susceptible to social surroundings
Self-protective 'withdrawal and social isolation' (FES)

Yarrows of all colours are *protective* and the *yellow* colour of Golden Yarrow flowers indicates that its protection extends especially to the *solar plexus chakra*. An overexposed and unprotected solar plexus means that our environment can too easily *dynamically imprint* on our being. In other words, we can become *over-sympathetic and over-identified* with our environment.

All Yarrow flowers are recognised for their finely-detailed geometric patterns (see 'Yarrow'), which interweave to form strong, enduring structures (FES). Traditionally, Yarrow herb has been used for its ability to stem bleeding. At an energetic level, Golden Yarrow flower essence *stems 'emotional bleeding,' sealing, protecting and stabilising the life force.*

The Golden Yarrow personality

Golden Yarrow is for those who sympathise too strongly with their environment. Emotional over-identification occurs with those around them, and this can create a sense of mental congestion, confusion and even deeply-felt pain (if pain is in the environment). Too often, this leads to attempts to dull or numb emotional sensitivity through use or abuse of alcohol or drugs. Another response is to retreat into social isolation, becoming more and more introverted. Or we become hardened and superficially insensitive, as do some healers and health practitioners desensitised by constant exposure to suffering. (see also Yellow Star Tulip).

Heightened sensitivity to the world around us may be used in creative and artistic ways but if we are unable at the same time to shut off or limit the input from our environment, the cost to our health can be great. Kaminski and Katz (1996) state that 'one of the greatest challenges in the life of the soul is that of learning to stay open and balanced, without compromising one's basic integrity and health.'

Benefits of taking Golden Yarrow

Golden Yarrow flower essence helps us to maintain our sense of Self and our identity whatever the surroundings. 'Golden Yarrow helps [us] build a [psychic] sheath which shields and protects' (Kaminski and Katz 1996) without dulling the sensitivity needed for creativity and self-expression.

Possible physical imbalances

The solar plexus has a strong influence on the state of our nervous system. Golden Yarrow flower essence helps protect, balance, and strengthen this energetic centre and as a result, has a beneficial and nourishing effect on the nervous system and general vitality.

Common uses

For emotional protection; for hypersensitivity to the 'emotional atmosphere'; to help balance creative work, rest and play; to protect from overstimulation; to 'cushion' against the harsh effects of the world; to provide a healthy buffer between you and the outside world; to help balance your 'gut' reaction to the world

Complementary &/or similar flower essences

Angelica, Arnica, Canyon Dudleya, Chaparral, Corn, Dill, Echinacea, Fringed Violet, Garlic, Indian Pink, Lavender, Love-Lies-Bleeding, Mallow, Mimulus, Mountain Pennyroyal, Mugwort, Nicotiana, Oregon Grape, Red Clover, St John's Wort, Sturt Desert Pea, Violet, Walnut, all the Yarrows, YES formula

Supporting the changes

- Develop methods of dynamic self-protection – visualise white light around you or use other forms of meditation or protective rituals.
- Maintain a balanced lifestyle, especially when it comes to getting enough sleep. Try not to inhibit your dream life with drugs or medication; dreams play an important role in healing the emotional body.
- A diet rich in nutrients for the nervous system, especially Vitamin B, is supportive.
- Integrate your creative work into a balanced daily routine. That way, you know when to start but, more importantly, you know when to stop because the boundaries between creative work, rest and play are well defined.

Gorse

Ulex europaeus   (Golden-yellow / Bach)

Positive state

'Light at the end of the tunnel'
Optimism

Negative state

No 'light at the end of the tunnel'
Hopelessness and despair

The growth pattern of the Gorse plant illustrates its healing qualities as a flower essence. During the coldest and darkest winter days, one or two Gorse blossoms remain in flower like the pilot light in a gas heating system, always on standby.

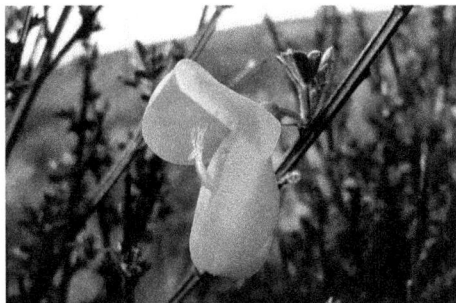

Just as a gas heater comes on when the switch is flicked, at the first sign of spring the Gorse bush *comes to life* and covers itself in an abundance of sunny, *golden-yellow* flowers, summoning forth all the other spring blossoms. The *flame of life is rekindled* and with it, the will to live. *Sustained hope* – 'the (sun)light at the end of the tunnel' – is symbolised by these few blooms that appear throughout winter. This symbol of *resilience* is *protected* by mighty spines that defend the plant and deter animals (Barnard 1988).

The sudden emergence of the flowers' golden-yellow radiance, like sunshine dispersing clouds, reminds us that Gorse flower essence can help us to *recover and lift* ourselves out of the darkest and bleakest times.

The Gorse state of mind

Dr Bach described those in the negative Gorse state as 'looking as though they needed more sunshine in their lives to drive away the clouds' (Bach 1987). If all seems lost and we are in despair, especially about the future, Gorse can arouse a glimmer of hope, reigniting our desire to carry on. It allows us to see obstacles as opportunities for growth and service.

Never forget the friend you have in Gorse flower essence during personal trials – when an illness persists for such a long time that you forget what it is to feel well; when you endure a prolonged emotional drought; when you lose your job or when any situation is imbued with a sense of hopelessness.

Benefits of taking Gorse

We can emerge triumphant after challenging times, displaying our true colours just as Gorse displays its golden radiance in spring. Gorse flower essence helps to reawaken our deepest survival instincts, carrying us out of the depths of despair into a full appreciation of life. It can help guide us to the light at the end of the tunnel via a path now 'lit up' by optimistic vision.

Possible physical imbalances

Dr Bach recognised a condition of chronic resignation and loss of heart which occurs in many people who have been ill for a long time. Gorse flower essence can help lift this impediment to recovery by reigniting optimism and the courage to fight on.

Common uses

For complete loss of faith in the future; for 'clouds on life's horizon'; for chronic resignation; to restore faith and hope; to rekindle the flame of life; to resurrect optimism

Complementary &/or similar flower essences

Agrimony, Baby Blue Eyes, Borage, Chrysanthemum, Forget-Me-Not, Foxglove, Gentian, Hibbertia, Honeysuckle, Hound's Tongue, Iris, Pansy, Scotch Broom, Self-Heal, Sturt Desert Pea, Sweet Chestnut, Waratah, Wild Oat, Wild Rose, Zinnia

Supporting the changes

- Actively seek something you can put your faith and energy into. Gorse will help clarify what this might be – a new creative outlet or interest, a new career path or a revitalised philosophical or spiritual perspective.
- Avoid doom and gloom merchants and gravitate towards people who are more optimistic and committed.
- Re-commit and say YES to life!

Harvest Brodiaea

Brodiaea elegans   (Deep purple / FES-res)

Positive state

Clear/broad vision
Mentally refreshed/lightness of mind

Negative state

Materialistically 'one-eyed'
Feeling mentally tired, uninspired, 'heavy headed'

Over the ages, the *violet/deep-purple* colour of Harvest Brodiaea flowers has been symbolic of spirituality. Harvest Brodiaea flower essence can help materialistic, overly sceptical or cynical people gain a more *spiritual perspective* or at least help them to become less cynical and more open to a philosophy of life that embraces something beyond the materialistic view. Harvest Brodiaea helps spiritualise the *mental body*, thus allowing a *spiritualisation of the intellect* and *'lightness of mind.'*

The bulb-like shape of the plant signifies its relationship with the pineal gland and the crown chakra or 'overseer' and also with the eye and insight. The flower essence helps to increase sensory perception overall, especially vision.

The Harvest Brodiaea state of mind

Harvest Brodiaea flower essence is useful when we have a heavy, overburdened mind and habitually 'overthink,' dwelling on things to the point where we become mentally bogged down. We are tired and unimaginative and need to be lifted out of the doldrums or we may be disillusioned with the overly materialistic focus that has ruled our life up till now.

It can also be helpful for those who have been rewarded for their intellectual gifts but who eventually begin to feel burdened and unfulfilled by what has become a lopsided way of thinking and living.

Benefits of taking Harvest Brodiaea

Harvest Brodiaea flower essence helps us draw on our right-brain faculties so that we can think more laterally and creatively. It spiritualises the intellect, loosening and lightening us up! It can help you to think beyond your usual constraints, uplifting your heart and mind to view your current circumstances more positively. Harvest Brodiaea allows you to stand back from the materialistic concerns of everyday financial, family and work worries and take a broader perspective on your life.

Possible physical imbalances

I have found that, when prescribed appropriately, Harvest Brodiaea flower essence can improve vision on a metaphysical level and also on a physical level, especially when there has been a tendency to depressive states of mind.

Common uses

To clear a 'crammed head' and stop overthinking; for times when, as the Monty Python character says, 'my brain hurts!'; to lighten up; to gain a perspective beyond the materialistic view; to expand your qualities of perception and intuition; to develop insight; to go 'beyond the brain' and beyond blue!

Complementary &/or similar flower essences

Angelica, Angelsword, Baby Blue Eyes, Borage, Chrysanthemum, Coffee, Fllaree, Forget-Me-Not, Garlic, Hibbertia, Hound's Tongue, Iris, Lavender, Lemon, Morning Glory, Mountain Pennyroyal, Nasturtium, Nicotiana, Onion, Peppermint, Queen Anne's Lace, Shasta Daisy, Silver Princess, Tall Yellow Top, White Chestnut, Zinnia

Supporting the changes

- Consider practising relaxation and meditation techniques to ease and 'unload' constant and unnecessary thoughts and worries from the mind.
- Seek out non-materialistic philosophies (or friends/persons who adhere to them).

- Engage in some regular 'grounding' in the form of physical work or exercise.
- Take a day off – take time out!!

Heather

Calluna vulgaris   (White / Bach)

Positive state

Considerate and understanding
Empathetic

Negative state

Self-absorbed
Seeking out anyone who will listen

Heather's straggling evergreen shrub is widespread on European mountainsides and boggy moors. From among its needle-like leaves bloom *pinkish-purple* flowers with a honey fragrance. The Scots have long used its stems for brooms and roof thatching and boiled the flowers to make a yellow dye. The *purple* colour of the flower relates to the *crown chakra* and symbolises the plant's influence on our own *spiritual journey.* The fact that purple is blended with *pink*, relating to the *heart chakra*, reminds us that this journey on Earth is best *shared empathetically* with the life journeys of others, not taken alone in a *self-obsessed* way.

The Heather plant lives comfortably in the wilderness and on infertile soils, being *self-reliant* and able to thrive where other plants may not. But Barnard (1988) gives us a clue to the negative Heather state by informing us that, during its long lifetime, Heather 'will *smother* all other plants and poison the soil with acidity, [preventing] other plants from living near it.' Those in need of Heather flower essence often send people running for cover to avoid being verbally buttonholed! The positive state enabled by using the flower essence is symbolised by the plant's *independence* and ability to survive alone.

The Heather personality

Heather flower essence can help when our need to share thoughts and feelings becomes a compulsion for us and a drain on others. In a desperate attempt to draw people closer for comfort and recognition, we succeed only in repelling them. Our anxiety urgently seeks expression and validation from others — it doesn't matter who. The relationship exists solely in terms of whether or not they are willing to listen to us.

Self-obsession about every detail of health, home, finances and safety has the effect of obscuring the overall picture. We can't see the wood for the trees, in our minds or in our lives. We have no ability to reflect in a meditative way and our awareness has become confused and agitated – our thoughts disturb us and others.

Heather people in the negative state can be hypochondriacs. They become the health practitioner's nightmare, giving long, detailed accounts of their medical history and complaints. Heather flower essence can help us gain a broader perspective on our state of health, allowing a much more holistic approach.

Benefits of taking Heather

Heather helps us to be more objective. The great sympathy and concern we have for ourselves can be transformed into an equal empathy for the plight of others. We can shift our inward-turned focus of concern and awareness outward, so as to be inclusive of those around us. When the heart chakra is balanced in this way, Heather people have a tremendous capacity for self-healing by healing others; they become the classic 'wounded healer.'

Possible physical imbalances

As mentioned above, people in need of Heather flower essence can be classic hypochondriacs, at times the health practitioner's nightmare, giving epic accounts of their medical history and complaints. Heather can help such a person gain a much more synthesised and holistic view of their own health, and this enables the health practitioner to assess their case more easily.

Common uses

For the self-obsessed; for those who buttonhole others; for hypochondriacs; for those who are a drain on others in their company; to help us listen to others with our hearts; to help us move from being a 'student' of our own health to becoming a teacher of health to others; to help us see our problems in a broader perspective

Complementary &/or similar flower essences

Angelica, Billy Goat Plum, Bleeding Heart, Calendula, Chrysanthemum, Crab Apple, Filaree, Forget-Me-Not, Hound's Tongue, Love-Lies-Bleeding, Quaking Grass, Sagebrush, Self-Heal, Shasta Daisy, Star Tulip, Sweet Pea, Zinnia

Supporting the changes

- Study holistic medicine or at least investigate its possibilities. This will help you develop a broader perspective on health issues and offer practical ways of improving your quality of life.
- Work with people in need – you will see your problems in a different light.
- Try practising meditation and other disciplines that integrate body and mind.

Hibbertia

Hibbertia pedunculata   (Yellow / Aus)

Positive state

Wisdom from experience
Warmth and spontaneity

Negative state

Uncomfortable unless they 'know it all'
Knowledge used to gain control; one-upmanship

Hibbertia flower essence *teaches us how to learn*. The *lower intellect* is about accumulation of knowledge for its own sake, whereas our *higher spiritual intellect* (as represented by the *yellow* flower colour) involves deeper understanding and *heartfelt wisdom*, which results from integration of the emotional body with the mental body. Hibbertia flower essence can help us combine our feelings and experience with our thoughts and knowledge to achieve a contentment and peace of mind that results from '*inner knowing.*'

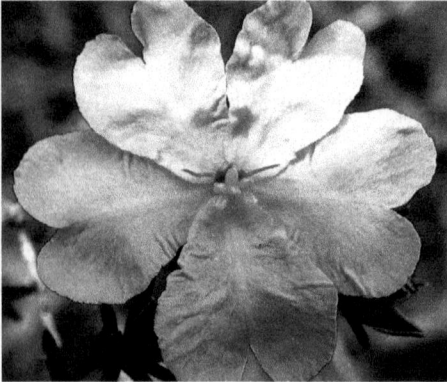

Ian White, who produced this flower essence, has drawn attention to the signature of the fallen flower petals, which form a *heart shape* on the ground.

This is a beautiful symbol of the heart connection and also a reference to the *grounding* of spiritual 'knowledge' in Earthly reality. The shiny green leaves (the colour *green* is also associated with the heart) contrast strongly with the bright *yellow* flowers (the colour associated with intellect).

There is a similarity to Californian Poppy in that both flower essences teach us not to look so much 'outside' ourselves for knowledge and wisdom but to '*venture inward.*' Where Californian Poppy lures us because of its ability to 'glitter like gold,' Hibbertia, often referred to by its common name of Guinea Flower, 'gleams like golden guineas.'

The Hibbertia personality

Hibbertia flower essence helps warm the 'cold' and clinical intellect. It enhances the role of the heart in learning and melts our mental defences, which inhibit us from getting a real 'feel' for things.

It is a suitable flower essence for those who tend to use their knowledge to gain intellectual 'one-upmanship' or as a weapon to get what they want. Unfortunately, this way of using the intellect also serves to protect them from fully feeling the joy of any situation, and their knowledge is used competitively rather than to further their learning. They safeguard themselves against ridicule and what they fear most – humiliation. As a result, they lack warmth, appear too intense or aloof and aren't enriched by experiences or the relationships that could stem from them.

The mental discipline required for the relentless pursuit of knowledge usually comes easily to the Hibbertia person – too easily in fact. They can become perfectionists who discipline themselves excessively.

Benefits of taking Hibbertia

Hibbertia flower essence helps us get out of our heads and into our hearts so that we can appreciate life from more than a one-dimensional, intellectual point of view. It enables a multidimensional perspective that incorporates our feelings and adds to the richness of experience.

Hibbertia helps to integrate intuition, gut feeling and heartfelt reactions with external knowledge. Peace and contentment of mind results from the confidence associated with inner knowledge.

Hibbertia flower essence can help us warm to life and the people around us, and this feeling becomes mutual.

Possible physical imbalances

According to Ian White, a classic Hibbertia man may be tall and thin with a tendency to lose their hair at the front. I have found that ailments of the head region ('above the shoulders') resulting from excess energy expended in 'overthinking' are common among my Hibbertia clients. These include sinus conditions, hayfever, post-nasal drip, recurring head colds and headaches (the head 'aching to go the way of the heart.') It is interesting to note that traditional Chinese medicine often describes nasal catarrh associated with sinus problems, as 'the heart trying to get into the head.'

Common uses

For the overly 'cerebral' person; for those who use knowledge as a weapon or for one-upmanship; for the person who needs to know everything before taking action and so never acts; to help trust your intuition or inner knowing; to enjoy experience by 'going with the flow'; to get better at acting in an impromptu or 'off the cuff' way; to display trust and warmth even when 'going in cold'

Complementary &/or similar flower essences

Angelsword, Baby Blue Eyes, Black Eyed Susan, Calendula, Californian Poppy, Chrysanthemum, Cosmos, Harvest Brodiaea, Hibiscus, Hound's Tongue, Lilac, Lotus,

Mallow, Manzanita, Nasturtium, Nicotiana, Oregon Grape, Shasta Daisy, Shooting Star, Star Tulip, Tall Yellow Top, Water Violet, White Chestnut, Zinnia

Supporting the changes

- Join a team or play a team sport and accept direction.
- Allow the occasional speech, social engagement or activity to be impromptu. Don't over-prepare – just let things develop and see where it takes you.
- Have a go at something you're not good at – take a risk and try.
- 'Get your hands dirty' and experience what you so often theorise about.
- Speak from the heart!

Hibiscus

Hibiscus rosa-sinensis   (Red / FES)

Positive state

Regained trust/belief
Open-minded, warm and receptive

Negative state

Guarded, often due to past emotional abuse or harsh treatment (FES)
Closed mind; 'lack of warmth and vitality' (FES)

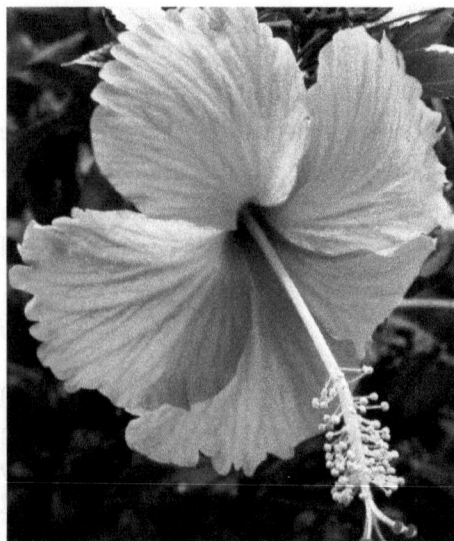

Hibiscus flowers' *reproductive organs, which protrude conspicuously* from the centre of five *red, flaring petals,* signify the plant's direct relationship with *sexual passion* and the *base chakra* and *sacral chakra*.

This may be an advantage for the plant when it comes to plant *interrelations* and celebrating its fertility in nature but from a human perspective, it also conjures feelings of *vulnerability* through over-exposure and lack of protection. In the negative Hibiscus state, you may feel that you are vulnerable to violation if you express yourself openly. This plant helps us safely develop *openness and trust* in our feelings and thoughts after trust has been abused or taken for granted. It can allow us to express our true *passion and warmth* (note the *brilliantly red* flowers) in intimate relationships.

The Hibiscus personality

Despite the emphasis placed by Kaminski and Katz (1996) on this flower essence's role in physical sexuality, my experience as a therapist leads me to believe that a description of the negative state of Hibiscus could be broadened to include psychological frigidity in the form of mistrust toward anything new, different or unfamiliar. We should consider Hibiscus when, after being emotionally hurt, we become overly cautious and guarded against further hurt. Even a fleeting gesture, insensitive comment or inappropriate physical contact can leave us feeling emotionally invaded or abused and can leave long-term emotional 'scars.' At a transpersonal level, women's consciousness suffers collective trauma as a result of 'the exploitation and commercialisation of female sexuality' (Kaminski and Katz 1996). As a coping mechanism, consciousness may split or disassociate from the passion, warmth and responsiveness that can be experienced through intimate relations.

I have encountered some clients who are cautious about accepting a regimen of natural therapy because it deviates from their familiar routine. They are uneasy, apprehensive and mentally unreceptive when faced with an opportunity to change their point of view. This does not come from intolerance, but rather from insecurity and a fear of letting down their mental and emotional guard, perhaps as a result of past experiences of being exploited.

Benefits of taking Hibiscus

Hibiscus assists in healing deep emotional wounds, allowing warmth of feeling once again to permeate and expand our perspective. While maintaining an ability to discern when it is appropriate and safe to be open and intimate with others, a more secure and open mind makes it possible to be more receptive to the pleasure of intimate relationships. A much greater potential for love and affection will result.

Possible physical imbalances

I have found that Hibiscus flower essence can help people to comfortably open their mind and become more receptive to natural treatment approaches which may be new to them and different from what they are used to. In other words, it can help them move out of what has been their comfort zone and benefit from something different and unfamiliar in the form of a new physical health perspective and regime.

Common uses

For mental and physical 'frigidity' or guarding; for the feeling of being 'once bitten, twice shy'; for warmth and receptivity in physical intimacy; for a vital responsiveness; to heal emotional wounds and learn to trust (again)

Complementary &/or similar flower essences

Baby Blue Eyes, Basil, Billy Goat Plum, Calendula, Crab Apple, Dogwood, Easter Lily, Flannel Flower, Hibbertia, Mallow, Manzanita, Mariposa Lily, Nasturtium, Oregon Grape, Pomegranate, Quince, Snapdragon, Squash, Star Tulip, Sticky Monkeyflower, Sweet Pea, Water Violet

Supporting the changes

- Consider engaging in a therapy such as Emotional Focus Therapy (EFT).
- Consider doing a personal development course that, while being supportive and nurturing, might challenge some of your personal beliefs.
- Choose your friends wisely and prefer those you can be at ease with. When someone close hurts you, acknowledge it to them immediately.
- Develop practical ways of protecting your natural emotional sensitivity, whether this involves visualising protective white light or physically going to your own special refuge for brief periods.
- Remember, you can recover fully from the 'once bitten, twice shy' syndrome, even years after it has developed.

Holly

Ilex aquifolium   (White / Bach)

Positive state

Positive thoughts and feelings
Open hearted love and generosity

Negative state

Thoughts of a jealous/envious or hateful/spiteful kind
'Prickly' and 'mean-hearted'

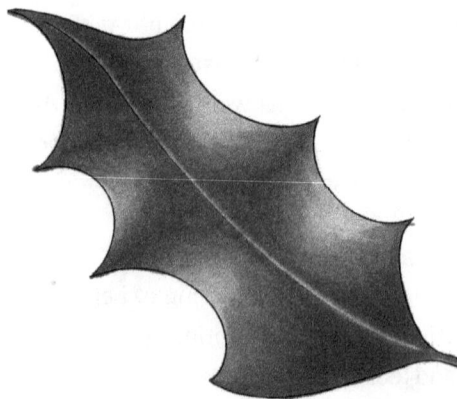

Holly is an evergreen shrub from the west of Asia and Europe, and its bright-red berries which appear in winter have come to symbolise Christmas. With *prickly*, leathery, glossy leaves and tiny fragrant flowers, it has a strong reputation in Druid, Roman and Christian folklore for *warding off evil* (Barnard 1988) or in new age terms, *protecting against negative thought forms.*

The *white* of the flower reinforces this reputation for *protection* and its hint of *pink* and *sweet scent* remind us of its ability to help *transform within* by *stirring the love in our hearts.* It grows with great determination and strength, forming *impenetrable* hedges. The flowering twigs are boiled to make the well-known Bach Flower Remedy, which helps transform the 'prickly' disposition of the negative Holly state into one of *unconditional love.* No other flower essence addresses such extremely polarised positive and *negative states of mind.*

The Holly state of mind

The negative Holly state illustrates the concept that emotion is an energetic force which should be in a constant process of transformation. When it stagnates, problems arise. Flower essences are a very good way to help get stagnant energy moving again and Holly is a prime mover in this sense. Holly flower essence enables a person to transform negative (maladaptive) emotional states into their positive (adaptive) opposites, forming a protective internal barrier against outward negativity.

Families typically experience many love-hate relationships which illustrate how emotions can undergo dramatic changes in the space of a few minutes. Brothers and sisters may be happily playing together one minute and at each other's throats the next. A minute later, the whole angry episode is completely forgotten and they are playing happily again. Healthy relationships allow emotions to remain in a state of flux but when feelings are permanently negative we face problems. At these times, Holly can help swing the emotional pendulum away from envy, suspicion, hatred and desire for revenge, towards feelings of love, compassion and trust.

Today's society is suffering an epidemic of envy, fostered by the media, towards those who are perceived to be better-looking or more successful. Holly flower essence can help transform the energy of this 'green-eyed monster' into creative positivity, bringing peace and contentment to our hearts.

Benefits of taking Holly

The Holly plant has always been a symbol of Christmas, a time dedicated to the emergence of new life from the darkness of winter (at least in the northern hemisphere where the tradition originates) and a celebration of our love and compassion for one another. However, all over the world Christmas also witnesses acts of violence and hatred – too often within families. Holly protects us against this kind of darkness and nurtures our heart-energy, allowing love to blossom so that we can fall in love with life again.

Possible physical imbalances

Negative and insidious, repressed emotions will eventually undermine one's physical health. If we let such feelings fester and 'eat away' at us for long enough they will inevitably lead to serious immune dysfunction in our physical body. Research in psychoneuroimmunology supports this.

Common uses

For acute feelings of jealousy, envy, vengefulness and hatred; for those moments when, metaphorically speaking, you feel you could 'just kill'; for protection against taking on the negative feelings of others (especially those people who are always 'glass half empty' types); to transform negative thinking with an 'injection' of positivity; to open our hearts to love

Complementary &/or similar flower essences

Beech, Bleeding Heart, Borage, Crab Apple, Dogwood, Garlic, Mountain Pennyroyal, Oregon Grape, Star Thistle, Star Tulip, Tiger Lily, Trillium, Walnut, Willow, Yarrow, YES formula

Supporting the changes

- Try to spend some time alone, away from negative influences, perhaps in the green of the countryside. However you create it, you need your space.
- Include more of the colours pink and green in your clothes and environment. These colours produce a feeling of secure space through their soothing, healing effects on the heart centre.
- Love yourself!

Honeysuckle
Lonicera caprifolium   (Red-white / Bach)

Positive state
Your heart IS in it!
Dynamic presence, enthusiastically involved

Negative state
Stuck in the past and an old paradigm
Nostalgic or homesick

Honeysuckle (the *caprifolium* variety) is known as red or Italian Honeysuckle. The very *fragrant* flowers are reddish on the outside then turn yellow after pollination. Like many *strong scents*, the aroma of Honeysuckle can trigger strong *emotional memories* and this reflects the Honeysuckle person's strong, *nostalgic* bond with the past. Plants with flowers that give off strong, *lingering* perfumes which *pervade* their surroundings are often helpful when dealing with issues relating to the need for *release from the past*. Barnard (1988) describes how the 'bursting *vitality of* the *blood red* corolla' of the flower grounds us in the *here and now!*

The Honeysuckle personality

In the negative state, Honeysuckle people have a belief that the past is much better than it actually was. The present can never live up to this imagined glory and so they never really live it. They view the present and the future negatively and resist any suggestion that their past ideal might fall off the pedestal on which they placed it.

Pining for the way we were at the beginning of a relationship or for how good it was in a past one; relentless homesickness after we have made a new beginning elsewhere; holding on to a past we shared with a loved one lost long ago; emotional attachments that persist past their natural time; clinging to old beliefs and thought patterns that have become obsolete – all these circumstances involving withdrawal from present reality call for Honeysuckle flower essence.

Benefits of taking Honeysuckle

Honeysuckle can heal the heart's disappointment, allowing it to gently open and receive life anew. Then we can experience the warmth and energy available in the present, reawakening our affection for life. The past comes to be valued as a learning experience but does not hinder living in the present or impede future progress. If you do bring back the past, it is with a positive aim in mind for the present.

Possible physical imbalances

In the negative Honeysuckle state, people often experience congestive symptoms in the head, which is working overtime to rule a heart that is being denied in some way. Conditions such as sinus congestion, persistent nasal discharge and post-nasal drip – 'inner tears' – and recurring head colds are common. As mentioned previously, Traditional Chinese Medicine regards sinus congestion as 'the heart trying to get into the head.' In other words, the heart wants to EMBRACE the NOW!

Common uses

For constant nostalgia; for homesickness; for those whose past has become a legend in their own mind; for those stuck in the good old days; to assist past-life and regression therapies; to help one become grounded in reality (and in the NOW); to integrate heart and head; to greet life with a dynamic and open heart; to become enthused again

Complementary &/or similar flower essences

Baby Blue Eyes, Blackberry, Bleeding Heart, Bottlebrush, Cayenne, Chrysanthemum, Clematis, Corn, Fairy Lantern, Forget-Me-Not, Golden Ear Drops, Red Lily, Rosemary, Sagebrush, Shooting Star, Silver Princess, Star Tulip, Sweet pea, Tall Yellow Top, Tansy, Walnut, Wild Rose

Supporting the changes

- Meditation and other practices that bring mental clarity will help centre the head and the heart in the present. Regression therapy may begin to resolve emotional attachments to the past so that the present can be experienced more fully.
- Grounding activities such as gardening or vigorous exercise will be of great benefit – anything to get the red blood of life flowing through us.
- Take the plunge into life! In one way or another we have chosen to be here (still).

Hornbeam

Carpinus betulus   (Yellow-green / Bach)

Positive state

Refreshed and enthusiastic
Stamina for getting the job done

Negative state

Tired, 'Monday morning' feeling
Pacing oneself to get through the day

Hornbeam's long, *drooping*, cylindrical flowers and smooth, *deeply furrowed bark* (which is *grey streaked* like the hair of an ageing person) could give a first impression of being *old, tired and worn-out*.

This is an apt description of the negative Hornbeam state. However, the lasting impression given by the tree is of *wisdom and endurance*, holding on to life with a *tenacious* grip. The wood of the tree is exceptionally hard, *strong and white* like horn or bone and can *withstand* much wear. Its *strength and utility* means that it is highly valued as a timber. This is the true spirit of the tree and using Hornbeam flower essence can allow us to tap into these qualities. Its characteristic *adaptability* is exemplified by the varied uses to which its timber has been put and also the way it can be trained to make arched walkways and tunnels sheltered by dense foliage (Barnard 1988).

The *yellow-green* (green + yellow = brown) flowers relate to the *Earth energy* (brown) of the *sacral chakra* and the *heartfelt commitment* to life (*green*) of the *heart chakra*. Using the flower essence brings a *recommitment* to life which in turn creates a sense of rejuvenation.

The Hornbeam state of mind

Hornbeam is for the 'Monday morning' feeling that pursues some people all day, every day. This flower essence is helpful for times when we wake and look towards the day and its commitments (and indeed life in general) with a feeling that we face an insurmountable obstacle. Everything is a chore and we fear that we will be unable to fulfil our everyday responsibilities. Nevertheless, once we are up and about, we somehow get through the day. ((Olive flower essence, for instance, is appropriate for times when we are unable to fulfil our commitments.) Much energy is wasted in concern about whether or not jobs will get done – we do them despite the fact that our minds are continually psyching us out and dissipating the precious energy we have left.

Consider Hornbeam when life becomes mundane and predictable, a tired old routine that does nothing for us and we feel we have nothing to offer. Hornbeam helps us get out of this rut, whether we have fallen into it from sheer overwork (for example in the case of a first-time mother on call twenty-four hours a day or a workaholic suffering from burnout) or in midlife if we start to think, 'I've done my bit and I don't know if I've got the energy or desire for what comes next!'

Benefits of taking Hornbeam

Hornbeam flower essence assists us in developing a fresh attitude and approach to life, bringing new energy to our interests, like the feeling of approaching an old problem after a holiday or a complete break. It doesn't 'teach an old dog new tricks' but offers a refresher course in the tricks you already know.

Possible physical imbalances

Hornbeam flower essence should be considered during rehabilitation and after illness, especially when you have 'never felt the same since.' It is a very handy remedy for chronic fatigue syndrome as part of an overall recovery package. It should be considered for depression and depletion of energy associated with lingering illness. For those who are very much 'in touch with their bodies,' it is useful when the warning signs of impending illness are sensed.

Common uses

For those who feel they lack the strength to cope with everyday tasks; for those who feel they need to pace themselves to get through the day; for the tired procrastinator; to help break out of a rut; to help bring vitality and freshness when life feels stale and mundane; to help regenerate vitality and spontaneity in life.

Complementary &/or similar flower essences

Aloe Vera, Blackberry, Borage, Cayenne, Chrysanthemum, Elm, Forget-Me-Not, Hound's Tongue, Indian Paintbrush, Iris, Larkspur, Macrocarpa, Madia, Morning Glory, Nasturtium, Olive, Peppermint, Silver Princess, Tansy, Wild Oat, Wild Rose

Supporting the changes

- Take more interest in your health and lifestyle. Investigate natural treatments and ease into a pattern of regular exercise.

- 'All work and no play makes Jack a dull boy.' Develop a better balance of work, rest and play, and redefine your priorities for quality of life.
- Take a break, or even better, take a holiday. If you can't, take Hornbeam instead!

Hound's Tongue

Cynoglossum grande   (Blue-white / FES)

Positive state

Vital, 'holistic thinking' (FES)
Uplifted, philosophical, imaginative

Negative state

Dull, insular, overly technical thinking
Overly material world view

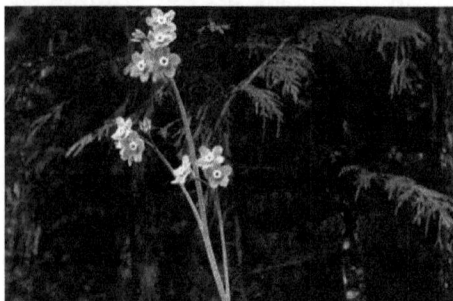

Hound's Tongue's *blue* flowers with *white* centres tell us about the possibility of experiencing an *enlightened* outlook from within what can otherwise be an overly *materialistic/ mechanistic perspective*. A more *holistic* and *philosophical* view can *'lighten us up'* from within, just as the bright blue Hound's Tongue flower lights up all around it when it emerges from the darkness of the forest in early spring. The flowers are projected upwards above the base of the plant on long stems so that they cannot become *too heavily Earth-bound* and are more able to capture the *light from the sky* above.

The Hound's Tongue personality

Hound's Tongue is the remedy to use when mundane reality seems your only lot in life. When you feel that all you ever do is change dirty nappies, feed hungry babies and fill your days with cooking, cleaning and washing followed by sleep (when you are allowed!) this flower essence can help to raise your spirits. Primary carers such as mothers of young children have discovered the benefits of taking Hound's Tongue.

Another group for whom it has proved useful are technically minded people such as scientists who spend their time engaged in focused, analytical thought but have reached a point where their work feels too clinical and 'vanilla.' Hound's Tongue flower essence can revitalise the thinking process for these people (Kaminski and Katz 1996), bringing vivid, creative insight to work which has begun to feel barren and uninspired.

Benefits of taking Hound's Tongue

With Hound's Tongue flower essence you can stand back a little, become more philosophical about life and see the bigger picture. It can 'help the soul to think in clear and specific ways about the spiritual dimensions of the physical world' (Kaminski and Katz 1996) at a time when you may feel 'Earth bound' like a grounded eagle. You will be able once more to review with wonder and awe the beauty around you and be uplifted to soar majestically.

Possible physical imbalances

Most people who benefit from Hound's Tongue flower essence also feel 'heavy' in the head. They may be suffering from sinus congestion, recurring head colds and/or a generally lowered immunity to infections at this time.

Common uses

For the 24/7 mother who has time for nothing else; for those weighed down and trapped in mundane thinking; to broaden and enlighten a narrowly-focused mind; to receive a 'ray of sunshine' in your life or work!

Complementary &/or similar flower essences

Angel's Trumpet, Angelica, Baby Blue Eyes, Chrysanthemum, Filaree, Forget-Me-Not, Gentian, Gorse, Harvest Brodiaea, Hibbertia, Hornbeam, Iris, Lady's Slipper, Morning Glory, Nasturtium, Pansy, Peppermint, Scotch Broom, Zinnia

Supporting the changes

- Read about positive philosophies that bring a sense of meaning to life.
- Get a new and positive perspective from a friend or counsellor.
- Engage regularly in some physical activity that you enjoy.
- Take time out to stand back from your life and review it.

Impatiens

Impatiens glandulifera   (Pale mauve / Bach)

Positive state

Relaxed; stopping 'to smell the roses'
Patient; process orientated

Negative state

Tense, irritable and 'time-challenged'
Impatiently goal orientated

There is no doubt that Dr Bach was very *single-minded and driven* to find a system of healing that would enable him to help his patients in a profound way and at a truly causal level. It is no surprise, then, that Impatiens was the first flower essence he developed in his system of healing. Impatiens is a tall, *imposing* plant found near Europe's rivers and streams, although it is native to the Himalayas (Barnard 1988). The ripe seed pods intrigue young children because they *burst open* at a touch – like those with a *'short-fuse' temper* when they are distracted from an immediate *goal* – a characteristic of those who need Impatiens flower essence! Most of the plant's flowers are a 'hot' red-mauve colour but Dr Bach specified that only the *pale mauve* flowers (signifying heart-soothing qualities) were to be used in preparing the flower essence. The *heart-soothing* colour and delicacy of these flowers conveys the potential *tolerant, gentle and relaxed* positive Impatiens state.

The Impatiens personality

Impatiens people in the negative state have too much to do and too little time to do it in. It seems that they arrive on Earth as interplanetary tourists, desperately trying to pack as much as possible into a whirlwind tour. They feel different, alone and held back by the pace of these backward Earthlings around them!

When we are in the negative Impatiens state we are driven by a constant sense of urgency with an insatiable desire for results. And while we may be capable of achieving these results, we suffer from overload and deadline delirium because of our inability to accept support from those around us. Our intolerance of and impatience with the slow pace of others' work prevents us from developing collaborative working relationships. 'Leave it alone! I'll do it. I'm the only one who can get the job done properly and on time!' is our attitude. It quickly alienates others, supporting our self-fulfilling sense that we don't belong here. The resulting mental and physical tension from constant activity can lead to many problems and make us vulnerable to exhaustion and burnout.

Benefits of taking Impatiens

In the positive state, Impatiens people have much to offer the world in the way of vision, inspiration and the ability to be self-motivated in the pursuit of goals. They are often the natural movers and shakers of the world, the reformers and transformers of society. With a little patience (and maybe a dash of Impatiens!) they can share these qualities and not feel so alone. Impatiens flower essence helps them to find that elusive peace of mind when they realise that we all may be on different paths but we are generally united in the direction we are heading.

Impatiens helps us accept that we all have an equal role in bringing the vision of a better world into reality. It can foster our sense of belonging to a place where we can relax and be truly at home.

Possible physical imbalances

Mental and physical tension can lead to many problems – indigestion through rushed eating, headaches and other body aches, insomnia and an inability to relax. Constant activity makes us vulnerable to exhaustion and burnout. In addition, some cases of female infertility respond well to Impatiens, where there is a need to slow down, BE more in the moment, less outcome-orientated, and therefore more inwardly receptive to the fertilisation process. (And this includes the partner and others who are close!)

Common uses

For a constant sense of urgency; for intolerance and impatience; when nothing happens fast enough; for the child who wants to be an adult now; for those who convert anger and frustration into busyness and hurry; for obsessively goal-oriented people; to help accept the natural pace of others and of life; to help learn to enjoy the process and not just the result; to help trust in life; to help find a home inside yourself and just Be!

Complementary &/or similar flower essences

Beech, Californian Poppy, Chamomile, Cherry Plum, Crowea, Dandelion, Indian Pink, Larkspur, Lavender, Passionflower, Quaking Grass, Quince, Rabbitbrush, Shooting Star, Snapdragon, Star Tulip, Tiger Lily, Vervain, Zinnia

Supporting the changes

- Persevere with relaxation and meditation techniques. They may seem totally unproductive and even a painful waste of time at first but they can change your life profoundly.
- Investigate philosophies that will help you understand that the process is as important as the goal. While everyone travels the path in their own way, we are all travelling it together.
- Join a team (but not as captain!)

Indian Paintbrush
Castilleja miniata   (Red / FES)

Positive state
Energy and exuberant activity (FES)
Creative and inspired work

Negative state
'Low vitality and exhaustion' (FES)
Creatively frustrated

Indian Paintbrush confirms, absolutely, that there is much in a name. When the *brush of creativity* is not sweeping through your life or work or when you feel that your creative endeavours are being thwarted professionally or personally, consider using Indian Paintbrush flower essence. The tips of the flowers resemble a *paintbrush* with a generous dab of *vibrant red* paint that symbolises the capacity of the essence to sweep creatively and artistically through those areas of life where more '*colour*' is required.

The *red* colour of the flowers relates to the capacity of the flower essence to stimulate the *base chakra*. Through this chakra we plant spiritual insight in the Earth, grounding it, so that it can be expressed in a *creative and desirable* form. Indian Paintbrush flower essence helps align the etheric, emotional and physical bodies which relate to the lower chakras, so that they can connect with the Earth. Just as we 'earth' electrical devices so that they function safely and efficiently, the base chakra 'earths' us so that we *resonate better* with the physical world and channel its power in a sustainable way.

The Indian Paintbrush state of mind

When your creative forces are not flowing because you feel inhibited by external obstacles, Indian Paintbrush flower essence can help. Creative block is often experienced as a loss of vitality or as a result of personality conflict in the workplace that restricts creative contribution. However, what happens outside reflects what is inside, and what seems to be an external restriction is often the manifestation of an internal block or inhibition.

In the negative state, Indian Paintbrush people have the inspiration but lack the dynamic, grounding energies of the lower chakras that make it possible to marshal the resources needed for physical expression of creativity. In contrast, those in need of Iris flower essence are bogged down and encumbered by Earth energy and lack the uplifting and directing effect that inspiration brings. It's as if, in the negative state, an Indian Paintbrush person knows what they want to buy but haven't got the money to spend, while an Iris person has plenty to spend but doesn't know what they want to buy!

Benefits of taking Indian Paintbrush

Indian Paintbrush flower essence enables you to access, ground and harness the 'horsepower' needed to reach your productive potential creatively. Indian Paintbrush helps you resonate better and connect with 'the physical world and the natural resources' (Kaminski and Katz 1996) needed for happy and creative functioning.

Possible physical imbalances

Those in the negative Indian Paintbrush state often have a sense of physical exhaustion. After taking the flower essence, energy and vitality begin to flow again along with the creative 'juices.'

Common uses

To clear creative block; to overcome external hurdles to creativity; to help conjure the energy and resources for creative expression; to enhance creative and artistic flair; to dynamically Do!

Complementary &/or similar flower essences

Aloe Vera, Blackberry, Californian Poppy, Cayenne, Coffee, Hibiscus, Iris, Larch, Madia, Nasturtium, Nicotiana, Paw Paw, Pomegranate, Red Grevillea, Red Lily, Shasta Daisy, She Oak, Snapdragon, Trumpet Vine, Violet, Watermelon

Supporting the changes

- Think about doing courses that help you to assert yourself effectively, along with those that facilitate the creative process.
- Political correctness, diplomacy and tact have nothing to do with the creative force itself but everything to do with how it is accepted in the world via proper presentation. Perhaps you need to get a manager, agent, publisher or adviser.
- Nurture your body, acknowledging that it is the physical instrument of your creative expression.

Indian Pink

Silene californica   (Red / FES)

Positive state

'Managing and coordinating diverse forms of activity' (FES)
Calm focus in the midst of heightened activity

Negative state

Psychically 'frayed at the edges'
'Inability to stay centred during intense activity' (FES)

From above, the Indian Pink flower looks like a rag *frayed at the edges* by what has happened to it. However, the whole plant stands proudly and singularly, growing *upright* from the ground to make a *strong statement of independence*.

When we feel that outside influences have encroached on our *personal space* to the point where we are *torn in many directions*, losing our orientation and focus, we should consider Indian Pink flower essence.

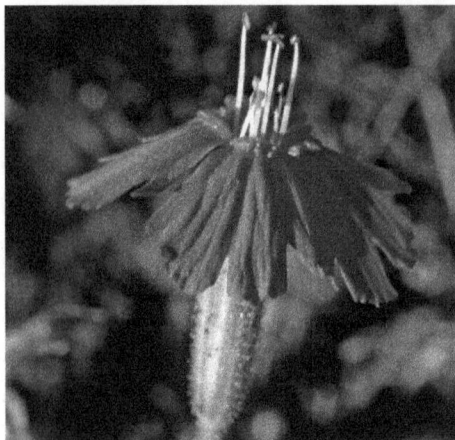

The flower's rich, blood-red colour is significant. It signals the flower essence's ability to address acute, *inflammatory, red-raw and 'angry'* reactions in the body and mind to stressors in the immediate environment. Its red colour also signifies its affinity to the *base chakra* and our primal *survival* instinct – the *'fight or flight'* response to heightened activity around us in our lives.

The Indian Pink state of mind

Generally, Indian Pink people live life to the full or have been thrust into the centre of activity, to the point where they eventually lose their internal calm and stillness and move into the negative state. 'Psychic forces ... are easily torn or shattered' (Kaminski and Katz 1996) – frayed at the edges – by too much external activity. The resulting feeling of being under threat causes tension, irritability and over-emotional responses which further deplete energy reserves.

Benefits of taking Indian Pink

With the help of Indian Pink flower essence we can regain composure and remain centred and focused amid intense activity and turmoil. It helps us to remain grounded and unscathed while negotiating daily stresses and pressures. Indian Pink can help to transform raw, instinctual reactions into passionate endeavour and constructive activity that is considerate of and sensitive to our surroundings. It can help soothe and calm a highly inflamed reaction to circumstances.

Possible physical imbalances

Heightened or inflamed mental/emotional responses to the environment often manifest on the physical level in the form of acute inflammatory reactions. (In my experience, Scarlet Monkeyflower flower essence is often indicated along with Indian Pink.) For example, skin conditions can tell us much about our internalised reaction to the external environment. After all, skin is the physical boundary and point of exchange between what is inside and what is immediately outside.

Adrenal fatigue may also develop as a consequence of being stressed over a period of time.

Common uses

For times of heavy involvement in many activities; to help with multi-tasking; when feeling torn between all the activities happening around you; to help ground and identify your 'still' centre; to remain calm amidst intense activity; to remain in the calm 'eye of the storm'; to maintain concentration and focus when pulled in all directions

Complementary &/or similar flower essences

Aloe Vera, Calendula, Californian Poppy, Canyon Dudleya, Chamomile, Chaparral, Cherry Plum, Corn, Dill, Echinacea, Elm, Fringed Violet, Garlic, Golden Yarrow, Impatiens, Lavender, Madia, Paw Paw, Pink Yarrow, Rabbitbrush, Red Clover, St John's Wort, Scarlet Monkeyflower, Shasta Daisy, Walnut, all the Yarrows, YES formula

Supporting the changes

- All flower essences that address issues relating to the base chakra can benefit from supportive measures that enable the user to properly ground and centre themselves. All activities that further this end, from physical exercise and gardening to relaxation techniques and meditation should be encouraged.
- Explore how you manage or express anger in life. Counselling in this area may be very helpful.
- 'If you can't handle the heat, get out of the kitchen!' Commit to change or at least take a well-earned break and create some space for yourself.

Iris

Iris douglasiana   (White / FES)

Positive state

Fulfilling creative lifestyle
Uplifted; 'inspired artistry' (FES)

Negative state

Bogged down – 'Wallowing in the mire'
Stuck and uninspired

In the wild, Iris plants prefer marshlands and other *wet, swampy*, open places. This beautiful flowering plant *emerges* from the swamp and signals the usefulness of Iris flower essence to *inspire* us to *rise up and out* of the doldrums when we feel *bogged down* by life and unsure about how we can bring about change. Iris is a much-loved flower with many cultural associations – in Greek mythology Iris is the goddess of the rainbow, a messenger who accompanied the *souls* of the dead, and the flower was placed on graves to symbolise *hope and redemption*.

The beautiful spectrum of Iris's *blue to violet* flowers vividly reminds us of its strong connection with the spirit – these colours represent the *upper chakras*, dynamic receptors of *inspiration* from our *higher Self* in harmony with the soul.

The Iris state of mind

Iris flower essence helps us to receive inspiration at crucial moments. It can help steer us towards an intuitively-perceived 'sign,' just as in the biblical story, the rainbow was a sign to Noah that the great flood was about to end. These subtle directives can help us live in a more creative and self-fulfilling way.

If your life seems mundane and dreary and you lack energy, motivation and direction; if you feel mentally flat and weighed down by the ordinariness of the world; if you are suffering from lingering 'winter blues,' mid-life uncertainty or just desperate for inspiration, consider taking Iris flower essence.

A good example might be the common scenario where a woman, having devoted her younger years to her family, passes through menopause. Although she has reached a period when there is more time for herself, she is depressed about her predicament, unable to identify things she might enjoy and finds former pleasures unappealing. If offered suggestions she may reply, 'Oh, I've tried that but didn't like it much,' or 'I know I wouldn't like that.' (Sometimes as the natural therapist in consultation with such a person I have felt the need for inspiration myself!) Iris flower essence can bring a much brighter perspective to this situation, along with inspiration to make a few innovative adjustments to life.

Benefits of taking Iris

Iris flower essence inspires a creative approach to life. (Indian Paintbrush relates more to periods of 'creative block' at work or in a chosen art form.) Kaminski and Katz (1996) state that 'Iris helps the inner life of the human soul harmonise with Soul of Nature, and in this way to become alive, vibrant, and truly "iridescent."' Iris can open us to a more inspired, creative level of awareness so that we develop a more innovative and fulfilling approach to our lives.

Possible physical imbalances

As a therapist, I have found that Iris flower essence can be a very helpful remedy for some depressions associated with menopause and/or midlife.

Common uses

When everything seems ordinary and mundane; for feeling uninspired by life; for times of feeling bogged down in a daily rut; for visionary inspiration in YOUR life; to add colour to your life; to be inspired and uplifted; to help develop a fulfilling and creative lifestyle

Complementary &/or similar flower essences

Aloe Vera, Angelsword, Blackberry, Borage, Cerato, Chrysanthemum, Coffee,

Filaree, Forget-Me-Not, Harvest Brodiaea, Hound's Tongue, Indian Paintbrush, Morning Glory, Nasturtium, Pansy, Peppermint, Pomegranate, Silver Princess, Tansy

Supporting the changes

- Explore different philosophical approaches to life, especially those of people you admire and respect. Read about how they negotiated periods such as menopause, midlife or a 'sea change.'
- Explore the 'Creative living' or 'Lifestyle' section of a bookstore, newsagency or library to get some ideas. What hobby might interest you?
- Get moving with some moderate but regular exercise – preferably every day.
- Take renewed interest in your diet, your lifestyle and YOURSELF!

Kangaroo Paw

Anigozanthos manglesii   (Green-red / Aus)

Positive state

'Cool' and comfortable
Socially adaptable and 'reads the room'

Negative state

Uncomfortable, awkward and socially 'green'
Socially insensitive (Ian White)

Kangaroo Paw is a relatively short-lived plant. It thrives after bushfires or land clearing. Over time, other long-lived plants crowd out Kangaroo Paw, which is not seen again until the next fire or clearing (White 2008). The plant displays the ability to *quickly adapt* and *fill a niche* in its environment. This reflects the positive aspects of the Kangaroo Paw personality which *blends* with and *understands the environment* (and the people in it) and is then able to *relax*, enjoy and benefit from it.

The flower is *red and green* (= brown) and these colours imply a close relationship with the *sacral chakra*, which governs how we relate on an *intimate* level with others – how *comfortable* and confident we are in developing warm *rapport and empathy* with those around us.

The Kangaroo Paw personality

Kangaroo Paw flower essence is useful for people who are socially 'green' (White 2008) and naïve and who find it difficult to mix and behave appropriately in social situations. Just as the Kangaroo Paw plant can comfortably move in and establish itself soon after the heat of a fire, so the flower essence can teach people who feel 'uncool' to become 'cool'!

Kangaroo Paw should be considered during phases of life when we feel particularly self-conscious and uncomfortable socially. Adolescents often feel this way, when peer group pressure to be 'cool' is at its most intense. It is also useful at times when we have simply lost touch with social etiquette and wish to develop more social sensitivity. This may be a result of being 'out of circulation' for a while. For instance, a mother who leaves the workforce to have a child may feel socially awkward when she returns to work or a divorcee may feel unsure about how to behave in new or revisited social circles. Or perhaps you have never felt enough at ease to fully enjoy other people's company. Interaction and conversation may feel forced and contrived so that you can't relax in company.

Benefits of taking Kangaroo Paw

In all social situations, Kangaroo Paw can help you to relax so that you can behave in a way that is appropriate to the situation, neither too formal nor too informal, striking a happy medium and achieving a comfortable rapport. The essence can help you to recognise the needs of others and relish the opportunity to engage in mutually satisfying communication.

Possible physical imbalances

Feeling socially inept may be accompanied by an experience of physical clumsiness which can intensify the feeling of being 'uncool.' A number of clients who have responded well to Kangaroo Paw flower essence have also reported that they have become less accident-prone, and this has been very good for their physical (and emotional) health!!

Common uses

For more confidence socially; for 'clumsy' teenagers (don't tell them that though!!); when coming back into social or professional circulation after being away for a while; for the feeling of being 'green' in a new job or social situation; for more 'savoir-faire' and 'je ne sais quoi' in social situations; to help you become more 'cool' and self-assured

Complementary &/or similar flower essences

Angelica, Buttercup, Calendula, Dogwood, Echinacea, Fairy Lantern, Flannel Flower, Garlic, Larch, Impatiens, Mallow, Mimulus, Oregon Grape, Star Tulip, Violet, Water Violet

Supporting the changes

- Meditation and relaxation techniques can help to raise your awareness and sensitivity, making you generally more receptive and relaxed.
- Involve yourself socially but choose the company you find most comfortable.

- Develop more centred, artful and coordinated movement through the practice of tai chi, yoga, pilates, dance and other exercises. In this way you will also improve physical flexibility.
- If you stumble or fall, get up and try again.

Larch

Larix decidua   (Red female & yellow male / Bach)

Positive state

Confidence and determination
Tries for 'personal best'

Negative state

Lacking confidence, conceding defeat
Won't try for fear of failure

Larch's pinkish-grey branches often droop 'in a languid manner and seem reluctant to straighten up with the determination needed for *strong growth*' (Barnard 1988).

Those in need of Larch flower essence *lack the confidence* to take the next step and try new things. Even the slender top of the trunk seems to *lack definite direction*, curving gracefully.

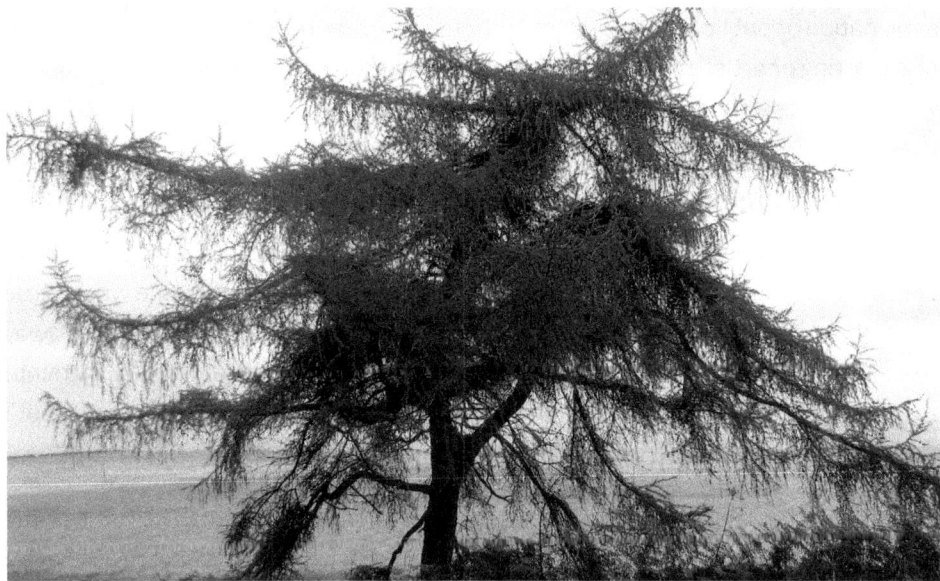

Larch is the only European conifer to shed its leaves in autumn. It is indigenous to hill and mountain areas in central Europe which have brief summer growing periods in which Larch *grows rapidly and strongly, grabbing its opportunity* before the long harsh winter sets in. Winter temperatures are so low the ground freezes and no water can be taken up into the trees, hence Larch must shed its leaves to survive (Barnard 1988). Its delicacy and apparently weak posture (seeming almost unable to hold itself up) hides its *resilient character* and ability to withstand extremes. Similarly, Larch people in the positive state are far more capable than they may feel or appear. Larch was originally introduced into England for its enormous value in providing timber for housing and shipbuilding as its wood is stronger and more durable than that of most other conifers.

Both male and female flowers are used in the flower essence preparation.

The Larch state of mind

At the heart of the negative Larch state is the fear of failure and if this fear is strong enough, failure usually occurs or is avoided only because no attempt was ever made. To quote Shakespeare: 'Our doubts are traitors, and make us lose the good we oft might win, by fearing to attempt.' The negative Larch state can lead to a stagnant existence in which one is repeatedly immobilised by fear. Creative capacities contract and personal growth is suspended (just as the larch tree suspends growth over the long harsh winter).

What appears as downright stubbornness may in fact be a refusal rooted in fear of failure. Young children sometimes illustrate this pattern well – refusing, for example, to read in class because of an overwhelming fear of failure and humiliation. This fear of failure and the judgement of others can be at the root of severe anxiety in anticipation of public speaking, examinations and other performances such as those of a sporting or artistic nature. Commencing a new job, changing direction in life and work, even prescribing your first flower essence are all situations that can bring up deep fears around adequacy and ability to perform a task.

Benefits of taking Larch

Larch can help us to access our unique creative talents, instilling strong self-belief. It can help us view setbacks and mistakes as valuable steps on the way to true mastery and direction in our lives. Larch flower essence moves the emphasis away from our fears about the expectations and judgements of others, towards an attempt to make our best contribution. In other words, Larch helps us to 'give it our best shot'!

Possible physical imbalances

Larch has an affinity for the sacral chakra located in the pelvic basin – the source of our strongest creative energies. When out of balance, this chakra can have a restrictive/inhibiting influence on the natural upward flow of creative energy towards the throat chakra and there may be congestive problems in the reproductive organs. This dynamic 'congestion' may lead to physical problems associated with the menstrual cycle, for example.

Common uses

For fear of failure; for fear of public speaking and for speech problems such as nervous stuttering; for more self-confidence; to encourage more creative self-expression and/or self-assertion; to encourage 'having a go' for 'personal best'; to self-appreciate and value one's contribution

Complementary &/or similar flower essences

Blackberry, Buttercup, Cerato, Elm, Indian Paintbrush, Iris, Kangaroo Paw, Mimulus, Pomegranate, Snapdragon, Sunflower, Trumpet Vine

Supporting the changes

- Personal development courses are invaluable, especially those that address assertiveness and develop communication skills.
- Activities that liberate creative energies are very valuable.
- Spend more time with people who appreciate your attributes and point of view.
- Above all, have a go!

Larkspur
Delphinium nuttallianum   (Blue-violet / FES)

Positive state
Altruistic, 'charismatic leadership' (FES)
Enthusiastic, generous and 'joyful service' (FES)

Negative state
Inflated sense of self-importance
Overburdened by sense of duty and obligation

After Achilles was slain at Troy, his mother offered her son's armour as a gift to the most deserving hero among the Greeks. The mighty Ajax, next bravest warrior to Achilles put his hand up to accept the honour but was rejected; the judges awarded it to the prudent Ulysses. As a consequence, Ajax committed suicide – a monumental 'dummy spit' that said 'Stuff you, I'll take my my talents elsewhere and see how you get along without me!' Larkspur flower essence is for those with a habit of self-aggrandisement who may be unwilling to serve if they feel they are not properly appreciated.

The ancient Greeks thought that the flower's spurred upper petals gave it the appearance of a dolphin's head and the plant's botanical name is *Delphinium*, meaning 'dolphin plant.' In traditional herbalism it has been used to kill parasites such as lice and mites. Sometimes people in need of Larkspur flower essence feel burdened by their duties and by parasitic 'hangers-on' who become dependent on them, having been drawn to their charismatic leadership and obvious capabilities.

The Larkspur state of mind

This flower essence is for people who feel overly dutiful and have a knee-jerk reaction of automatic responsiveness to demands made on them. They are often excellent leaders because they are able to respond quickly when action is needed. However, they may come to resent the fact that they always seem to be the ones who do the work, or they may react by becoming 'inflated with self-importance' (Kaminski and Katz 1996).

Unfortunately, the problem often lies in their over-responsiveness and inability to pause and ask, 'Is this going to benefit all of us? Should someone else take responsibility this time?' Too often the Larkspur person overdoes their duty – visiting elderly relatives, ringing friends they haven't spoken to for a while, cleaning up the kitchen after meals – before anyone else has had a chance to share the load.

Benefits of taking Larkspur

Larkspur flower essence helps you break patterns of over-dutiful behaviour so that you are able to act with a greater feeling of generosity, altruism and 'an inner joyfulness which energises others'(Kaminski and Katz 1996). Whether in the family, at work or in a community group, everyone learns to accept responsibility, inspired and motivated by your natural leadership qualities and charisma.

Possible physical imbalances

Larkspur people are often so busy fulfilling duties towards everyone else that they forget their duty to themselves. As a consequence their physical health suffers because their lifestyle does not take their own health needs into account. Larkspur flower essence will help to make them more aware of these needs and better able to find space in their busy lives to attend to them.

Common uses

For an over-dutiful attitude; for inflated self-importance ('a legend in your own mind'); for resentment of responsibility; to enable leadership roles to be taken on generously; to foster contagious enthusiasm; to bring joy into service

Complementary &/or similar flower essences

Borage, Centaury, Chicory, Elm, Fairy Lantern, Forget-Me-Not, Lady's Slipper, Lotus, Oak, Quaking Grass, Shooting Star, Sweet Pea, Trillium, Wild Rose

Supporting the changes

- Before you respond in a knee-jerk manner, 'reprogram' yourself to ask, 'Will my action benefit all of us? Would it be better to delegate? Would it be more useful to leave it alone?'

- Don't let the word 'should' rule your life.
- After taking the previous points into consideration, enJOY the opportunity to help and serve.

Lavender

Lavandula angustifolia   (Violet / FES)

Positive state

Calm disposition
Relaxed, mindful awareness

Negative state

Emotionally hyped
Nervous and 'strung out'

Lavender's *violet* colour relates to its affinity with the *crown chakra*, our direct connection with our *higher Self*. Lavender flower essence can enable the spiritual Self to integrate into and exert more influence over the *personality*. In this way we can temper *deep-seated or karmic patterns* that prevent personal and spiritual development, especially those that affect our *close relationships* with others such as our partners and children. For this reason, in my practice I have recommended Lavender flower essence for couples undergoing counselling, and for a parent who is having particular difficulty in their relationship with one of their children.

All the herbal healing qualities the Lavender plant is known for are also expressed in the flower essence: it *soothes nerves* frayed by *overstimulation* and *calms* emotional reactions. Commonly used today in perfume and soap and used by the ancient Romans to scent their bath water, the plant takes its name from the Latin *lavare*, meaning 'to wash,' referring to its literal and metaphorical ability to *wash away* the *clinging tensions* of the day. The herb grows all year round and flowers over the warm months.

The Lavender state of mind

Those in need of Lavender flower essence are usually sensitive and mentally active people who tend to become anxious and 'wound up' (Kaminski and Katz 1996). When work and everyday life puts pressure on your nervous system and you wish to develop a more meditative, less draining lifestyle, consider using Lavender flower essence. When the children are driving to you to distraction, take Lavender flower essence to help you step back a little and gain perspective and calm. Remember that Lavender helps establish emotional balance, especially between individuals who seem to be locked together in negative behaviour patterns.

Benefits of taking Lavender

Lavender flower essence can be taken as an adjunct to therapies for all sorts of nervous complaints, especially tension headaches and inability to sleep due to overstimulation during the day. The age-old folk remedy of putting a few Lavender flowers under the pillow to help let go of the day and have more restful sleep is still practised by many people, as is the use of Lavender oil vaporisers.

Letting go of the day and trusting that all will be well tomorrow involves trusting that you will receive benevolent guidance from your higher Self along the journey. I have seen in my practice how the flower essence can help you acknowledge and accept the likely deep (karmic) connection with your partner, your children (especially the one who is just like you!) and your friends and acquaintances. Personality conflicts and tensions then appear less significant amid the bigger picture.

Possible physical imbalances

As mentioned above, Lavender flower essence helps to ease the same nervous ailments as the essential oil. However, it does this by addressing more of the underlying issues, for example those that cause nervous tension or headache, rather than treating the acute problem as the oil does so well.

Common uses

To calm 'frayed nerves'; to help you learn to unwind after work; to help you gain better perspective during highly emotional times in relationships; for emotional and spiritual hypersensitivity; for 'empaths' (in combination with YES formula); to help LET GO of petty conflicts in your day

Complementary &/or similar flower essences

Aloe Vera, Angelica, Californian Poppy, Canyon Dudleya, Chamomile, Crowea, Dandelion, Dill, Echinacea, Elm, Filaree, Forget-Me-Not, Garlic, Golden Yarrow, Indian Pink, Passionflower, Pink Yarrow, Red Clover, St John's Wort, Vervain, Wedding Bush, White Chestnut, Yarrow, YES formula

Supporting the changes

- Relaxation and meditation techniques such as yoga and tai chi are ways of de-stressing and 'grounding' yourself, leaving you calm and emotionally balanced.
- Try meditation. It will not only help you relax and unwind but will allow you to stand back and gain a broader perspective on your life and those close to you. You may just see things in a new light.
- Eat foods that are rich in the Vitamin B group, drink calming, nervine herbal teas and avoid mood-altering substances such as sugar, coffee and alcohol. Get

THE **ESSENTIAL** FLOWER ESSENCE BOOK

sufficient sleep, which means having some sleep before midnight, and stick to a regular sleep pattern.

- Cool down!

Lemon

Citrus limon (White / FES-RL)

Positive state

Mentally tuned and toned
Mental clarity balanced with imaginative and artistic capacities (FES)

Negative state

Mentally 'turns to jelly' under pressure
Mentally fatigued – thoughts do not 'take shape'

Lemon's *yellow* colour symbolises the strong *invigorating* effect the flower essence has on the *mental sphere*. It tones your mind so that it can guide rather than suppress or control your emotions, helping to balance the *solar plexus chakra*.

We have all experienced the *astringency* of the sour fruit and this points to its capacity as a flower essence to *tone the mind* especially in times of intense emotion. If our *thinking is clear and defined*, our actions in the material world will be more conscious – *form follows thought*. Plutarch, a high priest in the temple of the Greek god Apollo, expressed it this way: 'An idea is a Being incorporated, which has no subsistence of itself, but gives figure and form unto shapeless matter and becomes the cause of the *manifestation.*' Lemon flower essence helps *clarify and crystallise thoughts* arising from their source in abstract impressions and collective primordial senses.

The Lemon personality

Those who can benefit from taking Lemon flower essence are otherwise intelligent and capable people who, for some reason, turn to jelly when they have to deal with a particular mental activity such as, for example, figures or statistics. They manage very well in many areas of life or with most aspects of a subject or discipline, yet lose their logic and rationality and become overemotional when dealing with some aspect of it. Although intelligent, they find it difficult to make a decision when emotions are high. Lemon flower essence can help such people come to grips mentally with this situation. The left-brain qualities used for mathematical, rational and logical thinking are enhanced and come into balance with right-brain qualities of abstract, intuitive and creative thinking and sensing.

Benefits of taking Lemon

Lemon flower essence is very much about balance. It helps balance the masculine and feminine, yin and yang, mental and emotional subtle bodies, and right and left-brain aspects of mental functioning. It helps us develop our 'emotional intelligence' so that we can think both logically and laterally, bringing mental clarity along with a strong imaginative and artistic capacity. Our ability to maintain an integrated mental overview is enhanced.

Possible physical imbalances

Lemon flower essence is useful as part of any overall refreshing/rejuvenating 'kickstart' health program. When appropriately selected it will de-stress and 'refresh' the energy meridians known in Traditional Chinese Medicine. A better energy flow makes muscular relaxation easier and enables better flow in the lymphatic and blood systems.

Common uses

As part of a 'spring clean,' detox program; to improve mental clarity; to mentally 'tone up'; as part of a study mix during examination periods; to mentally refresh and rejuvenate

Complementary &/or similar flower essences

Aloe Vera, Blackberry, Cayenne, Clematis, Cosmos, Hornbeam, Iris, Macrocarpa, Madia, Morning Glory, Nasturtium, Paw Paw, Peppermint, Rabbitbrush, Rosemary, Shasta Daisy, Silver Princess

Supporting the changes

- Participate in exercise and sports that rely heavily on good physical coordination such as tennis, swimming or soccer.
- The practice of meditation (or yoga and tai chi) has a balancing effect on the left and right sides of the brain and their associated capacities.
- All foods rich in potassium phosphate are good for mind power, for example olives, lentils, tomatoes, apples, lemons, dates, walnuts, onions, garlic and ginger.
- Take up juggling!

Lotus

Nelumbo nucifera   (Pink / FES)

Positive state

'Walking the talk', feet on the ground
Open minded and inclusive

Negative state

'Talking the walk', head in the clouds
'Spiritual pride'(FES) – inflated and insular sense of self

The Sacred Lotus has been revered by generations of poets, priests and philosophers throughout the Hindu and Buddhist worlds as a highly evolved plant associated with religious practices, culture and history. It also serves in a very practical way as a valuable source of food and medicine.

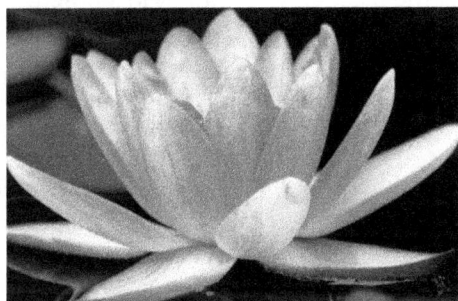

One of the flower's common names, the 'thousand-petal lotus', symbolises the 1000 *nadis* (subtle energy channels) of the *crown chakra*. The *opening of the lotus flower* is used as a metaphor for the moment of enlightenment, which occurs as a result of *balanced integration and awakening* of all the energy centres, culminating in the opening of the crown chakra.

Unfortunately, the quest for enlightenment often involves periods when we are unable to *integrate head and heart* and haven't yet learned to really *'walk the talk.'* Because of its strong resonance with the crown chakra, Lotus flower essence can help at these times, bringing it into *alignment* with all the other chakras below it and in this way *grounding* the spiritual path in Earthly reality.

Lotus acts as a bridge between the air and water elements, as indicated by the signature of the flower which sits on top of the water and opens to the air. Thus it links *sky and Earth*, intellect and emotion, thinking and feeling. Lotus flower essence enhances the action of other flower essences and/or homeopathic and herbal blends – this is referred to as a *synergistic action*. Another synergistic action of Lotus occurs when it is given with other flower essences that have brought about an *awareness crisis* in a person when, for example, they experience a temporary upsurge of basic, lower chakra-related emotions as part of the grounding and healing process. Lotus flower essence aids and *facilitates* a more comfortable and easy resolution in these circumstances.

The Lotus personality

Lotus flower essence helps balance the unfolding of subtle energies, especially when the higher chakras tend to dominate at the expense of the lower ones. This unbalanced state may manifest as a type of arrogance which causes us to believe that we are more spiritually evolved and therefore more 'spiritually correct or superior' (Kaminski and Katz 1996) than others – in this situation the ego has inflated faster than consciousness! Such a belief is an indication that we are not so much evolved as deeply isolated. To be effective, spiritual insights need to be grounded in the practicalities of everyday life. Those who benefit from taking Lotus flower essence can sometimes 'think right' but not quite feel right, often because of difficulty in acknowledging that they might be capable of 'crude and uncivilised' emotions such as anger. (Or, as one of my clients, a very gentle and refined elderly lady who benefited from taking Lotus flower essence, expressed it so eloquently, 'Oh you mean S.O.L.' When I asked what 'S.O.L.' meant, she replied very softly and deliberately, 'Shit on the liver.') Lotus flower essence helps us express the most basic emotions in a practical and creative way. It can help us strike the right balance between the influence of the more 'refined' upper chakras and the 'cruder' lower ones.

Benefits of taking Lotus

Lotus flower essence is often used to enhance the action of other flower essences in balancing the subtle energies. It can help us gain insight and supports personal development and meditative practices. Lotus flower essence aids the integration of spirituality in a balanced and practical way, incorporating the passion and potency of the lower chakras.

Possible physical imbalances

Subtle (not necessarily pathological) liver issues can occur in clients who may benefit from taking Lotus flower essence. When the liver, sometimes referred to as our 'emotional editor,' has come under stress through repression of genuine emotional reactions to experiences, people often have a bit of 'mud on the liver' or S.O.L from unexpressed frustration and anger caught up in the system.

Common uses

For 'spiritual correctness' or superiority; as part of your regime for removing 'S.O.L.'; to enhance the action of other flower essences; for support to 'free up' the action of other therapeutic, potentially cathartic, flower essences; to enhance meditative practices; to support personal growth in a practical way; to help you to 'walk the talk'

Complementary &/or similar flower essences

Blackberry, Californian Poppy, Impatiens, Lady's Slipper, Larkspur, Manzanita, Nasturtium, Shooting Star, Tall Yellow Top, Water Violet

Supporting the changes

- Read about the lives of hands-on/practical, spiritual persons such as Jesus, Florence Nightingale, St Francis of Assisi, Mother Teresa.
- Engage in grounding activities such as gardening, housework, pottery, playing with the kids and having fun.
- Consider the saying: 'Before enlightenment, chop wood and carry water; after enlightenment, chop wood and carry water.'
- Walk the talk!

Macrocarpa
Eucalyptus macrocarpa   (Red / Aus)

Positive state

Dynamic resilience and positivity
Revitalised reserves of energy

Negative state

Prolonged enervating stress
Physical and mental exhaustion

Macrocarpa has the broadest fruit and flower of all the eucalypts; the *deep red flowers* which concentrate the plant's most potent forces can measure over seven centimetres across. They *fling off* their seed caps when they bloom (White 2008) and this *strength* suggests the properties of the flower essence: *energy, vitality and passion.* The deep red colour of the flower denotes its influence on the *base chakra* and reflects Macrocarpa's potential for *stimulating and arousing energy.* Its strong affinity to the base chakra also results in a focused influence at the level of the adrenal glands which, in Traditional Chinese Medicine, govern the flow of *regenerative chi* or energy.

The Macrocarpa state of mind

Whether we are at the end of our mental and physical endurance or are just in need of a pick-me-up, Macrocarpa helps us regain strength and energy to carry on with renewed vigour. It may also help us to contemplate our lifestyle and motivate us to make changes that are more conducive to good health and wellbeing.

Benefits of taking Macrocarpa

Macrocarpa enhances resistance to stress by improving our natural resilience and increasing our energy and vitality on all levels. It can help restore our passion for life!

Possible physical imbalances

When appropriately matched to the individual, Macrocarpa flower essence's vital energy-conserving and concentrating effect can enhance natural immunity. It helps break the cycle of low resistance to infection that often develops when vital energies are scattered indiscriminately. Adrenal fatigue and resultant general physical fatigue may also be part of the picture for those who can benefit from taking Macrocarpa flower essence.

Common uses

For exhaustion on all levels; as a 'pick-me-up' during stressful times; to help you bounce back after prolonged stress; to restore your energy levels; to refresh, re-vitalise and re-enthuse

Complementary &/or similar flower essences

Aloe Vera, Cayenne, Garlic, Hornbeam, Honeysuckle; Hound's Tongue; Indian Paintbrush, Indian Pink, Iris; Lady's Slipper, Madia, Morning Glory, Nasturtium, Olive, Peppermint, Self-Heal, Tansy, YES formula

Supporting the changes

- Consider what got you into this state of energy depletion and work to change offending life choices, patterns and habits.
- Improve your diet – include foods rich in the B vitamins and consider consulting a health practitioner for expert advice.
- Break up your frantic lifestyle with periods of constructive or reconstructive quiet time. Engage in calming activities that encourage healthy reflection and debriefing on life issues. Consider relaxation techniques such as yoga, tai chi, meditation etc.
- Work smart and take time out for leisure activities you enjoy.

Madia

Madia elegans   (Yellow with red spots / FES)

Positive state

Attention and mental precision
'Disciplined focus and concentration' (FES)

Negative state

Easily distracted (FES)
Energies scattered; diffused concentration

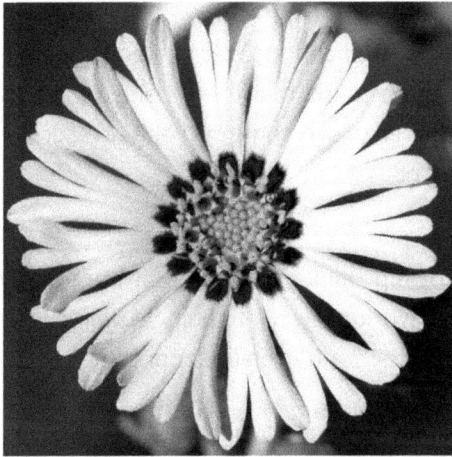

Tiny, *intricate red dots* on the yellow bloom symbolise the creative *attention to detail* which Madia flower essence helps to foster. The flowers close each day in the afternoon heat of the sun, just as we might take an afternoon siesta to rest and recuperate before starting work again with more *efficiency and accuracy*. The plant has a distinctive *stickiness* to it and Madia flower essence helps us *stick at* jobs – even those we've put off for a long time.

The Madia personality

Madia flower essence improves the *integrity of the mental body* so that it is less easily undermined and distracted by emotional needs and desires when there is a need for *disciplined* application. This allows more lasting *mental focus/concentration* and allows us to follow projects through to *completion*. When the mental body is strong, the desire for instant gratification is less likely to hamper our attempts to achieve important long-term goals.

Madia flower essence is helpful when we need to boost our concentration and focus in the short term, for example during study and examination periods, but also in the longer term when we need to remain clear about priorities. If we become distracted too easily, our energies are consumed by less fulfilling activities or those that offer immediate gratification. We remain busy and self-motivated but not satisfied with what we bring to fruition. We may develop a habit of 'splitting off' or becoming 'spacey' (Kaminski and Katz 1996) so that the mind wanders away from the job at hand. We find it difficult to stay in the moment and remain 'in the zone.'

If this is part of your pattern, consider Madia flower essence to help you keep on track as you work towards important goals in any sphere of life, whether in the short or long term.

Benefits of taking Madia

Madia flower essence helps you to be discerning and gives the clarity of mind needed to make decisions regarding when to delegate and how to prioritise for better energy efficiency. Often my clients have told me that while taking Madia they have got around to completing jobs they had put off for a long time such as painting a room or finishing an assignment and they are happier for it. Madia helps you focus and direct energy in a more disciplined and productive manner.

Possible physical imbalances

Madia will also help you to remain committed and focused on healthy eating and lifestyle habits. A number of my clients have found that it has helped them to maintain the mental energy and willpower required to overcome the habit of resorting to comfort foods to get them through stressful phases.

Common uses

To improve concentration on detail; to help maintain focus; as part of a study mix around exam times; to help you complete work/projects; to help discipline your mind against distraction; to help you remain 'in the zone' even under pressure

Complementary &/or similar flower essences

Cayenne, Clematis, Crowea, Dandelion, Dill, Filaree, Forge-Me-Not, Indian Pink, Jacaranda, Lemon, Paw Paw, Peppermint, Rabbitbrush, Red Lily, Shasta Daisy, Tansy, White Chestnut

Supporting the changes

- Meditation and other disciplines such as yoga or tai chi can help you to balance, centre and ground yourself.
- A time management course may prove helpful.
- Spend some time brainstorming what you want to complete or achieve over the next week, month or year.
- COMMIT to your goals!

Mallow

Sidalcea glaucescens   (Pink / FES)

Positive state

Trusting, personable and warm (FES)
Self-assured but open hearted

Negative state

Can come across as clinical and self-contained
Guards against insecurity by 'creating barriers' (FES)

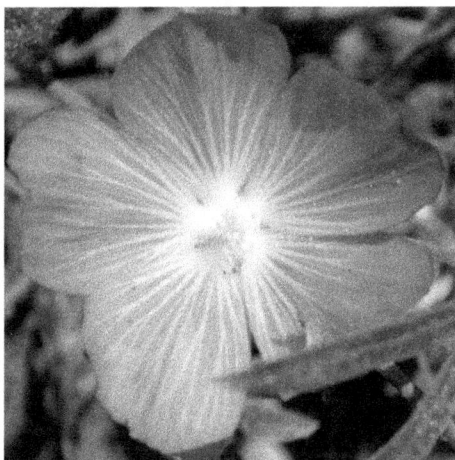

Mallow is from the *Malvaceae* family, which is famous for its soft leaves and healing properties. The name *Malva* comes from the Greek word *malakos*, meaning *soft and soothing* and the juice of the plants in this family is generally mucilagenous. The flowers are a *delicate pink* with veined petals giving them a *membranous* look. Membranes are important in keeping cells and organs in the human body in a *harmonious relationship – providing a soft but secure buffer that also allows beneficial exchange of nutrients etc.* It is no wonder the flower essence helps create harmony in relationships by allaying fears and helping people to be *open and transparent, warm, sharing and personable* with others.

In my practice, I have also found Mallow flower essence to be helpful for a number of clients who, as they have got older, have begun to lose *confidence* in their mental capacities, especially when they *'put up a front'* in order to disguise this loss of confidence.

The Mallow personality

Mallow flower essence helps soften the persona of those who give the initial impression of being very clinical and lacking in warmth. Mallow people often feel socially insecure or isolated (Kaminski and Katz 1996) and present in a very formal, self-protective manner, even when you have already met them on many occasions. This fear and mistrust may stem from incidents early in life but its effect in the present is to cause distance in existing relationships and often prevent new friendships from developing.

Benefits of taking Mallow

Mallow flower essence can help heal past hurts that, over time, have deeply undermined our confidence and left us defensive because we fear that others may take advantage of us if we drop our guard. It allows us to feel more secure about displaying our warm, friendly and endearing qualities. In this way it can help us to break down barriers we have created between ourselves and others.

Mallow enables us to develop more warmth in our friendships and personal relationships. As Kaminski and Katz (1996) put it, 'Mallow helps the soul learn to trust the feelings buried in the heart, encouraging the individual towards greater social involvement.'

Possible physical imbalances

Mallow flower essence has an important role to play in the ageing process. It can allow us to remain confident in mind and body as we relate more and more from the heart rather than the brain and/or the persona as we get older.

Common uses

For those who appear clinical and officious; to better balance right and left brain faculties; to operate from the heart as well as the head; to display the warmth within; to help you make friends!

Complementary &/or similar flower essences

Buttercup, Calendula, Dogwood, Flannel Flower, Hibiscus, Kangaroo Paw, Lotus, Mimulus, Nasturtium, Nicotiana, Pink Monkeyflower, Sage, Sticky Monkeyflower, Violet, Water Violet, Wild Rose, Zinnia

Supporting the changes

- Find a counsellor or therapist you are comfortable with to discuss earlier life experiences. Understand how these experiences have influenced your behaviour in the present.
- Read about emotional IQ. Investigate left and right brain qualities – exercise your right brain attributes.
- Join a team in which having fun is the main objective.
- Don't take yourself so seriously. 'Muck up' occasionally. Have some fun!

Manzanita

Arctostaphylos viscida   (Pink / FES)

Positive state

'Integration of spiritual Self with the physical world' (FES)
Warm and joyous embodiment

Negative state

Disembodied, averse to the physical body (and world)
Denial of body's needs – eating disorders

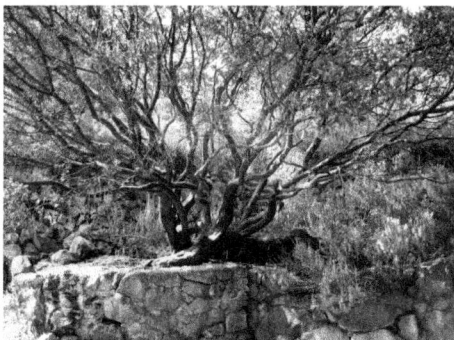

Manzanita's bloom is a *pinkish colour* implying its relationship with the *heart chakra* and its influence on *heart and circulation*. Whereas Lotus, with its strong connection to the crown chakra, affirms a conscious connection with life on Earth, Manzanita affirms a *physical* (heart) connection. It is a subtle and gentle reminder that *the body is the temple of the spirit* (Kaminski and Katz 1996). We can easily lose track of this on an unconscious level, with the result that our spirit feels *imprisoned by our physical body*, as if trapped!

Seeing our body as a temple of the spirit is further challenged in a society that places so much emphasis on having the stereotypical *perfect body* and sexualises the body in advertising and pornography (see also Pretty Face and Easter Lily).

Just as the strong Manzanita plant thrives and brings life to disturbed habitats, so the flower essence can make us feel strong in spirit and *physically* at *ease* in our body within the *coarse reality* of the physical world.

The Manzanita state of mind

If we have conscious or unconscious negative feelings towards our body or the physical realm in general (Kaminski and Katz 1996), Manzanita flower essence guides us to a more balanced view. Those with marked Manzanita tendencies may impose strict harsh diet or exercise regimes on their bodies, or at the other extreme they may be totally disconnected from bodily functions and needs. Eating disorders are often fuelled by rejection of our own physicality because it conflicts with the idealised image of a body that is perfect (and pure).

Benefits of taking Manzanita

Manzanita flower essence can help a woman to accept changes in her body, especially during pregnancy, so that she can welcome her beautiful baby with love. It has also been used to help mothers who are having difficulty breastfeeding, easing the process of opening and letting down the milk and making mother and child more receptive to physical nourishment and nurturing.

Manzanita flower essence can help us to see and respect our inner and outer beauty. It is particularly useful during adolescence, pregnancy, midlife and menopause. During these times when the physical body undergoes pronounced changes, Manzanita encourages us to comfortably negotiate the necessary psychological adjustments.

Possible physical imbalances

As mentioned above, eating disorders can be fuelled by an unconscious rejection of the body, which is exacerbated when we compare our own body with some socially constructed image of perfection. Manzanita flower essence can be helpful in establishing a better relationship, a more nurturing one, with one's body.

Common uses

To allow yourself to enjoy Earthly comforts; to follow health regimes that suit your needs; to understand that 'you are what you eat'; to improve body image; to enjoy the 'feel' of your body, after all 'you are (also) what you feel about yourself'; to nurture and love your body

Complementary &/or similar flower essences

Billy Goat Plum, Californian Pitcher Plant, Crab Apple, Fairy Lantern, Lotus, Mariposa Lily, Nicotiana, Pretty Face, Rosemary, Sweet Pea, Tansy, Watermelon, Water Violet, Wild Rose

Supporting the changes

- Engage in grounding activities such as working with earth in some form (gardening or pottery, for instance) or any other physical exercise such as bike-riding or bushwalking to get the blood flowing. This will make you aware of your body and give you a sense that it belongs to you.
- Don't undergo ridiculous 'make-overs' but do understand your best colours and wear what suits you without following fashion blindly.
- Take more interest in looking after your body – 'your temple for your spirit' – nurture it and love it.
- Appreciate and love your inner beauty.

Mariposa Lily

Calochortus leichtlinii (White/yellow centre/purple spots / FES)

Positive state

'Mother-child bonding; healing of the inner child' (FES)
Maternal warmth – receptivity to human and divine love

Negative state

Feeling unloved/unwanted as a result of early abandonment, abuse or trauma (FES)
Unreceptive to nurturing/mothering

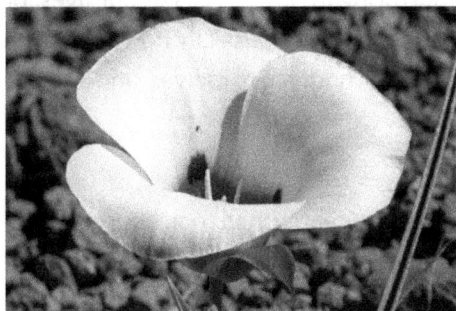

Mariposa Lily prefers rugged and mountainous environments and its *beauty emerges out of harsh terrain.*

Shallow roots, characteristic of the Lily family, connect this flower to its *harsh beginnings.* Despite the difficult environment from which it springs, the plant is able to *rise above* early limitations to *survive and thrive.* The flower opens like a *receptive cup* filled with an *abundance of light and support* – the universe provides what its Earthly beginning did not – the nurturing and love you deserve.

The Mariposa Lily personality

People in need of Mariposa Lily flower essence feel alienated from others or feel unwanted and unloved, often as a result of early disturbances in the bond with their mother (Kaminski and Katz 1996). They may have been rejected or traumatised or just deprived of love and nurturing and this has affected their ability to receive or accept love and kindness.

It is also useful for those of us who easily provide support and love to others but find it difficult to accept and receive love and support in return. Busy primary carers often fall into this category – eventually their ability to offer the love their loved ones need becomes eroded and so the cycle of neglect is perpetuated. Often the parent or carer is being asked to give something to others that they have never received themselves.

Benefits of taking Mariposa Lily

Mariposa Lily flower essence opens us to receive nurturing which compensates for past deprivations and feeds our souls in the present. The more we can release the pain and blame associated with past events, the more we feel connected and able to gain sustenance from Gaia – our Mother Earth, the archetypal mother. In my practice as a therapist, I once worked with a client whose only way of nurturing herself was to spend time alone. She came to see me during a period when her time and energy was in more demand than usual and she was finding it difficult to allow herself this 'luxury' time and her physical and emotional health suffered as a result. After taking Mariposa Lily flower essence, she became more receptive to the help and support of her co-workers and her environment in general. And despite the fact that she did not have much time to herself, she began to feel more secure and comfortable.

Possible physical imbalances

When our eating habits involve consuming lots of 'comfort' foods because we cannot obtain enough comfort and self-nurturing in other areas of our lives, or when we give more than we receive over a long period, Mariposa Lily flower essence can restore our capacity to properly emotionally nourish ourselves and receive nourishment from others and our environment.

Common uses

After early mother-child bonding trauma; after early childhood abuse; to heal the inner child; to enhance the capacity to mother and be mothered; to nurture and be nurtured; to be warmly receptive to divine love

Complementary &/or similar flower essences

Angelica, Baby Blue Eyes, Centaury, Chicory, Forget-Me-Not, Golden Ear Drops, Larkspur, Mallow, Pomegranate, Quaking Grass, Quince, Star Thistle, Tiger Lily

Supporting the changes

- Psychotherapy, Emotional Focus Therapy (EFT) or any type of regression therapy may be worth considering if the time and therapist are right.
- Learn to nurture yourself – have a bath, a 'playtime' or a good laugh.
- Create time for some indulgences (healthy ones!) every day. Allow yourself to be pampered.

Mimulus

Mimulus guttatus   (Yellow / Bach)

Positive state

Quiet courage and strength
Acceptance of life's inherent risks

Negative state

Mental fears
Dread of everyday things

Mimulus is often found clinging to the stones of riverbanks, *precariously hanging over* the water where it is constantly splashed and washed by the stream. The plant faces its fears and risks its future by releasing thousands of seeds into the water (Barnard 1988). Some seeds are washed away but others take root and form new growth.

The flowers are *yellow* in colour, which relates to our ability to express our *individuality.* Yellow signifies a relationship with the *solar plexus chakra*, and the solar plexus is certainly the area of the body where many people feel fear and anxiety, particularly *anticipatory anxiety* like *'butterflies in the stomach.'* The upright, bright yellow flowers represent our ability to *stand up and 'shine'* in life and display an *inner strength and security.* The flowers have five petals which are fused to form an open mouth, and this aspect of their signature relates to the capacity to *speak up for yourself.* At the same time, the flowers are delicate and are easily affected by chemical pollution or even the warmth of a hand during their preparation as a flower essence, indicating the capacity of the essence to foster *sensitivity and empathy.*

The Mimulus personality

Mimulus is part of the Monkeyflower family and essences made from this group are used to treat fears and intense emotional reactions of various kinds. (Scarlet Monkeyflower is used to reduce fear of intense emotions such as anger and frustration; Sticky Monkeyflower is used for fear of intimacy.) Mimulus flower essence is used to balance fears relating to individual assertiveness and autonomy – the capacity to step out into the world and be yourself. When we need Mimulus, our fear relates to something of a known origin, to a particular aspect of our life and environment such as fear of speaking in public; fear of a certain person; fear of travel; fear of animals (dogs, for example); fear of risk-taking or fear of any activity that someone else might take calmly in their stride. A Mimulus person in the negative state may shy away from anxiety-producing situations. Unfortunately, this means that personal power is given over to the object of their fear.

Benefits of taking Mimulus

When our fears restrict our experience of life, we should consider taking Mimulus flower essence. It can help us take the risk of living a fuller life and reaping its rewards. Mimulus encourages feelings of personal freedom through an increased willingness to accept life's inherent risks and vulnerabilities – after all, nothing ventured, nothing gained. Mimulus can help transform a shy and timid disposition into a more confident and courageous stance.

Possible physical imbalances

Fear that is intense and held-in can eventually have a negative effect on the kidneys and bladder. Problems such as bed-wetting are also a possibility – a child may be inwardly fearful during the day, unconsciously 'holding on' until in sleep they let go with the inevitable result. Nervous tension and related problems are common, manifesting in conditions such as nervous stomach, gut and bowel.

Common uses

For any fear of a known origin; for shyness, timidity and/or self-consciousness; for those who fear confrontation; for nervous dread of normal/everyday experiences; to improve self-confidence; for courage when facing everyday situations

Complementary &/or similar flower essences

Angel's Trumpet, Angelica, Garlic, Golden Yarrow, Hibbertia, Larch, Mallow, Mountain Pride, the Monkeyflowers, Oregon Grape, Red Clover, Rock Rose, St John's Wort, Sunflower, Trumpet Vine, Violet

Supporting the changes

- In order to safeguard their sensitive and delicate nature, Mimulus people need to take refuge on a regular basis in their 'sanctuary,' which can be anything from a favourite cubbyhouse to a temple. This sense of sanctuary can also be created internally through meditation and relaxation techniques or through creative visualisation.
- A balanced approach to diet and lifestyle is extremely important for the survival of those who are spiritually sensitive. Mimulus will help you tune in to the particular needs of mind and body in this regard.

Morning Glory

Ipomoea purpurea   (Blue / FES)

Positive state

Wide awake and refreshed (FES)
In touch with life's natural rhythms

Negative state

Dull, sluggish, feeling 'hung over' or 'jetlagged'
'Addictive habits' (FES); out of sync with natural body rhythms

Morning Glory flowers are sky-blue and the essence makes us feel as if we are *'under a clear blue sky'* – it *lifts us* mentally and brings *clarity* and strength to our *mental body*. The *nervous system* follows and is strengthened and *re-vitalised*, re-establishing contact with our health-inducing, *natural body rhythms*. Morning Glory flower essence *lights up* the nervous system – the conical shaped flowers dotted over the vine like Christmas lights symbolise the lit-up *acupuncture points* along the etheric energy meridians. This etheric *luminosity* is infectious and so can also have a positive influence on those around us. We can literally *'glow with good health.'* Morning Glory flower essence enables us to break addictive and energy-depleting habits, allowing us to become more in sync with our natural, energy-generating rhythms.

Morning Glory flowers open in the early morning and close as the day progresses. When we are properly attuned, our body rhythms will enable us to function at our optimum. Morning Glory can help us to become more of a *'morning person,'* working productively and then tapering off as the day draws to its close, enjoying the energy and health benefits of being in tune with the *rhythms of life*.

The Morning Glory state of mind

When the natural circadian (24-hour) rhythms of the body and mind are out of harmony because of irregular sleeping and eating habits or an erratic lifestyle, Morning Glory flower essence can be helpful. Night shift, JETLAG or too many late nights that result in a hung-over feeling, destructive and/or addictive habits are all signs of a need for the Morning Glory flower essence. Dependence on coffee, tobacco and other stimulants throws our body clock out, creating artificial cycles that compete with natural, healthy rhythms.

Benefits of taking Morning Glory

Morning Glory flower essence helps us to break free from energy depleting habits and behaviours by re-establishing normal body rhythms and improving energy levels, promoting vitality and freshness. Along with a number of my colleagues in natural therapies, I have prescribed Morning Glory flower essence as an adjunct to programs aimed at reducing sugar or caffeine intake, quitting smoking or breaking a dependence on alcohol and other drugs.

Possible physical imbalances

Morning Glory helps revitalise and detox a body that is run down due to unhealthy lifestyle choices and habits – especially coffee, nicotine and alcohol abuse and disturbances of the natural 24-hour rhythms of the body through late nights, air travel, shift work etc.

Common uses

For a continual 'Monday morning' feeling; for 'jetlag'; for coffee and/or nicotine dependence; for ill-effects of shift work; to get back 'in touch' with your body; to detox, refresh and re-vitalise; to re-awaken your natural energy and health-inducing body rhythms

Complementary &/or similar flower essences

Aloe Vera, Bottlebrush, Cayenne, Chaparral, Clematis, Coffee, Crab Apple, Dill, Hornbeam, Macrocarpa, Nasturtium, Nicotiana, Olive, Peppermint, Rosemary, Tansy, Walnut, YES formula

Supporting the changes

- Think about what got you into this state of energy depletion and work to change offending lifestyle, patterns, habits and foods.
- Improve your diet – include foods rich in the B vitamins. Consider consulting a health practitioner for expert advice.
- Break up your frantic lifestyle with periods of constructive or reconstructive quiet time. Calming activities that promote healthy reflection and debriefing on life issues is highly recommended – in other words become more mindful. Consider relaxation techniques such as yoga, tai chi, meditation etc.
- Wake up to yourself.

Mountain Pennyroyal

Monardella odoratissima (Violet / FES)

Positive state

Able to deflect and expel others' negativity
'Mental integrity', clarity and positivity (FES)

Negative state

Easily affected by the negative thinking of others (FES)
A mind congested or contaminated by others' negativity

Mountain Pennyroyal is for those who are *psychically congested* by *negative thought forms* absorbed from the surrounding *'atmosphere.'* Mountain Pennyroyal flower essence repels these negative thought forms just as its close relative Pennyroyal repels insects, leaving the *mind clear and positive*. Peppermint, another plant from the same family, also has a strong positive influence on *mental clarity*.

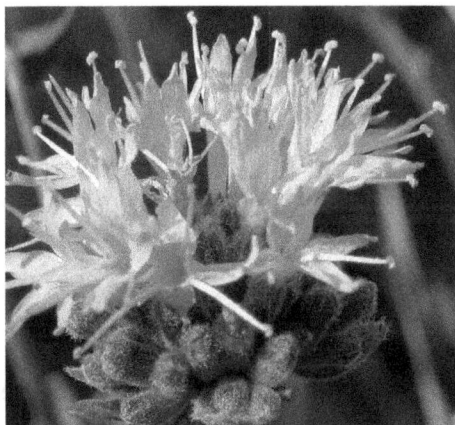

Mountain Pennyroyal flower essence *cleanses* our *'mental field.'* The plant's signature includes whorls of small violet flowers that extend outwards like 'feelers' able to receive from and transmit into the plant's *atmospheric 'field.'*

The *violet* colour of the flowers relates the plant to the *crown chakra* and our ability to stay true to our *higher Self* and not be thrown off track by negative external influences and distractions. Mountain Pennyroyal helps maintain the *integrity of the mental body*.

The Mountain Pennyroyal state of mind

Mountain Pennyroyal flower essence is good for people who are easily 'sucked in' by negative energy or negative exchanges and are especially sensitive to emotional negativity in their immediate environment. A client once told me, 'Every time I go to visit my mother I am determined not to get into an argument with her. But sure enough, within 20 minutes we are having words. Try as I may it always happens.' She took Mountain Pennyroyal essence for a few weeks and soon found that she was far more able to let her mother's comments and attitude go right on by. She said,

'After a while, because I had managed to stop taking her bait, she started to cheer up and talk about more pleasant things.'

If someone has grown up in a family where arguing and abusive behaviour is common, they may become programmed to accept it as the norm. Over time it begins to create damage in our aura and the essence of our being and even when we leave the situation we may still find ourselves vulnerable to the effects of negativity around us. (Some people may resort to using drugs, especially alcohol, as a way of temporarily numbing or de-sensitising against negativity in the environment.) Mountain Pennyroyal can help to heal old wounds so we can 're-program' our reactions to negativity in our vicinity. It no longer has the same negative impact.

The following subtle distinctions between some commonly used 'protective' flower essences may aid accurate prescribing:

- Mountain Pennyroyal flower essence repels negative thought patterns and negative thinking.
- Yarrow protects against negative and destructive energy in the general atmosphere.
- Pink Yarrow helps protect against negative emotions in others, especially those close to us.

Benefits of taking Mountain Pennyroyal

Mountain Pennyroyal flower essence helps strengthen us mentally. It improves mental integrity, which results in greater mental clarity and a more positive frame of mind (Kaminski and Katz 1996). We cannot be 'got at' so easily by those who in the past may have found us an easy target. With a more buoyant attitude we can deflect others' negativity with greater tolerance and good humour.

Possible physical imbalances

Any form of oversensitivity to one's surroundings will eventually compromise the immune system to some degree. Continued exposure to negativity in the environment will make one more susceptible on a physical level.

Common uses

For those who succumb too easily to negativity; for psychic attack and contamination; to deflect negative thought forms; to help cope (temporarily) with a negative work environment; to develop a psychic shield; to help re-program for mental positivity; to improve mental strength and integrity; for mental clarity; to remain mentally positive even under threat

Complementary &/or similar flower essences

Angelica, Angelsword, Arnica, Baby Blue Eyes, Borage, Calendula, Canyon

Dudleya, Chaparral, Crowea, Dill, Echinacea, Fringed Violet, Garlic, Golden Yarrow, Indian Pink, Peppermint, Pink Yarrow, Red Clover, St John's Wort, Star of Bethlehem, Violet, Walnut, Waratah, Yarrow, YES formula

Supporting the changes

- Develop methods of dynamic self-protection such as visualising white light around you or use other forms of meditation or protective rituals.
- Maintain a balanced lifestyle. It is very important to keep yourself grounded with activities such as gardening and outdoor exercise in open spaces full of greenery.
- A diet rich in nutrients for the nervous system, especially Vitamin B, is supportive.
- Limit your exposure to people who are always negative towards you and the world, and who have no intention of changing.
- Secure your hide-away haven for regular time out to regroup – your room, your study, your shed, YOUR SPACE!

Mullein

Verbascum thapsus (Yellow / FES)

Positive state

A clear sense of a guiding conscience
Honesty and integrity

Negative state

'Inability to hear one's inner voice' (FES) – confused
In denial of one's truth

Mullein is *tall and stately*, adorning the slopes of fields, railway embankments and waysides. It flourishes in arid situations and stands up to the heat of the sun. In its flower essence form, Mullein helps us to *stand up for what we believe as individuals*, despite external pressures and indoctrination. The yellow of the flower shows the plant's affinity to the *solar plexus chakra* which confers qualities of *individuality and the capacity to be true to Self*. Its stately appearance symbolises our potential to gain status through our unique statement to the world.

The Mullein personality

In the negative state, Mullein people are divided about who they really are and are easily defined by what others expect them to be. They are indecisive when they must make choices for themselves as they can't seem to connect with their own inner guidance or morality (Kaminski and Katz 1996). This can result in antisocial or negative behaviour especially when under the influence of peer pressure.

Furthermore, in the negative state, Mullein people don't have the moral fortitude to address negative traits such as their susceptibility to group pressure, as they don't really believe in or know themselves.

Benefits of taking Mullein

When we feel pressure to conform to something that does not feel right, Mullein flower essence helps us to hear clearly the voice of conscience so that we can respond to our internal sense of morality. It also helps us to patiently stand tall and firm as we consider the ethics of issues before us. Mullein helps us resist being swayed from what we believe in our hearts to be true. It helps us to display the courage of our convictions and follow our own moral beliefs. For this reason it is very helpful when experiencing our astrological natal Saturn return in our 28th year and again as we approach 60. This is a time when it is necessary to be deeply reflective about where we are in life and what we have become and offers an opportunity to confront our 'life issue' responsibilities. Have we been living in a way that is true to our life purpose? Mullein flower essence can give us that second (or third) chance to realign with our true Self.

By following the inner guidance of our personal truth, we can grow into and display our full potential. If we are honest with ourselves, the world will be honest with us.

Possible physical imbalances

Mullein flower essence helps you to stand up to social pressure, for example in relation to eating sweets, drinking alcohol, smoking and drug-taking when you are striving to maintain a healthy diet and lifestyle and/or 'stay clean.'

Common uses

For moral/ethical dilemmas, especially related to one's occupation; for midlife crises; for 'Saturn return' crises; to develop a conscience in some difficult area of your life; for courage to 'do the right thing'; to be genuine and true to your Self; for self-actualisation

Complementary &/or similar flower essences

Angelica, Californian Poppy, Cerato, Chrysanthemum, Deerbrush, Fairy Lantern, Forget-Me-Not, Golden Yarrow, Goldenrod, Lady's Slipper, Mimulus, Mountain Pride, Pink Monkeyflower, Purple Monkeyflower, Sagebrush, Scleranthus, Sunflower, Tall Yellow Top, Walnut, Wild Oat

Supporting the changes

- Meditation and practitioner-facilitated therapies such as Gestalt therapy or voice dialogue will be helpful.

- Spend time away from peers or friends when you begin to feel uncomfortable with their conversation or activities.
- Choose your friends wisely!
- Acknowledge your talents.
- Learn to think and speak for yourself.

Mustard

Sinapis arvensis   (Yellow / Bach)

Positive state

Understanding our 'dark energies' (our shadow side)
Positive outlook

Negative state

A dark cloud 'out of the blue'
Depression of unknown origin

Mustard's flower is yellow – a colour that stands for the sun and has a cheering effect, encouraging the perceptive faculties and allowing us to 'shine' in our interaction with others. As a flower essence, it is used for 'dark' depression that clouds our experience of the world and other people. Yellow is associated with the *solar plexus chakra* which, when balanced, facilitates the *spiritualisation of the intellect* or in this case the elevation of the mental body out of depression into a higher and lighter state. Our *perspective is elevated* to that of our *higher Self* as if, when a dark cloud passes between us and the sun, we are able to maintain a wider view, understanding that the darkness is only temporary – the cloud will move on to reveal the sun once more. Mustard helps us come to terms with our *'Shadow side'* by helping us to sense, even during times of depression, that this is a natural, temporary state that will not last forever. This *patient expectation of better times* is displayed in the *life cycle* of the Mustard plant. Julian and Martine Barnard (1988) describe how Mustard seeds 'lie dormant in the soil for many years in what is termed a natural seed bank: hundreds, thousands of seeds may be buried in a square metre of ground waiting their opportunity to grow when conditions are right.'

The Mustard state of mind

In life's darkest moments, and in lives that are full of such moments, this flower essence can help. Mustard is useful for those types of depression where, however frequently the darkness falls, there is no conscious warning. It is as if a black hole appears out of nowhere and disappears just as fast. Women may experience it regularly during their monthly cycle without ever having a sense of being prepared;

it may also come during certain seasons of the year. Because there is no feeling of impending gloom beforehand, it can make us feel like victims of a dark and unseen outside force. Depression arrives suddenly for reasons known only to the inner Self.

Benefits of taking Mustard

Mustard can help put us in touch with the deeper Self and its rhythms and energies. Knowing that the darkness is temporary, we feel less trapped and safer about facing eruptions from the Shadow side, even gaining some insight into their nature. These times do in fact provide great opportunities for soul-searching. As we acquire self-knowledge, mood changes become far less pronounced and more predictable. A more harmonious relationship between conscious and unconscious aspects of Self is established – we become a more whole person embracing all aspects of our being.

Possible physical imbalances

Think of Mustard flower essence for any illness that coincides with or directly follows the sudden onset of a depressed state. Although not an illness, PMS could be included here.

Common uses

For sudden depression and gloom that arises for no apparent reason; for a history of sudden periods of depression followed by equally sudden recoveries; to assist in developing a deeper understanding of Self and natural rhythms; to help shine in the world with the energy of the whole Self

Complementary &/or similar flower essences

Baby Blue Eyes, Black Eyed Susan, Borage, Chamomile, Cherry Plum, Garlic, Gentian, Gorse, Hibbertia, Hound's Tongue, Iris, Pansy, Red Clover, St John's Wort, Scotch Broom, Sturt Desert Pea, Sweet Chestnut, Waratah, Wild Oat, Wild Rose, Zinnia

Supporting the changes

- Make use of therapies which develop self-awareness, such as dreamwork, psychotherapy and meditation.
- Body-awareness is also helpful and can be developed through yoga, tai chi and breath work.
- Study the Jungian concept of the Shadow, that largely unknown area of the psyche where much energy is stored.
- Take over and take the plunge inward, toward insight and self-understanding!

Nasturtium

Tropaeolum majus   (Orange-red / FES)

Positive state

Enthused and joyful
Emotional warmth and vitality (FES)

Negative state

Mentally 'dry', colourless and flat
'Depletion of life-force and emotional verve' (FES)

asturtium is a sprawling annual admired for its *variety* of colourful blooms – variety is the spice of life. Their *orange/yellow/red* colours invoke the qualities of the life force and its energy through their strong association with the *intrapersonal base, sacral* and *solar plexus chakras*. They also signify the sheer *joy of life* – the flower essence can quite literally add emotional colour and 'inject fun' into a lack-lustre, *dry intellect*. The plant's *succulent* quality illustrates its ability to preserve the *water element*, supporting the *fluency of our emotions* and nurturing the deep spring from which *creativity* flows. Nasturtium's capacity to reconnect us with the *life force* results in increased *mental energy* and *passion* and restores our capacity for decisive action.

The Nasturtium personality

Nasturtium can add vitality, passion and feeling to life when we are drained because of an excess of mental activity or concentrated mental work. It adds emotional colour (the water element) to an otherwise 'dry' personality in which the mental (air) element dominates.

Nasturtium flower essence is useful for cerebral people who tend to live in their thoughts. This lopsided existence with an emphasis on intellect at the expense of emotion can be likened to an engine running without the lubricating effects of oil. The system eventually seizes up, resulting in mental and physical exhaustion. We get a sense of this in the 'flat' feeling that follows prolonged study. This essence can also be useful when the higher chakras have been overworked or abused through excessive meditation or overuse of the intuitive and creative processes.

Benefits of taking Nasturtium

When the Nasturtium plant is eaten it stimulates appetite and broadens tastes, and the flower essence can also stimulate our appetite for life, broaden personal tastes and add to the enjoyment and appreciation of living. Nasturtium flower essence helps to harness the energy of the lower chakras. This makes it possible to reconnect with the metabolic forces of life and warmth and the body's needs and sources of nourishment. Nasturtium helps add a new depth of awareness to our everyday experience. It grounds us so that we can obtain a deeper connection to the Earth (Kaminski and Katz 1996), integrating depth with breadth and qualitative with quantitative aspects of experience. The result is a more deeply felt experience of life and greater enJOYment.

Possible physical imbalances

General nervous system fatigue associated with a heavy mental workload or prolonged mental activity is often relieved by taking Nasturtium flower essence. It is particularly useful when common 'head' colds have followed this mental over-activity.

Common uses

For feeling emotionally flat and colourless; for overly dry intellectualism; for narrow-mindedness; for single issue obsession; to 'get out of your head'; for the courage to look outside the square; to open your mind and broaden your horizons; to enhance appreciation and enjoyment of life

Complementary &/or similar flower essences

Aloe Vera, Californian Poppy, Cayenne, Filaree, Harvest Brodiaea, Hibbertia, Hornbeam, Hound's Tongue, Indian Paintbrush, Iris, Lotus, Nicotiana, Peppermint, Rosemary, Shasta Daisy, Tall Yellow Top, White Chestnut, Zinnia

Supporting the changes

- Grounding activities as simple as walking or working with soil will enhance your ability to tap into the Earth's energy.
- When making personal decisions or considering something that is meaningful to you, ask yourself how you feel about it. Try not to rationalise or underrate your feelings.
- Take a rest from mental activities and get physical.
- 'Laugh your head off'!

Nectarine

Prunus persica   (Pink / FES-res)

Positive state
The 'calm after the storm'
Restored faith and TRUST

Negative state
For 'riders of the storm'
Anxious feelings of life 'out of one's control'

Nectarine was hybridised over 100 years ago as a cross between *plum* and *peach*. As you would expect, Nectarine flower essence has a broader action than that of Cherry Plum and Peach flower essences on their own and has qualities that relate to the mental and emotional states characteristic of both. Its appearance on Earth coincides with the transition from the consciousness of the Piscean age, one in which life consists of *crisis after crisis* and personal growth is gained only through adhering to the motto of *'no pain no gain,'* to the consciousness of the Aquarian age of growth that unfolds more organically, with less pain and *less catharsis*. Nectarine flower essence combines Cherry Plum's ability to help us recover *composure* and *calm, heart-centred consciousness* in the midst of a crisis, with pink flowered Peach's ability to help us open our hearts more; then we can display more compassion for our fellow humans, and by embracing them, restore our *faith and trust* in humanity. Like Peach, Nectarine's *pink* flowers attest to the flower essence's strong affinity to the *heart chakra* and its ability to help us become more *peaceful* and *emotionally balanced*.

The Nectarine state of mind

Like Cherry Plum, Nectarine flower essence is suitable when we have reached the end of our tether and feel we cannot go on. In the negative Nectarine state, too many things in life have been out of control for too long, so that we feel we cannot continue as before. It is the point where we finally say, 'No more. Enough's enough.'

Benefits of taking Nectarine

Nectarine flower essence helps us to regain peace and stillness of mind after enduring long-term stress and worry. Always think of Nectarine when you feel as though you have reached the end of your endurance after months or even years of angst. You are 'sick and tired of being sick and tired,' as they say, and are ready to regain the calm and composure that has eluded you for so long.

One of my clients was robbed at knifepoint while at work in his small business. He had previously worked as a security guard, so during the robbery he was able to act to prevent any harm coming to his shop assistant or himself. However, despite his cool demeanour during the robbery, the experience affected him profoundly. He felt that he never fully recovered from the episode and was obviously suffering from some PTSD. When he consulted me, matters were intensifying because of an impending court case. His wife complained that he had never before been so irritable and uptight. After taking Nectarine flower essence for a few days he felt calmer and more relaxed. His wife gratefully acknowledged this too.

Possible physical imbalances

All sorts of stress-related ailments are possible in the negative Nectarine state.

Common uses

For fears about doing something desperate; when you have 'reached the end of your tether'; when you feel that 'this is the straw that breaks the camel's back'; when desperate for change after prolonged stress; to maintain a 'cool head' in a crisis; for acceptance; to learn to live and work 'smart'; to help 'get a grip' on your life; to regain inner peace and TRUST in what may be.

Complementary &/or similar flower essences

Agrimony, Baby Blue Eyes, Cherry Plum, Chrysanthemum, Crowea, Indian Pink, Lady's Slipper, Love-Lies-Bleeding, Oak, Olive, Pear, Sagebrush, Star of Bethlehem, Sweet Chestnut, Waratah

Supporting the changes

- Seek professional guidance and emotional support.
- Establish a healthy, nourishing diet and lifestyle.
- Practise relaxation techniques or other activities that enable you to let go. Become familiar with how it feels.
- Affirm that things have turned around for the better.

Nicotiana
Nicotiana alata   (White / FES)

Positive state
Feeling alive! Your 'heart's in it'
Grounded and 'switched on' emotionally

Negative state
Your 'heart's not in it'; ill-at-ease
Desensitised and emotionally detached (FES)

Nicotiana (flowering tobacco) is a plant from the nightshade family that is well known to us because of worldwide *addiction* to nicotine through tobacco-smoking. The rise of this phenomenon has been rapid since the colonisation of the Americas and it has pervaded all levels of our society. Use of tobacco originated with Native American peoples long before Columbus and for them the lighted fire and spiralling smoke signify *dreaming*, enabling one's imagination to *spark up*. Healthy dream work and *reverie* can allow us to deal better with our day-to-day problems.

It is said that the ancients smoked mixtures of ingredients – of which tobacco was one – to induce a dream-like state in which they would become more receptive to *spiritual guidance* (Cunningham and Ramer 1988). Native American spiritual teachings counselled prudent and reverent use (often in combination with other healing herbs) in *peace* pipe ceremonies. Smoking was part of a group *bonding* ritual that facilitated a deep connection between people on a *'heart'* level. These deep feelings also enhanced the *connection with Earth and all life*. Unfortunately, smokers today use tobacco by itself to try to undo the overstimulation caused by our alienation from the environment, *numbing feelings* and emotionally detaching (Kaminski and Katz 1996). Initially smoking may *heighten* our daytime *perceptions* but ultimately, just as it deadens the taste buds, it *deadens* our other senses too! Loss of the purposeful, ritualistic and spiritual approach to smoking this plant coincides with a time of rapid growth of industry and technology and a changed relationship with the Earth. Earth and its resources have become objects of *exploitation* rather than being nurtured and treated with respect (Kaminski and Katz 1996).

The Nicotiana state of mind

People often smoke a cigarette in an attempt to relax and stay grounded, while at the same time trying to heighten their sensibilities and perception in order to cope better with everyday stresses and challenges. Unfortunately, smoking merely brings about a numbing of feelings and senses, which become blunted so that we are able 'to adapt and even thrive in the harder, denser world of modern technology' (Kaminski and Katz 1996). However, one does not have to be a smoker for this numbing to occur – a hardening has already occurred in the physical and etheric bodies of most modern people. Our machine-based culture damages our 'heart' connection with the Earth. Nicotiana flower essence is a great healer for the heart, allowing us to reconnect with the natural and nurturing energy of the Earth and life around us.

Benefits of taking Nicotiana

Nicotiana flower essence reduces the need to numb the feelings in order to cope and reduces the impulse to use recreational stimulants to self-anaesthetise in social situations or at work. Nicotiana helps restore our heartfelt energies so that bonding with others becomes more natural and comfortable. It helps us to naturally generate healthy energy in our hearts and gain emotional sustenance (which we would otherwise seek by having a cigarette). We can begin to FEEL more alive in our hearts and more at peace within ourselves, losing the need for artificial stimulants. Kaminksi and Katz describe how Nicotiana flower essence helps us to reconnect with our deep, heartfelt feelings and gives us 'our true connection to the Earth and all living beings.'

Possible physical imbalances

Nicotiana flower essence (as well as its homeopathic form, Tabacum) enhances the elimination of tobacco residue from the system. Once the residue of any drug of dependence is completely eliminated from the body, cravings for it decline dramatically.

Common uses

For feelings of detachment and isolation; for nicotine addiction; for the two polarities of feeling anxious/overstimulated or emotionally deadened; to get your 'spark' back; to put your 'heart' back into life; to feel ALIVE again; to FEEL at peace in your heart and on Earth

Complementary &/or similar flower essences

Agrimony, Aloe Vera, Angelica, Californian Poppy, Cayenne, Clematis, Corn, Dill, Echinacea, Flannel Flower, Forget-Me-Not, Fringed Violet, Fuchsia, Golden Yarrow, Indian Pink, Lavender, Lotus, Mallow, Manzanita, Morning Glory, Nasturtium, Quaking Grass, Red Lily, Shooting Star, Sweet Pea, Walnut, YES formula, Zinnia

Supporting the changes

- Re-establish your connection with the Earth. Walk along a river, take a drive in the country or immerse yourself in the greenery of parkland or gardens. Do some regular gardening!
- Relaxation, yoga, tai chi or meditation practices, especially when done in a group, will enable you to relax physically and mentally in company.
- Develop methods of dynamic self-protection such as visualising white light around you.
- Maintain a balanced lifestyle that fits with natural Earth rhythms, especially when it comes to getting enough sleep within a regular, daily time frame. Try not to inhibit your dream life with drugs or medication – dreaming plays an important role in healing the emotional body.
- Join a green group!

Oak

Quercus robur   (Red / Bach)

Positive state

Endurance and acceptance of limitation
Work/REST/play balance

Negative state

Quietly suffers
'Life wasn't meant to be easy'

The majestic English Oak is called the King of Trees. It was sacred to the Druids and was used to build England's navy and its great cathedrals, churches and halls. It is mighty and broad – *robur* means *'sturdy'* – and so *rigid* it will not bend with the wind (Barnard 1988). In the positive state, Oak people display the *strong and enduring* qualities of the tree. They work hard and never complain, reminding us of the Englishman and his proverbial *'stiff upper lip'*. They seem to have an endless supply of drive and *willpower* – signified by the red of the flower and its relationship with the survival instinct and determined qualities of the *base chakra*. The female flowers, which are used in the preparation of the flower essence, can help balance the masculine quality of determination to 'do and keep doing' with the feminine side's more receptive, contemplative understanding of the need for rest and to just 'BE' rather than always keep 'doing.' There are fewer female flowers than male flowers, and the female flowers are less conspicuous, hidden among the leaves. Similarly, classic Oak people *never complain* or draw attention to themselves, despite

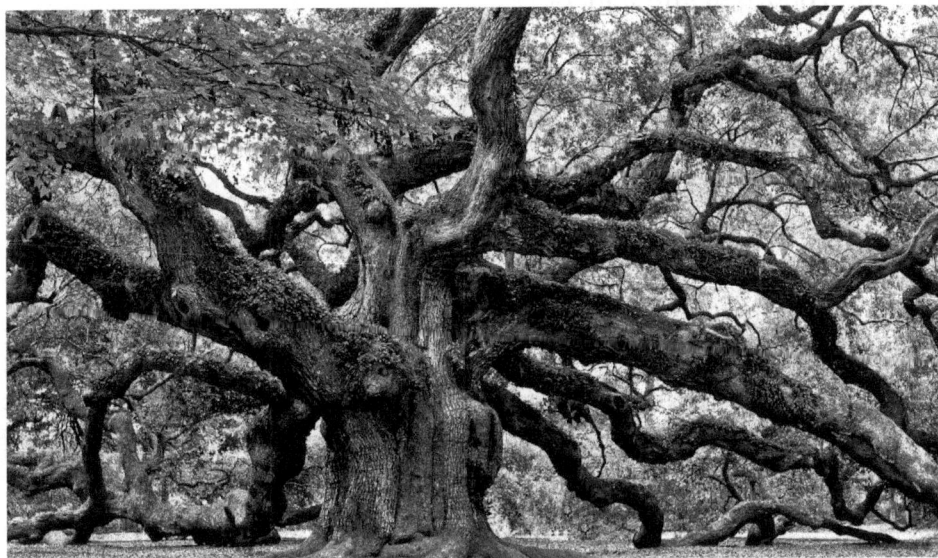

the fact that they may be in pain or stressed through overwork. Oak trees also excel in *tolerance and acceptance,* hosting hundreds of different insects, providing acorns as food for birds, rodents and pigs in olden times, sheltering a rich undergrowth of plants and allowing mosses and even seedling trees to grow on their branches (Barnard 1988). The Oak person, too, is only too pleased to share another's burden, helping friends without any expectation of reciprocation.

The Oak personality

Oak people often soldier on unnoticed, and this can lead to an ingrained belief that life must be a struggle. But there comes a time when they finally break down and cannot continue physically. Just as the tree's branches may crack under too much strain, Oak people sometimes break (down), become ill, or show themselves to be in need of help. Their lack of concern for their personal wellbeing means that their health is jeopardised and eventually they have no other choice but to slow down and STOP.

Benefits of taking Oak

Before an Oak person reaches a stage where physical exhaustion and breakdown becomes inevitable, Oak flower essence can help them be more reflective and direct their strength and determination towards their own healing. By using the remedy, the Oak person is freed to share their problems with others, to receive assistance and lighten their load. Life becomes easier and their capacity to enjoy it is reawakened. Oak flower essence fosters a more balanced perspective on life, which includes a realistic acceptance of our limitations. The remedy helps us to step back, take stock and consider alternative solutions.

Possible physical imbalances

Oak flower essence is useful for people who have a stoic attitude during illness, enduring their pain silently. Musculoskeletal health complaints can become chronic as a result of this unrealistic 'no complaints and soldier on' mentality. In other cases, the cumulative effect of many ailments forces them to seek help.

Common uses

For the silent sufferer who plods on regardless; for the battler whose health finally falters after years of neglect; for those who never complain despite difficult circumstances; for the dependable 'draught-horse' type who is finally getting tired; to help feel more deserving of the good things life has to offer; to help ask not what you can do for your country, but what your country can do for you!; to help you just BE and enjoy life

Complementary &/or similar flower essences

Agrimony, Centaury, Dandelion, Elm, Flannel Flower, Hornbeam, Larkspur, Manzanita, Nectarine, Pine, Quince, Rock Water, Vervain, Vine, Zinnia

Supporting the changes

- Set aside an hour or two for yourself every week and spend it doing something you really want to do, for no other reason than to indulge yourself. You deserve it!
- Ask yourself more often, 'How do I feel about this?' Respond to the needs that arise from your reflection. Meditation and relaxation techniques will assist this process.
- It's OK to ask someone for help!

Olive

Olea europaea   (White / Bach)

Positive state

Sustained, dynamically-applied effort
Revitalised and peaceful

Negative state

Too tired to complete tasks
Exhausted on all levels

Olive, slow-growing and *long-lived*, has been cultivated since ancient times for its fruit and oil. When cut back to a stump, new stems emerge from the wood of even the oldest trees. The Olive tree continues to flower and bear fruit generation after generation, even in the last years of its 'old age.' For this reason it is regarded as an inexhaustible *reservoir of energy*. A great *condensation of energy* occurs, as represented by the presence of an extremely *concentrated* oily substance in the dense fruit. The Olive fruit is the plant's focal point, packed full of complex nutrient substances, making it a *dynamic and compact* natural food supplement. The creamy white flower clusters (another expression of *density and concentration*) are used to make the essence which is a wonderful *remedy for exhaustion*.

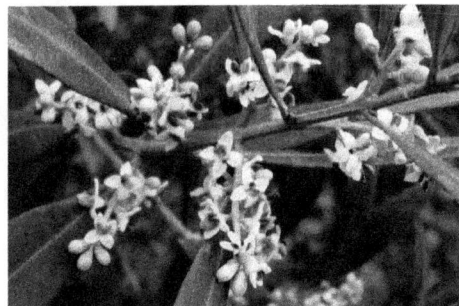

Olive flower essence helps people when they need to *focus energy intensely*

to achieve results and helps those who have become exhausted and drained of energy through intense activity. It enhances the ability to sustain focused energy without becoming enervated when working on a particular problem or purpose in life.

The flower essence helps those who are over-tired, 'extended to their limit', burnt out or over-achieving to *peacefully surrender* and start *'rehab.'* Olive has been a symbol of peace throughout the ages. When people offer an olive branch it indicates that they have relented and decided to do or say something to show that they want to end a disagreement and make peace. In the Bible we are told of how the Olive plant survived the Great Flood when the dove – another symbol of peace sent out by Noah – flew back with a sprig of leaves from the tree. The world was again at peace as the heavy rains ceased and the waters receded to expose the now-regenerating land. The Earth was now in recovery!

The Olive state of mind

Olive people tend to get exhausted on all levels – physically, emotionally, and mentally. Their complete lack of energy undermines any attempt to exert themselves in mind or body and means that their condition is actually made worse by thinking about it. Any exercise of the will is short-lived and they are slow to recover.

It is especially useful for those suffering exhaustion as a result of being thwarted in their concentrated attempts to solve a problem or achieve a purpose.

Benefits of taking Olive

Olive flower essence helps restore vitality at the deepest level at which energy and inspiration has its source. When energy is dissipated or lost over a period of time, Olive can help strengthen and reintegrate the subtle energetic bodies, *concentrating energy resources* and restoring our dynamic presence in the world. Olive can be used to treat exhaustion resulting from prolonged periods of stress on both mental and physical levels, such as that experienced by a mother after having a baby, or during and immediately after examinations or intense work periods. Use it as a support during intensive training for any event that requires endurance and quick recovery, and for all situations that place excessive demands on mental and physical resources.

Possible physical imbalances

Physical fatigue is always present in the negative Olive state, and this lack of vitality undermines natural immunity and leaves us susceptible to infection. When sickness occurs, full recovery from illness may be hampered if we are still severely run down, even if an infection is brought under control. Olive flower essence can help restore vitality so that complete recovery can occur.

Common uses

For convalescents; for rehabilitation after an incapacitating accident; for complete physical and mental exhaustion; for insomnia from overtiredness; as a support during times when endurance is tested; to help when intense focus of energy (physical or mental) is required; to help increase (physical or mental) resilience

Complementary &/or similar flower essences

Aloe Vera, Blackberry, California Pitcher Plant, Cayenne, Dandelion, Forget-Me-Not, Hornbeam, Macrocarpa, Madia, Morning Glory, Nasturtium, Nectarine, Peppermint, Silver Princess, Tansy, Wild Rose

Supporting the changes

- Rest at every opportunity – sleep, if possible. Learn to include more relaxation and play in your life. Schedule breaks during periods of intense work.
- Engage in energising but not exhausting activities such as gentle aerobic exercise or walking. Meditation and relaxation techniques, yoga and tai chi will strengthen body and soul.
- Maintain a healthy and nutritious diet. Look after yourself!

Onion

Allium cepa   (Greenish-white / FES-res)

Positive state

Foresight
Clarity about the way forward

Negative state

Lacking insight
Uncertain about the next step in life

The Onion plant has hollow, juicy shoots for leaves and a sphere of *greenish-white* flower heads. The most recognisable aspect of the plant signature is the bulb with its compact *system of layers* which grows at the base of the plant.

Each layer of the bulb can be *peeled away* to reveal another until eventually the *sweet heart* is revealed. In the same way, we get to the *heart of Self* by coming to know and understand ourselves better as we peel away and work through the mental and emotional *layers of our being*. Another aspect of the plant's signature is its *pungent odour* when crushed, which we have all experienced when chopping and preparing this vegetable for cooking. It causes *tears*, pointing to the *release* of emotion from a *stirred heart*, signifying that the *eyes of the heart* are now open

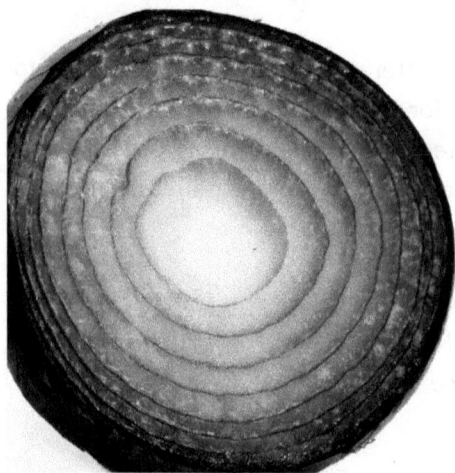

to '*see*' more clearly the next important step in life's journey. The *green* tint of parts of the flower further relates it to the *heart chakra*, while the *whiteness* of other parts emphasise its role in the release and *cleansing of old emotional pain and sadness*, opening the way for *pure insight*.

The Onion state of mind

Onion flower essence is needed when we are unsure about what the next step should be. Often we reach a stage when our next move, even after much deliberation, remains uncertain. This is not necessarily because we have an overwhelming number of options (as is the case with Wild Oat or Shasta Daisy) or because of change or crisis (as with Walnut) but is due to uncertainty about what is required next. Unlike the Walnut situation, where we need to make a decision after *thinking* it through, the Onion state of mind needs to make a decision that is *felt* in the heart. An emergency unit doctor needs to make quick, clinical decisions that have immediate, quantifiable, potentially life-saving results for patients but a holistic health practitioner in a practice in the suburbs needs to make mindful decisions that have a qualitative impact both immediately and in the long term, and this latter process is facilitated by Onion flower essence.

Benefits of taking Onion

As mentioned above, the analogy of peeling off the skins of an Onion is relevant. With the flower essence we peel away our current layer of understanding in order to see and understand at a deeper level. The essence helps us to dissolve restrictive barriers, especially emotional ones, that have protected areas of naivety in our lives until now, which no longer serve us. By getting to the heart of things and sensing the root causes of our problems we can apply these new insights and make progress. For this reason, Onion can be particularly useful in counselling and/or psychotherapy. It helps us to have a better 'felt' sense of where we are in life and recognise clearly what the next move entails.

Possible physical imbalances

Traditional Chinese Medicine informs us that sinus and 'head colds' indicate the 'heart trying to reach the head.' Onions have traditionally been used as an expectorant and the homeopathic form of the plant is prescribed for many upper respiratory ailments, especially when there is much sneezing. It can feel so good to have big sneeze!

Common uses

When the way is lost; unsure about next step; for the 'Where to now?' feeling; for indecision; for lack of foresight; to gain insight; to get a better life perspective; for a holistic view; to sense what does and doesn't need to be done next; for patience in anticipation of change

Complementary &/or similar flower essences

Almond, Angelica, Apricot, Black Eyed Susan, Blackberry, Boab, Californian Poppy, Cayenne, Chestnut Bud, Coffee, Deerbrush, Filaree, Foxglove, Golden Ear Drops, Impatiens, Iris, Lady's Slipper, Love-Lies-Bleeding, Mullein, Queen Anne's Lace, Scleranthus, Shasta Daisy, Silver Princess, Star Tulip, Walnut, Wild Oat

Supporting the changes

* Seek out 'active listening' or 'heart to heart' counselling with an appropriate person.
* Meditation is an excellent way of 'going inside oneself' to reach your 'heart.'
* Take regular time out from your busy schedule to reflect on life.
* Stop and listen to your heart!

Oregon Grape
Berberis aquifolium   (Yellow / FES)

Positive state
Trusting others' goodwill (FES)
Inclusiveness (FES)

Negative state
Socially paranoid (FES)
Fear-driven defensiveness which ostracises others

Oregon Grape's flower is bright *yellow*, which reflects its connection with the *solar plexus chakra*. The state of the solar plexus influences how well we present ourselves in the world, and whether or not we are able to *stand out confidently as individuals and 'shine.'* Solar plexus consciousness relates to the transition from *intra-*personal aspects of our being (as represented by the chakras below) to the *inter-*personal aspects of our being (the chakras above). Oregon Grape flower essence helps us to step forward confidently without *projecting* our own *internal fears* onto others.

The Oregon Grape personality

People who benefit most from Oregon Grape flower essence have ungrounded fears about the reactions of the bunch (of grapes!) they hang out with – especially peers. They fear the worst in terms of emotional hostility from those nearby and may be paranoid about how people around will react to any expression of individuality on their part. Kaminski and Katz (1996) tell us that 'these patterns were learned in childhood from the family or culture, and have not been healed,' leaving individuals 'set up' to expect the world to be hostile, unfair and unsafe. This fear can become a self-fulfilling prophecy – we look for ill will in the world and that is what we find, and this cycle of alienation can leave us with a tendency to avoid full involvement.

Benefits of taking Oregon Grape

Oregon Grape flower essence helps us re-establish and develop trust in the goodwill of others. It heals past emotional wounds – unresolved scars left from seemingly unfair experiences in an unjust world. But as Oregon Grape nurtures our potential to trust, our focus shifts to the positive intentions of others and creates situations of goodwill and loving inclusion (Kaminski and Katz 1996). We learn that trusting in the goodness of others allows us to be nourished by the milk of human kindness.

Possible physical imbalances

I have found that inflammatory skin conditions such as eczema are not uncommon among those who respond well to Oregon Grape flower essence. The skin often gives clues about our internal reaction to the external environment.

Common uses

For social paranoia; for fearing the worst in others; when anxiously anticipating emotional hostility from others; for projection of our fears onto others; for inner confidence; to be more comfortable in social situations; to be warmly self-assertive; to trust in the good will of others

Complementary &/or similar flower essences

Angelica, Aspen, Baby Blue Eyes, Buttercup, Calendula, Garlic, Golden Yarrow, Hibbertia, Mallow, Mimulus, Quaking grass, Red Clover, Shooting Star, St John's Wort, Star Thistle, Sunflower, Sweet Pea, Violet

Supporting the changes

- Study Carl Jung's concepts of projection or transference, in which we see others as the cause of our difficulties.
- Learn meditation or deep relaxation techniques. Let go and let the good in.
- Learn to trust!

Pansy

Viola tricolor   (Violet/yellow / FES-res)

Positive state

Optimism with broad/inclusive thinking
Wellness health model

Negative state

Pessimism with insular/exclusive thinking
Disease medical model

The wild Pansy, original ancestor of the garden plant, is regarded as a weed in fields and gardens. It is also known as Heartsease as it was thought to soothe the pain of a broken heart. The name Pansy comes from the French *pensées*, or *'thoughts,'* and for centuries a gift of pansies has meant, 'You are in my thoughts' in the language of flowers. It is no coincidence that Pansy flower essence has an influence on our thought forms. It stimulates the *mental body*, magnifying and improving the *quality of thought forms* we create. This gives protection against negative thinking (in the 'ether' around us), maintaining the *integrity of our thought patterns*.

This protective quality is particularly useful against the *mindset* that develops when we become *over-identified with our illness*. Pansy is also protective against group hysteria associated with contagious diseases such as winter influenza and with other illnesses such as cancer or HIV/Aids. Pansy flower essence can help us adapt and change our thinking without being overly influenced by the attitudes of the surrounding culture. Just as the plant displays its independent nature in the wild as the first flower to bloom in disturbed ground, so the flower essence can help us to *think 'outside the square'* in relation to health issues.

The Pansy state of mind

The negative Pansy state can be seen when someone has endured a long-term illness or health condition that affects the way they see the world. Limitation and compromised wellbeing can come to seem like their lot in life; they forget how they felt or thought when they were well.

Benefits of taking Pansy

Pansy flower essence can remind someone who has been unwell how to think outside the mental inhibitions of their illness so that they can be more open to the possibility of being well. This is not a false hope for a sudden or complete recovery but an opening and elevation of the mind to a different perspective on one's health and wellbeing. This change in perspective can help us transcend our over-identification with a diagnosed clinical condition or medical label.

Pansy flower essence can help clear a pathological way of thinking that has developed around the experience of a chronic health condition. It transforms the 'ill-fated' or 'doomed' mentality that causes us to self-identify as a victim of disease and limits hope and so potential for recovery. This is especially true in relation to diseases such as epidemic flu, HIV/AIDS and cancer, which can generate widespread paranoia, but is also true of any illness where there is a 'general consensus' about a negative outcome.

Negative thinking can affect our natural immunity in an insidious, undermining way, as psychoneuroimmunology studies testify. Pansy flower essence can help uplift our depressed attitude and resigned mindset to allow a broader and more creative view that also encompasses the potential for wellness and happiness.

Possible physical imbalances

Pansy essence relates to the mindset associated with disease rather than to any one disease in particular. Pansy should always be considered when there is strong fear of 'catching' a disease or resignation about ever being free of a disease.

Common uses

When over-identified with your disease; when resigned to never recovering; for those who have lost sight of what it is to be well; to protect against negative thinking associated with a disease; to remain positive; to be open and receptive to a 'wellness' health model

Complementary &/or similar flower essences

Angel's Trumpet, Borage, Cayenne, Crab Apple, Echinacea, Filaree, Garlic, Gentian, Gorse, Hound's Tongue, Heather, Hibbertia, Iris, Morning Glory, Mountain Pennyroyal, Red Clover, Self-Heal, Shasta Daisy, Tansy, Waratah, Wild Rose, Willow, YES formula

Supporting the changes

- Explore different philosophical approaches to life, especially those of people you admire and respect. Read examples of successful and natural negotiation of serious disease.
- Seek out the 'Creative living' or 'Lifestyle' section of a bookstore, newsagency or library to explore new (or long lost!) horizons.
- Take renewed interest in your diet, your lifestyle, your overall health – NOT just your disease! Consider consulting a holistic health practitioner.
- Aspire to WELLNESS.

Passionflower

Passiflora caerulea (Mauve / FES-res)

Positive state

'Bigger picture' – emotional IQ
Integrated feeling/thinking; passion

Negative state

Overly intellectual and objective
Thinking dominates feeling; impassive

Passionflower originates from the tropical Americas, where the Aztecs used the flowers and leaves as a *sedative*. Missionaries compared the intricate structure of the pale mauve, sweetly scented flowers to that of Jesus' crown of thorns, and the Passion of Christ gave the common name to the vine.

Passionflower essence unites our consciousness with our *spiritual body*, allowing us to perceive the *'bigger picture'* and see personal sacrifices in a wider context, sometimes referred to as 'Christ consciousness.' In Greek mythology, Chiron the 'wounded healer' is another figure who embodies this type of consciousness, teaching that through healing others we may heal ourselves.

Herbalists still value Passionflower herb for its use in treating insomnia and *disturbed sleep patterns*, and Passionflower essence confers the spiritual confidence that helps us to let go and let (our) God in, especially when retiring to sleep at night. The essence helps us overcome fears and resistances to *higher states of consciousness* through which, for example in our *dream life during sleep*, we receive *spiritual insight*.

Recent scientific studies have put the herb in the same category as St John's Wort in terms of its ability to help alleviate depression. For many people, depression occurs when they are unable to find their *'passion'* in life; Passionflower essence aligns the *crown chakra* to enable it to shed 'light' (or *grace*) and recognition on one's *true calling*.

The Passionflower personality

Passionflower essence is suited to strong-minded, rational people who have reached a stage where their emotions and passions can no longer be denied. The essence can help them to accept their feelings and integrate them better into their thinking.

Passionflower people may be successful academically or in other fields where a very astute and keen mind is required. They may have grown up in a home where family members seldom expressed their feelings, relating mainly on an intellectual level. For such people, restless sleep with an increased awareness of dreams is a telltale sign that they could benefit from taking Passionflower. After taking Passionflower, sleep becomes more restful and peaceful, as one becomes more receptive and comfortable in the 'dream life.'

Benefits of taking Passionflower

Passionflower adds spirit and passion to an overly academic or clinical approach to life. It can help a person to process buried emotions at a manageable pace, often during their dream life while asleep. Their emotional life can be integrated into their consciousness without strain on the nervous system. Emotional IQ is improved and intuitive qualities are enhanced.

Possible physical imbalances

Some of the plant's herbal qualities are passed on by the essence, such as improved quality of sleep (especially when dreams have been vivid and disturbingly persistent) and lessening of nervous tension. I have also found in my practice as a therapist that in some cases it can help people reach acceptance of their ailments so that they learn to live with them better – especially in the area of pain management (also consider Love-Lies-Bleeding).

Common uses

For overly 'cerebral' or academic people; for restless sleep disturbed by dreams; to help contact your 'feeling' side; to broaden your mind beyond your brain!; to discover your passion; to increase your emotional IQ; to trust your intuition

Complementary &/or similar flower essences

Black Eyed Susan, Chrysanthemum, Harvest Brodiaea, Hibbertia, Hibiscus, Hound's Tongue, Iris, Lotus, Mallow, Mugwort, Nasturtium, Nicotiana, Shasta Daisy, Tall Yellow Top

Supporting the changes

- Explore the world of the arts (healing arts included) and find something that ignites your passion.
- Work in a group with an altruistic purpose that you can align with.
- In your leisure time do some things that use different skills or parts of your brain from those you usually use at work.
- Throughout the day, repeatedly ask yourself, 'How do I feel about this?'
- Meditate.

Paw Paw

Carica papaya   (Cream/yellow centre / Aus)

Positive state

Discerning decision making
Calm, open and decisive

Negative state

'Gut-feeling' indigestion – 'burdened by decision-making' (Ian White)
Information overload

Paw Paw and papaya fruits contain the enzyme papain which breaks down protein. Papain herbal supplements are commonly sold in health food stores to assist people who have digestive problems, especially where there is difficulty digesting protein. Paw Paw as a flower essence helps people 'digest' what is happening in their lives and *assimilate information* presented to them. *Discernment* and better *decision-making* follows, just as the human digestive system breaks down the food we eat, discerning which parts can be assimilated and which should be excreted. (Many people report that the fruit smells a little like vomit, reflecting the fact that, like our stomach contents, it is rich in *digestive enzymes*.)

The fruit not only aids digestion but also speeds up digestive tract transit time to the point where some people get diarrhoea when they eat it. In keeping with this aspect of the plant signature, Paw Paw flower essence helps release blockages to *assimilation*, making it possible to *let go* of what's no longer needed and make room for *new ideas and experiences*. It can help us to *resonate* with what is best for us in our lives.

The tree produces male, female and hermaphrodite flowers. It is interesting to note that even today some people are born as hermaphrodites – that is, they have physical characteristics that belong to both sexes. Furthermore, some reputable psychological research findings have shown that as few as 30% of the population are absolutely certain about their sexual identity as either heterosexual or homosexual and the remaining 70% are *unsure and/or fluid*. My experience in practice, which is supported by that of some of my colleagues, is that Paw Paw flower essence can assist some people who are experiencing an identity crisis of this kind by allowing them to be more *comfortable with and accepting of* their sexual orientation.

The Paw Paw state of mind

Consider Paw Paw flower essence when changing jobs, coming to terms with new technology or feeling overwhelmed by new information you need to take in.

Paw Paw flower essence treats gut-feeling 'indigestion' and can bring calmness and clarity to your thoughts as you absorb new and challenging experiences.

Benefits of taking Paw Paw

Paw Paw flower essence helps us to assimilate and integrate information, concepts and ideas. It is particularly useful during times of intense study and during times of change when the right moves or decisions are crucial for future happiness. It strengthens intuition and helps us find solutions to our problems. Consider using Paw Paw when you are struggling with major life decisions or feel baffled and bewildered by a subject you are studying and have trouble with 'assimilation and integration of new ideas' (White 2008).

Possible physical imbalances

As a therapist I have found that a mix of Paw Paw, Chamomile and Dill flower essences is very useful for babies who suffer from colic or who seem overwhelmed, finding it difficult to digest and adjust to their 'new' life. Taken over a few days, this combination often helps the infant settle in and feel more at home on Earth. The parents often find it helpful too!

Common uses

For information overload; when learning new jobs; during intense study periods; for assimilation of new information and experience; for better 'vision' regarding where you are at; to help you resonate with what is right for you; for discernment in decision making; to enhance your intuition

Complementary &/or similar flower essences

Californian Poppy, Chamomile, Chaparral, Corn, Crowea, Dill, Filaree, Indian Pink, Iris, Lavender, Madia, Rabbitbrush, Scleranthus, Shasta Daisy, Star Tulip, Wild Oat, YES formula

Supporting the changes

- Attend to lifestyle and diet, focusing on balance.
- Integrate contemplative practices such as meditation, yoga or tai chi into your daily routines.
- 'Unclutter' and make some space in your life!

Peppermint

Mentha piperita (Reddish-violet / FES)

Positive state

Mentally refreshed and clear-headed
Conscious and alert

Negative state

'Mental lethargy' (FES)
Dull minded (FES)

Peppermint is a very popular herb and has a long history: the ancient Egyptians cooked with it; the Chinese and Japanese used it in medicines; Greek athletes rubbed it into their muscles before competitions; the ancient Romans used it in garlands to stimulate *clear thoughts* and enhance *inspiration and concentration*.

The *reddish-violet* flowers symbolise the ability of the essence to attune the *base chakra* with the *crown chakra*, just as the earth wire of a radio receiver (base chakra) ensures that the signal can come in loud and clear (crown chakra). Peppermint flower essence facilitates the soul's inspirational energy flow into our conscious being, giving us purpose and the ability to *'get moving'* when we are feeling sluggish and stagnant.

People have often benefited from taking Peppermint flower essence after engaging in taxing mental work, especially the type that has a monotonous, repetitive quality. Astrologically, it can also be thought of as being useful for the cloudy, confusing effects of Mercury in Retrograde. When thoughts are repeatedly turning back on themselves like a recording stuck on a short loop, the flower essence can help to restore *mental momentum and quickness of thinking* that will break the loop and make it possible to *start afresh and move forward*.

The Peppermint state of mind

Peppermint flower essence can be useful when your body feels lethargic and sluggish and your mind is numb or apathetic. This state is often induced by excessive study and concentration, especially of a repetitive kind, and the remedy is very useful for students who are studying for exams and the teachers who are correcting students' work.

Benefits of taking Peppermint

Peppermint flower essence helps clear the head. It lightens up and clears a mind that is dull and congested from excessive mental work. I have often prescribed it for teachers and students at the end of the semester when 'brain fag' sets in.

Peppermint can help promote a more active and alert state of mind for students, academics, desk workers and anyone who needs mental inspiration.

Possible physical imbalances

Those who can benefit from Peppermint flower essence often have digestive problems and may crave a quick fix from 'pick-me-up' foods that ultimately render them even more sluggish.

Common uses

For a sluggish mind; for those mentally weary after prolonged, repetitious mental work; to provide a spark in your life; to 'get into gear'; for a natural mental quickening; for mental clarity

Complementary &/or similar flower essences

Blackberry, Cayenne, Clematis, Coffee, Forget-Me-Not, Harvest Brodiaea, Hornbeam, Hound's Tongue, Indian Paintbrush, Iris, Lemon, Morning Glory, Nasturtium, Silver Princess, Tansy

Supporting the changes

- Take more interest in your health. Investigate natural treatments and ease into a pattern of regular exercise.
- 'All work and no play makes Jack a dull boy.' Don't get stuck in a rut. Develop a better balance of work, rest and play and redefine your priorities for quality of life.
- Redesign your study/office, move the furniture and change your perspective.
- Take a break. Do something different. Freshen up!

Pine

Pinus sylvestris (Red female & yellow male / Bach)

Positive state

Wisdom gained from lessons learned
Forgiveness of self and others

Negative state

Guilt and regret about the past
Self-reproach

Pine trees have an upright, elongated shape and their vertical growth far exceeds their width. The leaves are pointed, thin and needle-like and the tree's aroma *sharply pervades* the immediate environment.

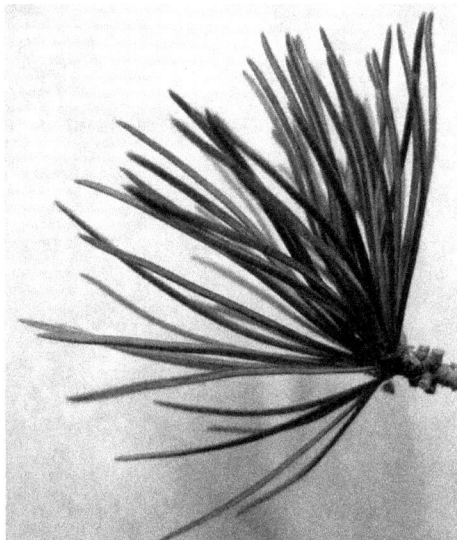

These qualities reflect the ability of the flower essence to enable us to be more *direct* and able to break free of the emotional *shackles of the past* and in particular, *guilt* about past 'mistakes.'

Pine has been on the Earth for a very long time. It has the ability to propagate itself and survive in a range of environments including difficult climates and terrains. Pine has always been recognised for having the capacity to carry on and thrive under almost any circumstances – hence the many Pine plantations that have been grown all around the world. I remember my botany lecturer at university saying, 'If any plant could survive a nuclear holocaust, it would be Pine.'

Sadly, at present many of us have lost our deep understanding of the Earth and at some level we 'pine' for what we have lost, *regretting our past* indiscretions against nature, which individually and collectively have left a legacy of *guilt*. Pine flower essence can help us to let go of the past and *move on* without being inhibited by previous tragic mistakes or errors of judgement.

Today, Pine oil is used commercially as a disinfectant and Pine flower essence acts as an *'negative emotion disinfectant'* which can be used whenever we feel burdened by regret about our actions, or non-actions, and what has transpired in our lives.

The Pine personality

In the negative state, Pine people regret the past and cling to it in the hope that it can be changed. The past will never change but our attitude towards it can. If our attitude and perspective doesn't change, we condemn ourselves to a life of guilt and self-reproach.

It is difficult to succeed in the present if we continue to relive the failures of the past. In fact, some of us may adopt a perfectionist approach to life as a way of undoing the damage done by past imperfections. But by setting ourselves unrealistically high standards and goals, we inevitably fall short and perpetuate our feelings of failure and guilt.

Benefits of taking Pine

Pine flower essence helps us to see the past more positively, viewing our 'errors' of judgement and behaviour as points on a timeline that serve as a learning curve. This allows us to adopt a more progressive approach that brings the desire and ability to move on and forward.

Possible physical imbalances

As Pine self-reproach eats away at the mind, the body often follows in sympathy. I have found in practice that this over time can lead to auto-immune type diseases, especially of an inflammatory rheumatic nature, but also of the lower bowel or colon – an area of the body which may give us indications about one's ability to let go of the past.

Common uses

For over-dutiful people who feel guilt-ridden over some failure of obligation; for those who easily take responsibility for the failings of others; for the self-reproachful perfectionist; for strong feelings of guilt (or resentment towards whoever you believe is making you feel that way?!); to help let yourself off the hook; to forgive yourself and others; to appreciate wisdom gained and move on

Complementary &/or similar flower essences

Arnica, Baby Blue Eyes, Cayenne, Crab Apple, Dogwood, Golden Ear Drops, Honeysuckle, Larkspur, Pink Monkeyflower, Sage, Sturt Desert Pea, Walnut, Willow, Yerba Santa

Supporting the changes

- Do some research into concepts such as personal evolution and karma.
- Practise forgiveness of self and others through counselling, meditative disciplines or any other means available to you. This will enable you to view your life with more balance and optimism.
- Work to construct an environment – family, friends, occupation – that will appreciate, respect and reinforce your talents and abilities.
- Always remember, you're allowed to make mistakes.
- No one's perfect!

Pink Yarrow

Achillea millefolium var. rubra (Pink-purple / FES)

Positive state

'Self-contained consciousness' (FES) while maintaining empathy
Emotional clarity

Negative state

Overly sympathetic – 'psychic sponge'
Lacking emotional boundaries (FES)

P lants of the Yarrow family, including Pink Yarrow, *protect against negativity* in the immediate environment. The colour of *Pink* Yarrow signifies its relationship with the *heart chakra* and its 'protective' qualities regarding those to whom we are closely *emotionally attached*. It acts like an energetic *emotional buffer* between us and our loved ones – *emotional boundaries* become better defined. Pink Yarrow protects against *negative emotions*, while (White) Yarrow provides protection against radiation, geopathic stress and other negative factors in the physical environment (Kaminski and Katz 1996). Please refer to the Yarrow and YES formula entries for in-depth descriptions of the various Yarrow qualities.

The Pink Yarrow personality

Pink Yarrow flower essence assists people who are emotionally oversensitive and act like 'psychic sponges,' absorbing everyone else's feelings. Kaminski and Katz (1996) speak of how in the negative state we can too easily engage in 'overly sympathetic identification with others' and take on board all the problems of partners, family members, colleagues, close friends or clients.   P i n k Yarrow flower essence can be very useful for children who outwardly appear to have weathered a family upheaval such as a marriage break-up better than any of their siblings. As a result, parents may confide in these children because they don't show signs of distress or 'act out' in the way other siblings may do to protect their own 'emotional space.' However, after a while the child may show a tendency to get sick more often and parents may begin to suspect that the child has in fact been affected more deeply than their calm exterior might indicate.

When a child takes this essence, parents should be prepared for the child to speak up more and be more reactive as they sort out their genuine (primary) emotional responses to changed circumstances.

Benefits of taking Pink Yarrow

Pink Yarrow flower essence has a strong affinity to the heart chakra. It helps strengthen personal emotional boundaries that protect us from the negative feelings of those close to us. It helps us develop a better sense of emotional clarity in our relationships, to take stock and consider feelings while setting up safe boundaries between self and loved ones.

Possible physical imbalances

When emotional boundaries are weak, the physical boundaries of our natural immunity may become weakened. Our mucous membranes may become compromised, making us more vulnerable to viral infections, allergies or more chronic immune dysfunction.

Common uses

For the 'psychic sponge' amongst friends and loved ones; for emotional oversensitivity; to prevent 'bleeding into another's wounds'; to help you distinguish between others' 'stuff' and yours; to help develop better emotional boundaries, especially in relationships; to strengthen one's natural emotional immunity

Complementary &/or similar flower essences

Angelsword, Bleeding Heart, Boab, Canyon Dudleya, Echinacea, Fringed Violet, Garlic, Golden Yarrow, Indian Pink, Love-Lies-Bleeding, Mountain Pennyroyal, Red Clover, St John's Wort, Walnut, Yarrow, YES formula

Supporting the changes

- Develop methods of dynamic self-protection such as visualisation of white light, meditation or protective rituals.
- Maintain a balanced lifestyle, especially when it comes to getting enough sleep. It is important to keep yourself grounded through activities such as gardening, pottery and outdoor exercise in open spaces full of greenery.
- Be very conscious of the people that you emotionally react to strongly.
- Secure your hide-away haven for regular time out to regroup – your room, your study, your shed, YOUR SPACE!

Pomegranate
Punica granatum (Red / FES)

Positive state
Emotionally inclusive – embracing all aspects of your life
Clear, creative direction in life (FES)

Negative state
Emotionally exclusive – divided allegiances
Confusion over family/career balance (FES)

Traditionally, the Pomegranate has been a seen as a symbol of *feminine fertility and creativity* because the fruit is thought to resemble the *uterus*, and the *rich red* colour of both flowers and fruit symbolises the *life-giving blood* that flows to it. In Greek mythology the goddess Hera is sometimes depicted holding the red fruit, *full of seeds*, representing positive femininity and *womanhood*. Pomegranate flower essence relates to the capacity for *creative expression*, especially for women.

Within the fruit, each of the many seeds is separated from the rest inside a capsule of red, juicy flesh surrounded by a membrane.

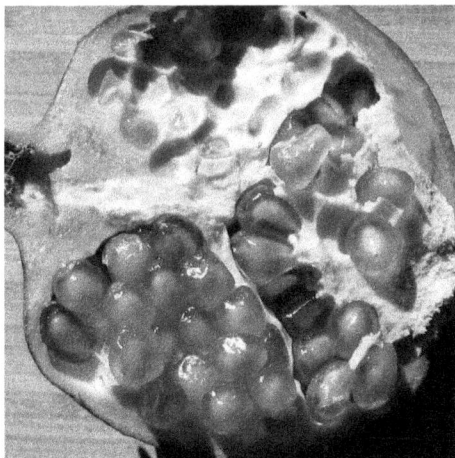

The colour is also symbolic of *passion and basic emotion* – qualities associated with the *base chakra* – and the compart*mental*isation of the seeds is symbolic of the way we often compartmentalise these types of *powerful feelings*. This may occur because we don't know how to integrate strong emotions appropriately and creatively in our everyday life. And if we do, indulging in our *creative passions* may be seen by some as being selfish and/or irresponsible. Pomegranate flower essence can help us learn valuable lessons and grow from our experiences where we have to negotiate a balance between personal needs and the *greater good* of the relationship, the family, the group, the community or society.

Pomegranate flower essence can help when there is a need for separation and balance between potentially conflicting roles. For example, parents, and especially mothers, need to constantly 'put on different hats' – *'compartmentalising'* life as they move between roles of nurturing parent at home and career and/or creative person out in the world. Kaminski and Katz (1996) tell us that Pomegranate can help to achieve creative balance between procreation and creativity and between *family and career*.

The Pomegranate personality

Having to make a choice between raising children and pursuing a career has been, and still is, a common dilemma for many women, and now the same is true for an increasing number of men. A dilemma exists for many men, for instance, between demands made on their contribution at work and the need to BE and contribute more at home. Both men and women can benefit from Pomegranate flower essence when they feel that their responsibility to provide loving and 'hands on' support for loved ones overwhelms or restricts their capacity to contribute outside the family, especially in relation to fulfilment of personal passions and ambitions.

Benefits of taking Pomegranate

Today, Pomegranate flower essence is mainly used to help bring balanced, creative expression to our lives. It is indicated when creative focus is blurred by conflict between the needs of career and home, creation and procreation or personal and global responsibilities. When you are torn between traditional values of family/home and creative/productive service in the outside world, Pomegranate will help you reconcile this within yourself.

Possible physical imbalances

In my experience as a natural therapist, a number of women have benefited from taking Pomegranate flower essence who have had a history of health issues relating to their menstrual cycle and reproductive organs, accompanied by a sense of resentment and frustration about 'that time of the month.' Pomegranate can help women come to a better understanding and acceptance of this important aspect of their lives, which in turn brings an improvement in physical symptoms.

Common uses

For emotional secularism; for being torn in your allegiances; confusion between family and career, personal and global needs; for frustrated creative expression; for emotional inclusiveness – the world is your home; for the right balance in one's life

Complementary &/or similar flower essences

Aloe Vera, Alpine Lily, Calla Lily, Elm, Fairy Lantern, Hibiscus, Indian Paintbrush, Iris, Lady's Slipper, Larch, Mariposa Lily, Quince, She Oak, Tiger Lily, Watermelon

Supporting the changes

- Study the concepts of yin and yang, anima and animus, and the importance of goddesses in mythology. Learn to understand and better appreciate the feminine principle.
- Recognise and learn to respond to your body rhythms and cycles – men have these as well. Tune in to them to make them work for you, rather than being at their mercy.
- Nurture yourself so that you can help to sustain others.
- Fully embrace all aspects of your life!

Pretty Face
Triteleia ixioides (Yellow, brown stripes / FES)

Positive state
Self-acceptance – 'warts and all'
'Beauty that radiates from within' (FES)

Negative state
Feels unattractive (FES)
Obsessed with aspects of personal appearance

Pretty Face's name says it all! The flower has a pretty and striking 'face' whose external beauty immediately attracts attention. The plant represents the world view that places emphasis on *external appearance* as an indicator of *inner beauty*. This approach is widespread in many societies.

The *yellow* colour of the flower relates to the *solar plexus chakra*, whose condition reflects how confidently we *'shine'* in the world.

Pretty Face flower essence helps us to communicate the *beauty within* us irrespective of outward appearance and gives access to our real and *enduring personal beauty*.

The Pretty Face state of mind

Western societies place great emphasis on external presentation: 'It needs to look good to sell'; 'Stay young and beautiful if you want to be loved and admired'; and most destructive of all, 'You need to stay young, fresh and sexy if you want to serve any useful purpose.' These attitudes put great pressure on all of us, and especially on women, to maintain an attractive personal appearance. The cosmetic and dieting industries have done very well as a result of this over-identification with physical appearance.

Pretty Face flower essence can be helpful in many different situations – for those born with physical deformities or unsightly features who are especially challenged to find their own inner worth and goodness (Kaminski and Katz 1996); for those who feel an excessive need to groom and alter their appearance and for those who fear ageing and the wrinkles (or lines of wisdom!) that go with it.

Consider Pretty Face when you over-identify with your physical appearance or are overly self-conscious and easily lose your connection with the real, sustainable and lasting beauty within.

Benefits of taking Pretty Face

Pretty Face flower essence helps us move beyond our over-emphasis on superficial things, allowing our inner beauty to shine out.

Possible physical imbalances

People who have suffered from long-term skin conditions often respond well to Pretty Face flower essence, when their appearance has become a focus of insecurity. It is also useful at times when we become acutely aware of the ageing process that is occurring in our physical bodies, especially approaching midlife.

Common uses

For poor body image; for obsession about one's external appearance; for those who 'judge a book by its cover'; to see through the superficial; to see and feel the beauty within; to accept yourself as you are; to be comfortable in your body

Complementary &/or similar flower essences

Billy Goat Plum, Buttercup, Chrysanthemum, Crab Apple, Heather, Manzanita, Sagebrush, Sunflower

Supporting the changes

- Forget about 'keeping up with the Joneses'!
- Cultivate relationships with people who accept you the way you are.
- Nurture and nourish your body by recognising its needs.
- Never judge by appearances.

Quince

Chaenomeles speciosa (Red / FES)

Positive state

Empowering others through nurture (FES)
Ability to provide loving guidance

Negative state

Denial of feminine/nurturing side (FES)
Overly authoritarian – autocratic

The red colour of the flowering Quince blossom reflects its relationship with the *base chakra* – the source of *personal power* and ability to assert one's will. The higher octave of the base chakra is the *heart chakra*, which is the source of *love and service*. Quince flower essence can help us to reconcile these apparent opposites and achieve a balance between the need for power (*the will*) and the ability to *love and nurture* (the *heart*); between *'tough love'* and the need to be kind; between directing things to suit ourselves and being directed by the *needs of others*.

The Quince personality

Quince flower essence is of great value to primary carers such as single mothers, who must strike the difficult balance between ruling with authority and nurturing with love (Kaminski and Katz 1996). Any parent or carer (or boss) who fears that they may lose their authority if they appear too 'soft' can benefit from taking Quince. It can also bring balance when, as a parent alone for long periods with children, you develop a tendency to appear strong and authoritative at the expense of your 'feminine' or nurturing side.

Benefits of taking Quince

Quince helps people reconcile affection and gentleness with discipline and authority, allowing them to show that love requires strength and vice versa.

A husband and wife I know ran a large, busy restaurant. The wife managed the staff and everyday running of the kitchen while her husband attended to the orders, general business and accounts. Their shop was held up and robbed, and about a month later, the wife came to see me about her health. She told me how difficult it had been for her to get all the staff to resume their normal routine and responsibilities. She understood and accepted that everyone needed time to adjust after the shock and trauma of the robbery and she had, as she put it, 'let things go a little.' As a result, many of the staff had fallen into bad habits and this was starting to affect the restaurant's service and presentation. She didn't know how to approach her staff – she took pride in treating them just like family – but needed to help them 'get their act together.' Quince flower essence proved beneficial, helping her achieve the required blend of managerial authority and generous understanding. She and her staff began to function smoothly once again.

Possible physical imbalances

I have observed that those who respond well to Quince flower essence sometimes have a history of hormonal imbalance or imbalance that manifests around menopause, when a woman's relationship with her feminine side is revisited.

Common uses

To soften your attitude; for those who operate only from a position of power – 'I'm in charge – do it because I say so!'; for fear you will lose control of a situation; to give more latitude; to develop a win/win attitude; to show more heart; to empower through loving and nurturing

Complementary &/or similar flower essences

Baby Blue Eyes, Bleeding Heart, Calendula, Calla Lily, Chicory, Flannel Flower, Larkspur, Mallow, Mariposa Lily, Pomegranate, Snapdragon, Squash, Star Tulip, Tiger Lily, Vine

Supporting the changes

- Study the concepts of yin and yang forces in Chinese medicine, the anima and animus in Jungian psychology and the importance of balance between them.
- Nurture yourself so that you can provide sustenance for others.
- Be empowered and empower with love.
- Open your heart.

Rabbitbrush

Ericameria nauseosa
(formerly *Chrysothamnus nauseosus*) (Yellow / FES)

Positive state

Integrated understanding of many simultaneous events
'Acute sensory perception' (FES) encompassing the 'big picture'

Negative state

Overwhelmed and overstimulated by details and events
Distracted, easily side-tracked, scattered

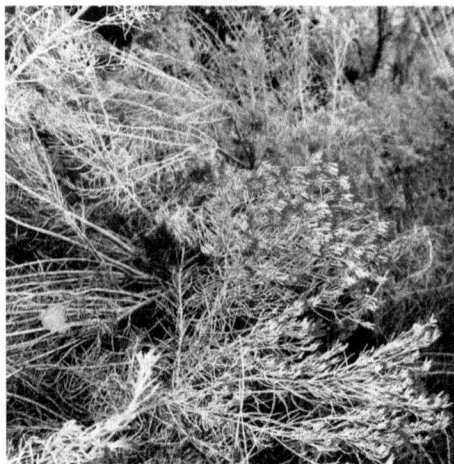

abbitbrush at first glance looks untidy, *scattered and erratic* – its growth is all over the place and Rabbitbrush flower essence is useful for minds that fit this description.

The plant's yellow flowers signify its association with the *solar plexus chakra* and how we take in and *'digest'* the world around us. If we are too easily thrown by activity in our environment we become *overwhelmed*, stressed and *mentally scattered*. Rabbitbrush eases the *overstimulated* solar plexus area, helping people to *focus* and have an inner sense of the job at hand so that they don't become *distracted and easily side-tracked*.

The Rabbitbrush state of mind

Rabbitbrush flower essence is helpful when studying complex subjects and for people in busy workplaces who are constantly subject to a variety of demands. It can be of use for anyone who feels overwhelmed, distracted and mentally scattered by details and differing perspectives that need to be considered at the same time.

Benefits of taking Rabbitbrush

Rabbitbrush helps us spread our attention in order to integrate our understanding of many simultaneous events. As Kaminski and Katz (1996) put it, it takes a special gift to be able to maintain both 'focused attention to detail, and a wide ranging perspective which can encompass the "big picture."' Rabbitbrush can help us remain focused and not become flustered or overwhelmed by activity around us or details that need our attention. If you have ever seen a radio presenter at work, you will have been struck by the number of activities they attend to at one time. An experienced presenter remains in complete command of the situation despite this pressure. They listen to talkback callers while deciding which music to play, preparing for the next advertisement and taking note of directions from their producer.

Rabbitbrush helps us develop and maintain an active and lively consciousness and an alert and flexible state of mind. A useful study mix is Rabbitbrush in combination with Shasta Daisy, Madia, Lemon and Elm.

Possible physical imbalances

Constant mental stress can lead to many physical problems ranging from headaches and digestive disturbances to general nervous tension and other nerve-related issues.

Common uses

For scattered thinking; for inability to focus and concentrate; when your life is 'all over the shop'; as a study aid; to help you multi-task effectively; to focus your attention; for a dynamic and flexible state of mind

Complementary &/or similar flower essences

Blackberry, Californian Poppy, Clematis, Corn, Cosmos, Crowea, Dill, Elm, Filaree, Indian Pink, Jacaranda, Madia, Paw Paw, Peppermint, Red Lily, Rosemary, Shasta Daisy, White Chestnut

Supporting the changes

- Study time management and goal-setting and learn how to prioritise activities.
- Integrate relaxation, contemplative time or meditation techniques into your busy life.
- Tidy up your desk or workplace and de-clutter your home environment.

Red Chestnut
Aesculus cornea (Pink-red / Bach)

Positive state
Projecting love – empathy
Emotional security about loved ones

Negative state
Projecting fear – sympathy
Over-concern for others

Red Chestnut trees are smaller and *less robust* than White Chestnut trees and are thought to be the result of a chance hybrid between a White Chestnut and a Buckeye Chestnut. They produce masses of deep *pink-red* flowers that are gathered in early summer and boiled to make the Bach flower remedy (Barnard 1988). The pink-red flower colour shows a simultaneous relationship with both the *heart chakra* and the *base chakra*. *Emotional attachment* (heart) and *fear* ('base' survival instincts) combine to create *fear and anxiety about the welfare of others*, especially your loved ones. When the Red Chestnut is in bloom the whole tree seems lit up by its flowers, radiating an impression of warm strength which is the polar opposite of fearful concern. In this way it shows the possibility of a positive combination of love (pink/heart chakra) and power (red/base chakra).

The *deeply furrowed trunk* is symbolic of the *worry lines* that can develop in the face of an *overly concerned* parent, carer or partner. It is interesting to note that the Red Chestnut tree rarely grows in the wild and seems to prefer the safe environs of a garden or grove to unprotected life 'out in the jungle.'

The Red Chestnut personality

People in the unbalanced Red Chestnut state can become withered by worry and anxiety about the welfare of those close to them. They have overactive and outward-directed heart chakra energy that takes the form of exaggerated sympathy (as distinct from empathy) for others.

An example of this state can be seen in excessively anxious parents who feel continual fear for their children's safety when the children are not with them. Their thoughts are constantly focused on the worst that can happen to friends and loved ones. These anxieties may become self-fulfilling as they wait for what they believe is the worst inevitable outcome. Julian and Martine Barnard (1988) put it this way: 'If in our minds we anticipate misfortune, then we help to create the pattern that brings misfortune about.' Red Chestnut people feel great relief when their child returns from school safely, their partner returns from work without being involved in a car accident or when close friends make contact again after a period of absence.

Benefits of taking Red Chestnut

Red Chestnut flower essence can heal the heart and soothe excessive anxiety. By calming mental fears we can free ourselves to radiate harmonious and comforting thoughts towards our loved ones and friends. This flower essence allows us to step back far enough from others' mental and emotional troubles to be of help. We are freed to empathise with those close to us without losing our sense of proportion and personal power.

THE **ESSENTIAL** FLOWER ESSENCE BOOK

Possible physical imbalances

With all that heart energy (associated with the thymus gland) being directed outwards, the natural immunity of Red Chestnut people to surrounding stressful influences can easily become depleted. Burnout, adrenal fatigue and increased susceptibility to infection is common.

Common uses

For projection of fear onto others; for the anxious over-protective parent or friend; for the co-dependent health practitioner or social worker who is overly concerned about clients' welfare; for the over-sympathetic person who finds another's slightest distress gut-wrenching; to bring about transformation through empathy rather than stagnate through sympathy

Complementary &/or similar flower essences

Aspen, Bleeding Heart, Centaury, Chicory, Crab Apple, Crowea, Filaree, Mountain Pennyroyal, Pink Yarrow, Red Clover, Vervain, Walnut, White Chestnut

Supporting the changes

- Meditation, creative visualisation, positive affirmation, yoga and tai chi help centre and focus your energies so that you can develop a greater sense of self-awareness and a positive outlook.
- Spend a bit more 'ME' time alone and get to know yourself and your own needs.
- Try to give the person you are concerned about a bit more personal space.

Red Clover
Trifolium pratense   (Red / Bach)

Positive state
Securely anchored amid the 'storm'
Calm self-awareness during emergency/crisis (FES)

Negative state
Loss of Self 'in the crowd'
Highly susceptible to group panic/mass hysteria (FES)

Red Clover has a compact and ovoid flower head which In some ways resembles garlic, onion and waratah flowers. Like Red Clover, these three flower essences also help to integrate all levels of our being from the subtle to the gross, enabling them to *come together* as a *unified whole*. Red Clover helps us to *'get our act together'* under extreme pressure and in mentally or physically *highly charged* and/or threatening situations.

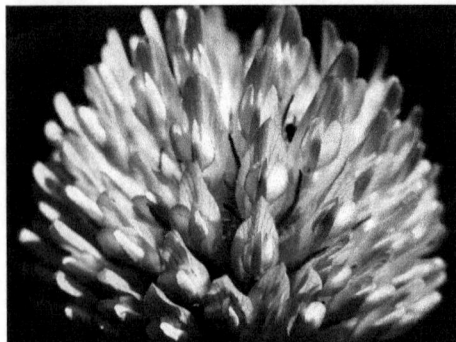

Red Clover flower essence *spiritualises the emotions* (and by contrast, many essences made from yellow flowers help to spiritualise the intellect) and this makes it very useful in situations of mass hysteria or panic. The *red* of the flower points to its affinity with the *base chakra* which when balanced has a grounding effect. This allows us to filter emotion absorbed from the atmosphere, transforming and re-releasing it and in this way breaking the emotional chain reaction.

The *spiritualisation of emotion* also makes it possible to gain a better understanding and acceptance of personal emotions through a *deeper sense of their purpose*, especially within relationships, including between partners or client and therapist.

The Red Clover state of mind

Kaminski and Katz (1996) tell us that people who can benefit from Red Clover flower essence are those whose 'ability to maintain [a] sense of individuality can be severely challenged in adverse situations, particularly where conditions of strong "mass consciousness" prevail.' Red Clover helps heal underlying and often unconscious fears of personal or existential annihilation by 'grounding' and strengthening us from within. This in turn improves the integrity of dynamic personal boundaries.

Consider Red Clover flower essence if you easily lose your personal identity in group situations or 'go with the flow' too willingly. Red Clover is useful when we experience a fearful sense of being overwhelmed that can develop into a panic attack. Red Clover helps defend us from becoming vulnerable to mass hysteria associated with sporting events, political and religious rallies, crowded airports and shopping centres and, of course, crisis situations (Kaminski and Katz 1996). Red Clover flower essence is also useful for animals when they are confined in an uncomfortable or fearful group setting – in this situation it can help to prevent contagious panic from developing.

Along with other therapists, I have found that Red Clover is a very important flower essence in its ability to quell fears that surround certain illnesses, from the latest 'flu' strain to cancer and HIV/AIDS. People who benefit from Red Clover flower essence are particularly susceptible to media scare campaigns. Red Clover may also be useful for those afflicted by these illnesses, protecting them against the negative and debilitating effects of panicky responses around them, especially the often-hysterical reactions of family and friends.

Benefits of taking Red Clover

Red Clover flower essence helps ease our susceptibility to fear when we find ourselves embroiled in situations where emotions run high, and helps us to remain grounded and anchored. In the midst of raging emotional storms we can find an inner calm and poise that provides an objective viewpoint. For panic attacks and other nervous complaints presenting acute symptoms, always seek medical advice if necessary and then consider Red Clover, especially in combination with other emergency flower essences such as Rock Rose, Star of Bethlehem, Cherry Plum and Nectarine.

Possible physical imbalances

Herbally, both Red Clover and Garlic are used as blood cleansers to improve natural immunity, and these qualities are transferred to the flower essences. From a psychosomatic perspective, our natural immunity to disease can be negatively affected by fear of disease itself. (The hormone produced in our bodies when we are stressed and fearful is cortisol and this is known to suppress our immune response.) Red Clover flower essence should be considered when there is a need to ease this fear. Also, anyone who easily absorbs negativity from their environment will be susceptible to some physical effects. Inability to resist or repel negativity in the emotional environment may manifest as lymphatic congestion. The lymphatic system acts like a 'rubbish disposal system,' processing toxins that accumulate in the blood.

Common uses

For panic attacks; for deep seated fear; to protect against mass hysteria; for strength/protection in crowds; to improve multi-dimensional immunity; to 'cleanse' after being in negative situations; to keep your dynamic integrity on all levels

Complementary &/or similar flower essences

Angel's Trumpet, Angelica, Arnica, Californian Poppy, Canyon Dudleya, Chaparral, Cherry Plum, Corn, Dill, Echinacea, Garlic, Indian Pink, Mimulus, Mountain Pennyroyal, Oregon Grape, Pink Yarrow, Rock Rose, St John's Wort, Violet, Walnut, Waratah, all the Yarrows, YES formula

Supporting the changes

- Make use of grounding and aura-protecting exercises such as work and play involving earth; practise creative visualisation and meditation.
- Consider bathing in, vapourising or wearing protective essential oils such as sandalwood, juniper and vetiver when going into emotionally charged situations.
- Cleansing diets, supervised or professionally guided fasts, exercise and massage should be considered to maintain the healthy functioning of the lymphatic

system and elimination of toxins from the body.
- Find a safe, secure and comfortable place that you can retreat to when necessary.

Red Grevillea
Grevillea speciosa (Red / Aus)

Positive state
Undaunted, free
Independent, receptive to change/new possibilities

Negative state
Subdued by environment, stuck
Dependent, fearful of change

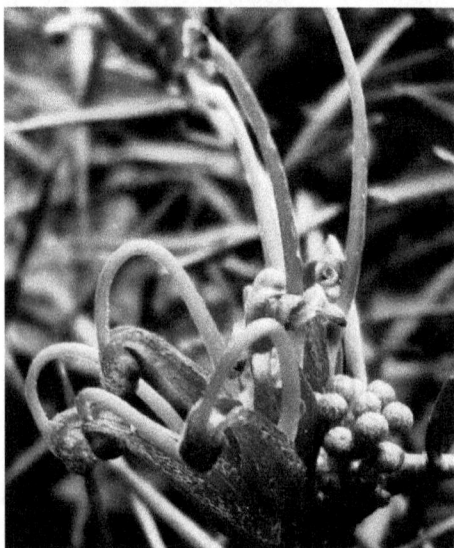

Red Grevillea's *red* tubular flowers first appear in large, *tightly bound*, circular clusters at the ends of branches or among the leaves. As they bloom, the flowers *unfold* like a clenched fist *opening* and becoming a *receptive* open hand.

This is symbolic of the flower essence's ability to assist release and *transformation of fears* that prevent us from opening up to new experiences or *new perspectives*, especially in personal relationships. Its decorative and showy flowers point to the *bold and fearless self-expression* that can be encouraged by the essence.

The Red Grevillea state of mind
Fear of change creates dependence, and dependence creates fear of change. For example, if we have a strong fear of change, we tend to remain dependent on long-established relationships and unsatisfactory living situations because of the security provided by their constancy and familiarity. We may even remain in situations that are emotionally abusive and mentally demoralising rather than face changing things. Or we may feel stuck (White 2008) in stagnant situations in which we no longer belong, unable to perceive a way out. Even when it becomes clear to us what our next move should be, we may be paralysed by our fear about what others will think or what their reaction might be.

Benefits of taking Red Grevillea

Red Grevillea flower essence helps to restore a sense of inner assurance, enabling us to be confident about following our true path in life and become less sensitive to the judgements and reactions of others. It can conjure in us the strength and courage to take decisive action to improve our situation (White 2008). What had seemed unattainable suddenly seems within our grasp.

Possible physical imbalances

Suppressed emotional oversensitivity and fearful attachment to a familiar environment can manifest physically – the body 'going out in sympathy' – as allergies and intolerances to food and other environmental factors. When we do not feel nurtured by our immediate and intimate environment, we may somatise this response and develop allergic and inflammatory reactions to it.

Common uses

Stuck in abusive relationships; for co-dependence; too reliant on an unsatisfactory source; too attached to other people's judgement; for the strength and courage to be bold; to dare!; for autonomy

Complementary &/or similar flower essences

Almond, Blackberry, Borage, Cayenne, Centaury, Iris, Mimulus, Oregon Grape, Sagebrush, Sweet Pea, Walnut, Waratah

Supporting the changes

- Try to take some time out of your normal routines and relationships so that you can catch a more objective glimpse of your life. Professional counselling may achieve the same end. This will allow you to establish personal priorities without undue influence by others.
- Assertiveness and self-esteem courses are invaluable, as are any activities that help you develop effective communication skills.
- Spend more time with people who encourage and support you to explore new experiences and be yourself.
- Do some research on dependency and co-dependency in relationships.
- Dare to be!

Rescue Remedy™

Star of Bethlehem, Rock Rose, Impatiens, Clematis and Cherry Plum in combination (Bach Flowers)

'When all else fails, or nothing else prevails.'

This jewel among the Bach Flower combinations was the product of Dr Bach's intuitive genius, with a perfect blend of qualities that make it a potent and yet gentle formula. Its multi-faceted nature also makes it accessible to the 'selective sensitivity' of all humanity. Rescue Remedy™ will help in all emergencies. It gives support in accident and trauma and helps to bring calm in situations where there is fear and panic. It helps to soothe the shell-shocked, settle the hysterical, consolidate the shattered and centre the disorientated. Rescue Remedy has a place in all homes!

Rescue Remedy can be used in emergency situations then followed later by specific flower essences based on your personality type to help you cope better in the future.

In research I conducted under supervision at Victoria University, I found that the most significant results (improvements) were gained in the anxiety/tension aspect of participants' profile of mood states (POMS) results, with other significant results obtained in all other areas (see the 'Contemporary Research' section of this book).

OTHER COMBINED REMEDIES:

Combining more than four flower essences is sometimes appropriate when prescribing for very general emotional or mental states and specific circumstances (as is the case with YES formula). Not all flower essences in each combination will elicit equally sensitive responses within the individual but they will have a cumulative (synergistic) effect.

Rock Rose

Helianthemum nummularium (Yellow / Bach)

Positive state

Mental calm and clarity
Transcending fear in order to 'shine'

Negative state

Terror/panic
Immobilised by fear

The *bright yellow* of the Rock Rose flower is paler around the edges and more concentrated towards its centre, which is emphasised by numerous, radiating, golden-yellow stamens. This paler periphery, intensifying towards a rich, golden centre, can be seen to represent the way in which someone who is overcome by *fear* may *withdraw* into themselves. Fear is a *contractive force* in energetic terms, as evidenced by a range of responses when we are fearful: we *'pull our head in,'* retreat, clam up, find a corner to hide in, breathe shallowly, tighten our abdomen etc. The opposite of this behaviour is to *stand strong* and be *unafraid to shine* – positive qualities related to a balanced *solar plexus chakra*, represented by the yellow colour of the flower.

The botanical name is derived from the Greek *helios* meaning 'sun,' while *nummularium* comes from a Latin word meaning 'coin-shaped' – the flowers shine like golden coins in the sun (Barnard 1988). Rock Rose flower essence helps us to *transcend fear* so that we can *shine* with the *radiance* of gold.

The Rock Rose state of mind

The negative Rock Rose state is an all-encompassing panic that involves intense anxiety and confusion. These are the qualities we associate with absolute terror: when a child has awoken from a nightmare, frozen with fear; when a first-time mother-to-be suddenly becomes afraid of labour and early motherhood; when a war veteran relives combat experiences. Rock Rose flower essence also helps to alleviate terror in anticipation of future events such as examinations, public performances, losing a job or having your worst nightmare come true.

Benefits of taking Rock Rose

Rock Rose flower essence can help prevent panic attacks and aids quick recovery when they have occurred. Panic attacks may continue while taking Rock Rose but they progressively become less intense and easier to manage. Like other flower essences, Rock Rose never suppresses feelings but helps us to work through difficult emotions until they are integrated within our whole emotionally balanced being. Free of excessive fear, we can live fully and feel at peace with ourselves and the world.

Possible physical imbalances

In the negative state, Rock Rose people may be prone to nervous digestive disorders, because the stomach is an area that reflects how we 'greet' each upcoming moment in time. The flower essence can be a useful supportive measure during the treatment of ACUTE and rapid onset physical problems that are associated with anxiety.

Common uses

For panic attacks and nightmares; for adrenal fatigue experienced by thrill-seekers or big event performers; for extreme anticipatory anxiety; for courage; to 'shine' through life's challenges

Complementary &/or similar flower essences

Angelica, Aspen, Borage, Cherry Plum, Garlic, Mimulus, Oregon Grape, Red Clover, Rescue Remedy, St John's Wort, Waratah

Supporting the changes

- Relaxation and meditation techniques, yoga and tai chi are all ways of developing inner calm, control and self-assurance.
- Grounding exercises and activities are recommended.
- Professional guidance and counselling may be considered.
- Creative visualisation may protect the solar plexus chakra – the centre where experiences of fear and terror are focused.

Rock Water

Spring or well water known for its healing qualities   (Bach)

Positive state

Flexibility and open-mindedness
Adaptability

Negative state

Obsession with ideals
Rigid formality

Rock Water, like the element of water everywhere, represents *movement, fluidity and emotional freedom and spontaneity*. These attributes describe the positive aspect of Rock Water flower essence. A steady stream or flow of water will, over time, etch its mark on even the *hardest of rock* and painlessly alter the most *rigidly held structures*.

No matter how *set, stuck and hardened* you have become on any level of your being, Rock Water can help *free you* from forms of *self-imposed bondage*, for example a tendency to become *'slave to a cause.'* Water will always follow the *'path of least resistance'* to its destiny of unification. Rock Water people hunger for unity through a shared ideal but in the negative state, often only manage the opposite, *alienating* themselves and meeting strong resistance when trying to put this ideal into practice.

The Rock Water personality

Rock Water people in the negative state place a rigid external ideal or set of beliefs before their own internal needs. For the sake of a way of living that has idealistic appeal they will sacrifice and deny desires and feelings. Unfortunately this behaviour is often viewed by others as self-righteous martyrdom, serving only to alienate them and their cause from family, friends and associates.

A classic Rock Water case history may look like this: A client comes to me for a consultation and lists major concerns about his general health. He describes his daily routine: He gets up at exactly 6.02 a.m. and begins the day with a 20 minute meditation; at 6.22 a.m. he goes for a brisk 15-minute walk; at 6.37 a.m. he schedules a bowel movement in which complete evacuation takes place (stressing that the quality of the whole day is dependent on this process); breakfast is a large bowl of muesli made from exactly weighed amounts of raw ingredients – the recipe comes from a book that outlines the rest of his regime – and so on, until bedtime at precisely 10.02 p.m. Needless to say this textbook lifestyle takes more from him than it gives. He, and to a lesser extent everyone around him, has become a victim of his own rigid regimentation. He has given up all his freedoms in pursuit of a way of life which (he believes) has worked beautifully for someone else.

Benefits of taking Rock Water

Rock Water can help us let go of much of our obsessive and/or very strict behaviour, allowing us to develop a more flexible approach that can accommodate spontaneous needs and desires, in this way making a place for enjoyment and pleasure.

Possible physical imbalances

The rigid mental make-up of the negative Rock Water state will eventually manifest structurally in the body. A range of complaints commonly develop, from muscular tension and stiffness through to rheumatic and arthritic conditions. Headaches – the head aching to follow the heart – are also common. Behaviours involving loss of control after over-control in the negative state may become a pattern, for example binge-eating after long periods of dieting and abstinence.

Common uses

For the perfectionist; for the martyr who sacrifices self as an example to all; for the fanatical idealist; for the workaholic; for the creature of habit; to enhance flexibility and adaptability; for a 'holiday' on the inside; to help bring back the JOY in our lives

Complementary &/or similar flower essences

Beech, Centaury, Chicory, Crab Apple, Dandelion, Dogwood, Elm, Filaree, Impatiens, Lady's Slipper, Larkspur, Lotus, Manzanita, Oak, Quaking Grass, Shooting Star, Sweet Pea, Vervain, Vine, Wild Oat, Willow

Supporting the changes

- Engage in physical exercise that improves suppleness, such as flexing and stretching exercises, yoga, tai chi. Do it purely for enjoyment!
- During the day, ask yourself regularly, 'How do I feel about this?' and try to follow your instinct whenever possible.
- Break some habits by taking a holiday.

Rosemary

Rosmarinus officinalis   (Violet-lavender / FES)

Positive state

'Warm physical presence' (FES)
Vitality; 'switched on mentally'

Negative state

'Forgetfulness' (FES); cold extremities
Vagueness; 'lights on, nobody home'

As herbal tincture or essential oil, Rosemary is used to stimulate circulation to the *extremities*, particularly the head. Historical records from ancient Greece, where Rosemary was used to strengthen *memory*, indicate that students wore sprigs of the herb in their hair while they studied. It stimulates a sense of *wakefulness and alertness* by spreading and *stimulating* the flow of blood throughout the body, just as when we exercise. Rosemary flower essence helps the *life-force energies* to expand throughout the body, giving us a sense of being physically grounded, *awake and clear-headed*.

The violet colour of the flower signifies its influence on the *crown chakra* (and pineal gland) which *'sheds light on the subject'* – where you are that subject! As a consequence you experience a *greater clarity* of mental perception. The flower is capable of blooming in the midst of thorny, tangled undergrowth, signifying how it can help us develop our capacity to *think our way through* puzzling mental issues.

The Rosemary state of mind

When we feel vague and forgetful, 'not really here,' as if our thought processes can't be properly relayed by the brain, we can benefit from taking Rosemary flower essence. The mind may remain disassociated from the physical body, not properly grounded in the present, as a result of childhood abuse or other karmic reasons (Kaminski and Katz 1996). Rosemary can assist us to feel more 'comfortable in our bodies' and physically present rather than 'a million miles away.'

Rudolf Steiner, whose work became the basis for Anthroposophy, described children with relatively cold hands and feet as 'sensitives' who are taking a little longer to incarnate fully into their physical bodies. In my experience as a therapist, many clients who take Rosemary flower essence report that their hands feel warmer and that overall they have a greater sense of physical warmth and presence.

Benefits of taking Rosemary

After taking Rosemary flower essence, a greater sense of 'warmth and full-bodied presence' (Kaminksi and Katz 1996) is accompanied by a more alert, dynamic and less forgetful mental disposition. One feels more mentally clear, 'switched on' and relaxed.

Possible physical imbalances

Those who can benefit from taking Rosemary flower essence often have a history of feeling cold, especially in the extremities, and may experience some difficulty with memory, most likely due to sluggish blood flow to the brain. I'm confident that experience and research will confirm other beneficial effects on the circulatory system.

Common uses

When feeling vague; for 'out of body' feelings; for poor concentration and memory; when studying; for better concentration and alertness; for 'BEING IN THE NOW' as well as 'being in the know'!

Complementary &/or similar flower essences

Arnica, Blackberry, Californian Pitcher Plant, Cayenne, Clematis, Coffee, Corn, Crowea, Echinacea, Forget-Me-Not, Honeysuckle, Lemon, Manzanita, Morning Glory, Mugwort, Nicotiana, Peppermint, Red Lily, St John's Wort, Shooting Star, Wild Rose

Supporting the changes

- Engage in as many grounding activities as possible, such as working with earth in some form (gardening or pottery, for instance) or any other physical exercise such as bike-riding or bushwalking that gets the heart pumping, making you aware of your body and giving you a sense that it belongs to you.
- Avoid spending too much time in meditation or other passive, mental activities.

- Get back in sync with your body's natural circadian rhythm. Have adequate sleep, including at least an hour before midnight and go to bed and get up at the same time each day when possible.
- Remind yourself to SWITCH ON!

Sagebrush
Artemisia tridentata   (Yellow / FES)

Positive state
Self-realisation – being true to self
Deeply receptive to positive transformation (FES)

Negative state
Self-delusion
Weighed down by obsolete and 'dysfunctional aspects of one's personality' (FES)

Sagebrush's whole plant has strong antimicrobial qualities and has a long history of use as a first-aid, disinfectant and *cleansing* wash by Native American peoples including the ancient Anasazi and present-day Paiute, and by Oregon farmers. The smoke of its burning leaves has been used in rituals to *clear the air* of pestilence and the *spirits of the dead*. Its cleansing, *purifying* ability is emphasised by its traditional use in saunas and Native American *sweat lodges*.

Plants with a strong aroma have a proportionally strong influence on our emotional aspects, especially those that linger, and Sagebrush has the effect of encouraging us to *let go of emotional dysfunctionality or 'baggage,'* purifying and decongesting the emotional body to allow personal growth.

The Sagebrush state of mind

We have reached a Sagebrush time in our lives when we feel the urge to cleanse ourselves of dysfunctional aspects of our history, surroundings or personality. If we have identified too closely with our material possessions, lifestyle or social status, thinking they were integral to who we are, Sagebrush can help us to modify our attachment to these things that have kept us out of touch with our true Self. If we do not make this shift voluntarily, 'often, the Higher Self intervenes by setting up a condition to cleanse the false persona through illness or misfortune' (Kaminski and Katz 1996).

Sagebrush flower essence is also useful when we want to change the way we have been behaving in relationships, helping us to resist habitual patterns of response to expectations we no longer feel able or willing to meet.

Benefits of taking Sagebrush

Sagebrush helps us to acquire a clearer sense of our true and essential Self in freedom of spirit. Recognising what is essential to our soul frees us to release what isn't essential (Kaminski and Katz 1996) so that we can resist pressure to remain the same.

Our higher Self intervenes throughout life. Synchronistic situations arise and at these times Sagebrush can help us gain a deeper awareness of a Self that is ever capable of transformation and change.

Possible physical imbalances

Sagebrush's traditional use in cleansing and detoxifying rituals is significant. When taken as a flower essence it can enhance the action of blood-cleansing and detoxification herbs, diets and fasts.

Common uses

For change that is overdue; to let go of emotional 'baggage'; for a personal identity crisis; to stop deluding yourself; for greater Self-awareness; for a personal 'growth spurt'; to clear the way for change for the better

Complementary &/or similar flower essences

Agrimony, Angel's Trumpet, Black Eyed Susan, Bleeding Heart, Bottlebrush, Chaparral, Chrysanthemum, Goldenrod, Larkspur, Mallow, Morning Glory, Mullein, Pretty Face, Red Grevillea, Sunflower, Walnut

Supporting the changes

- Take particular care with your health during times of internal disruption when you are questioning your path. Fundamental issues relating to diet and lifestyle often need to be addressed.
- Nurture relationships with people who really allow you to be your Self and love seeing you succeed at it.
- Meet new people and try new activities. Expose yourself to different and fresh perspectives on life.
- Don't resist change – feel the freedom!

Saguaro

Carnegiea gigantea   (White, yellow centre / FES)

Positive state

'A sense of tradition' (FES)
Connected to the wise one within

Negative state

'Conflict with images of authority' (FES); 'rebel without a cause'
Feeling 'on the outer'; alienated

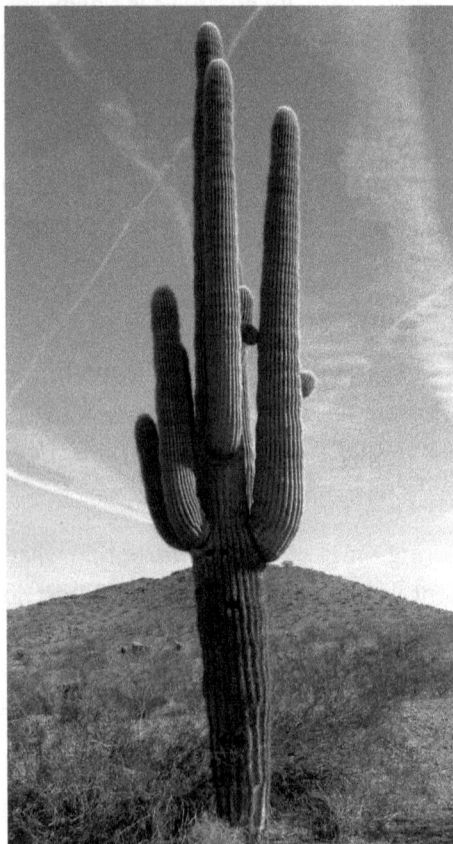

Saguaro cactus is huge and *awe-inspiring*. Its statuesque presence in the desert landscape reminds us of the human qualities of *strength and wisdom* acquired through age.

It *survives* in the toughest of environments for *hundreds of years*. It has *permanency* like the inner *truth* within us to which the Saguaro flower essence helps us better connect.

The Saguaro personality

Saguaro helps those with a rebellious personality to conform to their better nature and innate higher wisdom (Kaminski and Katz 1996). Some of us react negatively and/or rebel against things because we are confused and unsure about their worth.

Saguaro helps us develop a sense of internal authority that allows us to recognise what is right for us within the bigger picture. Unless we can connect with our inner sense of guidance and direction, we may be too strongly influenced by established authority and its representatives in our lives – father-figures, bosses, government or religion – responding by being either too submissive or too resistant. In each case our whole life is organised around reaction. Kaminski and Katz (1996) describe how Saguaro can help us to 'establish a more conscious relationship to elder authority and guidance' and remove confusion and pointless rebellion from our nature.

Benefits of taking Saguaro

Saguaro is particularly useful during adolescence and midlife (the 'second adolescence') when family upbringing and cultural traditions come under rigorous scrutiny. Acknowledging, understanding, accepting and drawing strength and stability from our roots and connections with the past, especially those of family and heritage, frees the soul to change, flourish and evolve more peacefully.

Possible physical imbalances

As a therapist I have found that Saguaro flower essence can be useful for clients who experience resistance and resentment, having discovered that they have inherited a significant illness or predisposition to it. It can help people in this situation reach a level of acceptance (NOT resignation!) and take positive action to live better with illness or the threat of illness. Recovery and prevention then becomes more of a possibility.

Common uses

For the rebel without a cause; for a positive relationship with inner and outer authority; to understand sacred wisdom; to respect the wisdom of elders; to build on lineage and tradition; to trust inner wisdom and guidance

Complementary &/or similar flower essences

Angelica, Baby Blue Eyes, Cerato, Chrysanthemum; Forget-Me-Not, Goldenrod, Mullein, Pomegranate, Quaking Grass, Sage, Shooting Star, Sagebrush, Silver Princess, Sunflower, Sweet Pea, Tall Yellow Top, Tansy, Tiger Lily, Wild Oat

Supporting the changes

- Study the concepts of karma and self-determination, and the Jungian concept of synchronicity.
- Investigate your genealogy. Rediscover, accept and respect your roots.
- Never say 'No' until you have really considered why not!

St John's Wort

Hypericum perforatum   (Yellow / FES)

Positive state

Confident and secure
Sunny disposition

Negative state

Feeling vulnerable; 'deep fears' (FES)
Disturbed sleep/dreams (FES)

St John's Wort loves dry and sunny positions and the upright stem branches at the top so that the flowers get *maximum sun*. The flower petals tend to curl back, so as to gain maximum *exposure* to the sun. The Latin word *perforatum* has the same origin as our word 'perforate.' John on the staff of the Flower Essence Society (www.flowersociety.org) says: 'If you look at the leaf in the sunlight it looks like it's filled with thousands of little pin-pricks. These are actually oil glands and they leave translucent holes in the chlorophyll of the leaf, *absorbing light*, sort of 'pulling it in.' This *perforated* aspect of the plant's signature also points to the flower essence's ability to *heal holes* in the *etheric body*. The *nervous system* is the main physical link with the etheric body, so it is not surprising that the homeopathic medicine made from St John's Wort – *Hypericum* – is used for treating *damaged nerves and puncture wounds* as a result of *trauma* or medical procedures.

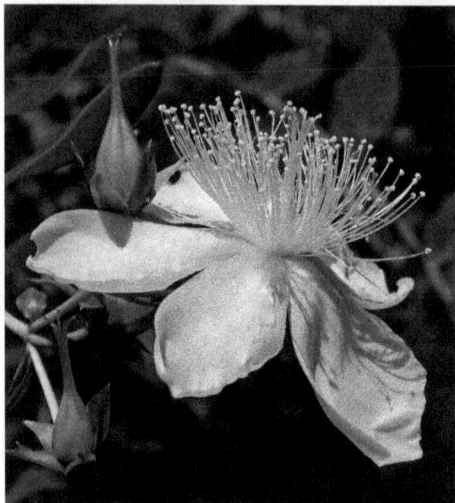

One aspect of the doctrine of signatures relates to the way in which a vulnerability in humans (in this case being *'too open and exposed'*) corresponds to a particular strength in a plant – in this case, St John's Wort's unique *receptivity* to the sun's healing rays. St John's Wort can help us transform over-exposed openness into a *dynamic capacity to soak up healing energies* from our surroundings.

This *protective* quality was recognised by the ancient Greeks, who believed that the fragrance of St John's Wort would repel evil spirits. Christian priests in the Middle Ages continued the tradition, performing exorcisms using the plant, and conferring its common name by association with St John the Baptist, because in the northern hemisphere it blooms in June, on or around St John's Day.

St John's Wort should also be considered when we feel exposed on a subtle level, when sleep is disturbed by vivid and *cluttered dreams* or even *nightmares* due to expansion of the emotional body during sleep. As a therapist, I have found that this often occurs in pregnant women when the aura is naturally in a more *expansive state* because it is enhanced by the presence of the child's soul-being. Many expectant mothers report a much more active and *vivid dream life* and St John's Wort flower essence can enable them to have more settled and *restful sleep*.

The St John's Wort state of mind

People who benefit most from taking St John's Wort flower essence are not necessarily timid and frightened – more often the contrary is true – but at some level they feel excessively vulnerable. The only clear evidence may be their disturbing and fearful dreams, during which they process fears which the waking mind represses.

Benefits of taking St John's Wort

St John's Wort can help to allay deep-seated fears, especially of unknown origin, so that you feel more internally secure and protected. It is excellent for easing night terrors and intense dreams that disrupt sleep in children and adults. It is extremely useful for those experiencing a feeling of vulnerability or 'thin skin' for no apparent reason. Also, St John's Wort may help us feel more secure during psychoanalysis or regression therapies when deeply entrenched fears may surface.

Possible physical imbalances

Some people who have benefited from St John's Wort flower essence also have a history of underlying adrenal/kidney health issues. This is consistent with Traditional Chinese Medicine, which relates emotional states of fear and anxiety (especially when repressed in any way) to the adrenal/kidney energy meridians. A sense of dread, coupled with unrestful sleep, puts the adrenals under constant pressure through the 'fight or flight' mechanism, and adrenal fatigue then becomes a definite possibility.

St John's Wort flower essence is also worth considering as an adjunct to other therapies such as light therapy used for Seasonal Affective Disorder (SAD or 'winter blues'). The photosensitising qualities of St John's Wort are an expression of its ability to make us more permeable to 'light' in all its dimensions. Kaminski and Katz (1996) remind us that 'just as flowers need sunlight to grow, so also the soul needs light – both physical and spiritual – to flourish.' St John's Wort flower essence can safely augment our receptivity to light in its full spectrum. (NB: St John's Wort flower essence can be prescribed safely in conjunction with conventional antidepressants as only an infinitesimal physical quantity of the flower is used. However, the herbal preparation should be avoided when taking certain antidepressants. Speak with your health practitioner.)

Common uses

For feeling vulnerable; for a sense of dread; for repressed fears; for SAD; for disturbed dreams and nightmares; to gain a confident awareness; to 'brighten and lighten up'; to gain strength from your surroundings

Complementary &/or similar flower essences

Angelica, Arnica, Aspen, Canyon Dudleya, Chamomile, Chaparral, Dill, Echinacea, Fringed Violet, Garlic, Indian Pink, Mountain Pennyroyal, Mugwort, Mustard, Red Clover, Rock Rose, Violet, all the Yarrows, YES formula

Supporting the changes

- Meditative techniques and creative visualisation of white light may strengthen your sense of security.
- Avoid mood-altering drugs – even caffeine, alcohol and sugar – and avoid becoming emotionally overstimulated before bedtime.
- Consider working with a health professional in dream analysis or regression therapy to resolve long-standing and deep-seated fears.
- Protect yourself by engaging regularly in simple grounding techniques and activities.
- Get a bit of sun!

Scarlet Monkeyflower
Mimulus cardinalis (Red / FES)

Positive state
'Clear communication of deep feelings' (FES)
Genuine passion and emotional spontaneity (FES)

Negative state
Sudden, disproportionate anger surges/outbursts
Repressed anger/passion (FES)

Scarlet Monkeyflower's *scarlet-red* colour is stirring and stimulating, an effect that is commonly associated with the *base chakra*. It is representative of *intense and raw emotions* that emerge from within us. On close inspection, the flower has a white projection emerging from its intensely coloured depths, symbolising the emergence of pure inspiration and insight out of fiery, *passionate and instinctual* responses to life.

The Scarlet Monkeyflower personality

In the unbalanced state, Scarlet Monkeyflower people feel anger and frustration that is often expressed indirectly or in sudden, inappropriate outbursts. They might keep a lid on disturbing emotions until, under pressure, they finally explode in a fit of rage (Kaminski and Katz 1996). Afterwards, frightened by the intensity of their anger and its effect on others, they repress these powerful emotions once more and so the cycle continues.

Benefits of taking Scarlet Monkeyflower

Scarlet Monkeyflower essence breaks the cycle of repression followed by eruption of volatile emotions so that strong feelings can be better integrated and expressed. By bringing insight and acceptance to frightening or overwhelming emotions we become comfortable with expressing strong feelings and reach a more authentic and spontaneous level of communication with others.

I once worked with a man who was having some difficulty expressing his true feelings to his wife. Their discussions became heated as his wife expressed anger and frustration while he became more and more detached, responding to her by saying, 'Be rational. I'll speak to you when you settle down.' These comments aggravated the situation, acting as a passive-aggressive provocation. His wife could express her intense feelings but he couldn't and the situation frightened him. He would go into a heavy silence in which nothing got resolved. At other times, however, he would express disproportionate anger and frustration over small incidents.

After he began taking Scarlet Monkeyflower essence, he felt more comfortable acknowledging his feelings and was less intimidated by his wife's ability to express strong emotion. As a result, he became better at articulating what he felt, and his wife became less frustrated with his responses and remained calmer during their discussions. The dynamic between the partners changed and so did the way they related, especially in potentially heated discussions on issues crucial to their relationship.

Possible physical imbalances

Inflammatory responses, especially of the skin, can often be a physical expression of emotions a person is either unaware of or finds difficult to articulate. Scarlet Monkeyflower essence can be very helpful for acute 'flare-up' complaints of this kind, by helping the person be more aware and more comfortable with fully experiencing strong emotions. In my practice I often prescribe it in conjunction with Indian Pink in such cases.

Common uses

Sudden, disproportionate, angry outbursts; discomfort about expression of anger; to shed light on your (emotional) shadow side; to be comfortable expressing your passion; for emotional spontaneity; to learn to embrace and enjoy strong and passionate feelings

Complementary &/or similar flower essences

Black Eyed Susan, Californian Pitcher Plant, Chamomile, Cherry Plum, Fuchsia, Impatiens, Indian Pink, Lotus, Snapdragon, Sturt Desert Pea

Supporting the changes

- As with all flower essences associated with the base chakra, 'grounding' exercises such as yoga, tai chi and invigorating physical exercise are extremely important. Those who benefit from using Scarlet Monkeyflower essence will find that if they are grounded in this way, they will be less subject to extreme emotional reactions.

- Counselling, psychotherapy and related body therapies in which feelings are explored and worked with may be worthwhile.
- Pursue interests and work that provides an outlet for your creative passions and urges.
- Never discount what you feel.

Scleranthus

Scleranthus annuus (Green / Bach)

Positive state

Conviction and self-determination
A clear sense of how to make the right decision

Negative state

Mental confusion/uncertainty
Indecision/changeability

When I look at the Scleranthus plant I always get a sense that it *can't make up its mind* whether to flower or not. Unlike the flowers of many other plants, the Scleranthus flower is almost *indistinguishable* from the tangled stems of the plant, which seem to grow in all directions.

The five-pointed sepals could be *mistaken* for petals but the minute flowers in fact have no petals and do not make any *definitive statement*, whereas other plants receive and broadcast emotional states which they *express* and display through the colour of their petals. It is interesting to note that Wild Oat also lacks petals and the essence relates to similar qualities of *confusion and indecisiveness* in relation to life direction or vocation (Barnard 1988).

People who benefit from taking Scleranthus flower essence often go *unnoticed* because of their inability to be decisive and 'take a step forward.' It is no coincidence that the plant is also easily *overlooked* because of its inconspicuousness. The colour of the flower is *green* – the primary colour associated with the *heart chakra*, which when activated can provide insight that transcends *mental chatter and debate* and can give *clear direction* in our daily actions.

The Scleranthus state of mind

People in the negative Scleranthus state cannot make up their minds, though their emotional indecision and confusion is often internalised and kept hidden from others. Scleranthus people are often inconspicuous and taken for granted in the family or group, going along with whatever is decided by others. They never challenge the status quo because they never resolve their own mental uncertainty and ambivalence about life. This manifests physically, emotionally and mentally as indecisiveness and changeability or in extreme cases, dramatic mood swings.

We are often torn between two apparently opposing options. This can mean that we hesitate until the opportunity for decision-making has passed or until someone else makes the decision for us. Either way we are left feeling powerless. Even when no decision is required we still agonise over issues at home or at work, creating a confused state of mind. Scleranthus flower essence can make it possible to choose between two tasks, both of which are urgent, by opting for the one we prefer, completing the task quickly and with little effort.

Benefits of taking Scleranthus

Scleranthus flower essence raises our awareness of what feels appropriate. Instinctively we sense the right options, and even more importantly, differentiate between situations in which we need to do something from those in which we don't. This brings a new balance to our lives.

Here is an example: Shirley was the youngest of three siblings. The older two were boys and her father had made all the decisions for the family. When she came to see me as an adult, she said she had never independently made a major decision for herself. She had four young children and was already experiencing stress-related health problems. In addition, she now had to decide how to respond to her husband's wish to have another child. I suggested she take Scleranthus flower essence and the remedy helped her make her own decision, one that she felt comfortable and clear about.

Possible physical imbalances

Imbalance and vacillation can easily manifest at the physical level as hormone imbalance and fluctuation, often as a result of the condition of the thyroid. Scleranthus flower essence should be considered for any physical or glandular condition with a marked, cyclical or changeable/swinging pathology.

Common uses

For dramatic mood-swings; for constant hesitancy and indecisiveness; for mental confusion and ambivalence; for dependence on another as 'decision-maker'; for calm clarity about when to take action and when to refrain; to grab opportunities when they arise; for self-determination

Complementary &/or similar flower essences

Blackberry, Bottlebrush, Calla Lily, Cayenne, Cerato, Iris, Larch, Madia, Mullein, Paw Paw, Pomegranate, Quince, Red Grevillea, Saguaro, Shasta Daisy, Silver Princess, Tansy, Walnut, Wedding Bush, Wild Oat

Supporting the changes

- To raise your awareness of the tensions and imbalances in your life, start a diary to gain an overview of the daily ups and downs.
- Study your natural biorhythms and cycles. Instead of being their victim, compensate for them or better still use them to your advantage.
- If you can't understand what your head is saying, see how your heart feels.

Scotch Broom

Cytisus scoparius (Yellow / FES)

Positive state

Seeing difficulties/challenges as opportunities for growth
'Positive and optimistic feelings about the world' (FES)

Negative state

Discouraged and disheartened
Pessimism about the world (FES)

Scotch Broom's branches bear numerous *golden-yellow* flowers that bring cheer to hillsides, forest glades and heaths in early spring. *'Cheer'* is the key word, expressing the essence's ability to help develop a more *positive outlook*. The large, pea-shaped flowers are the most outstanding and *uplifting* feature of the plant.

The Scotch Broom state of mind

Scotch Broom flower essence is useful when we are feeling down or pessimistic about our personal future in a world that doesn't seem to have much of a future either – or so it seems to us when we are in the negative Scotch Broom state. Scotch Broom pessimism is universal as well as personal; bleakness and despair is felt not only about our own prospects but also about the world (Kaminski and Katz 1996). In this state of mind we seem to focus on the darker side of the 'world psyche.' The obstacles in our lives seem too big to overcome and we wonder whether there is any the point to the struggle, when another obstacle is sure to be just around the corner. Kaminski and Katz (1996) describe the attitude as, 'What's the use? Why try?'

I especially enjoy prescribing this flower essence at an initial consultation when it is indicated for the client. Often it seems to help a person over their first hurdle in healing – the leap of faith in Self and its ability to heal, along with a renewed belief in the world. It is rarely required at the second consultation as almost invariably the client's attitude has changed to a more positive one.

Benefits of taking Scotch Broom

Scotch Broom flower essence helps us see the challenges of life as opportunities for growth and development (Kaminski and Katz 1996) – although I never say that to someone who is still in the negative Scotch Broom state as they are likely to dismiss this approach as 'new age' optimism at that stage! Positive philosophical viewpoints are best communicated later, when a more hopeful vision of the world has re-emerged.

Possible physical imbalances

Scotch Broom flower essence can help bring a more positive attitude in situations where the challenge of an illness seems insurmountable – and a changed perspective can in itself improve the prognosis.

Common uses

Discouraged and disheartened; depressed by world events; pessimistic about the world; to see challenges as opportunities for growth; to promote a positive attitude; to evoke hope and optimistic feelings about the world

Complementary &/or similar flower essences

Baby Blue Eyes, Borage, Buttercup, Chamomile, Garlic, Gentian, Gorse, Hibbertia, Hound's Tongue, Iris, Mustard, Pansy, Red Clover, St John's Wort, Sweet Chestnut, Wild Oat, Wild Rose, Zinnia

Supporting the changes

- Surround yourself with uplifting people, music, movies, television programs, colours and books.
- Protect yourself with positive thoughts and cheering visualisations during meditation.
- Develop a sense of humour about life and its challenges. Enjoy some comedy and laugh more!

Self-Heal

Prunella vulgaris   (Purple/ FES)

Positive state

Free flow of inherent, health-generating forces (FES)
Self-responsible for personal health and wellness

Negative state

Unable to access innate self-recuperative powers
Projection of responsibility for health onto others (FES)

Once again, so much is contained in a name! In the past, Self-Heal was commonly used externally and internally in herbalism, especially for treating infections and was particularly valued for treating skin conditions. It is a member of the mint family that grows all over Europe in pastures, woods and meadows and has become naturalised in America and Australasia.

Self-Heal essence helps us to access the qualities of *self-sufficiency, self-reliance, autonomy* and *independence* – not through aloofness or distance but through *harmonious connection with our surroundings*. The flowers grow in bunches and this highlights this quality of being able to live in close, harmonious connection with others.

Its signature as a skin-healing herb can give further insight into its action. Skin forms the membrane of exchange between us and our surroundings; it is the largest organ in the body and, when functioning well, can absorb healing agents through its pores, repel unwanted microbes and accept beneficial ones. This process is like the transpiration of oxygen and other gases in the alveoli of the lungs, which form part of our internal 'skin'; the skin generally is regarded in Traditional Chinese Medicine as the 'third lung.' Self-Heal flower essence can help us to access and absorb the life force or prana through our inner and outer 'skins,' so that our *innate Self-recuperative powers* can be re-ignited.

The *purple* colour of the tiny, bunched flowers relates to the *crown chakra*, which when open allows energy to flow in for expression of *your truth and healing*. Self-Heal flower essence helps you become more aware of what is true for you and therefore more able to sort through input from others such as health professionals so that you can make the best choices for your own healing. Your acceptance of greater *responsibility* and discernment is rewarded with feeling personally empowered and more autonomous with regard to your health.

The Self-Heal personality

Self-Heal flower essence is particularly recommended for people who have doubts about their own recuperative powers and/or hand over total responsibility for their health to doctors, counsellors and healers (Kaminski and Katz 1996). People who are so unwell or unhappy that they have forgotten what it's like to be well, or who have become dependent on outside influences to make them feel good can be helped by Self-Heal flower essence.

Benefits of taking Self-Heal

Self-Heal is used to help people remember that they can play a part in their own healing and awaken their Self-recuperative powers, Self-belief and inner motivation to be more personally proactive in getting well. Because of this quality it is often prescribed in conjunction with other flower essences and complements

THE **ESSENTIAL** FLOWER ESSENCE BOOK

natural healing approaches.

Naturopathic philosophy has the fundamental belief that there is an inherent Self-healing ability in all of us. Just as a cut finger can heal itself, so our emotional and spiritual wounds can be healed through dynamic inner forces; sometimes we just need to reconnect with this power. Once you really believe that there is a possibility of getting well, you've taken a first and vitally important step towards better health and wellbeing.

Possible physical imbalances

As mentioned above, Self-Heal flower essence can restore a person's faith in their ability to heal themselves and so awaken their innate recuperative powers through self-belief, inner motivation and taking responsibility for getting well. This facilitates all other healing modalities and approaches.

Common uses

Lost faith in recovery; totally dependent on health practitioner; re-establishing contact with innate healing potential; for self-belief in one's ability to recover; empowered and responsible for one's own health and wellbeing

Complementary &/or similar flower essences

Aloe Vera, Arnica, Borage, Californian Pitcher Plant; Cayenne, Crowea, Echinacea, Garlic, Gentian, Gorse, Morning Glory, Nasturtium, Pansy, Scotch Broom, Tansy, Waratah, Willow, YES formula

Supporting the changes

- Consider how you create your own reality through your thoughts, beliefs, attitudes and behaviours.
- Start taking real responsibility for your health by attending to lifestyle and diet, and include more movement and exercise.
- Take time to identify your health goals.
- Remember the Star Wars injunction – 'May the Force be with you always!'

Shasta Daisy

Chrysanthemum maximum (White/yellow centre / FES)

Positive state

Synthesis and integration of ideas; holistic view
Emotional intelligence; 'gut' sense

Negative state

Collecting bits of information; fragmented view
Over-intellectualisation (FES); overly 'cerebral'

Shasta Daisy's *yellow centre* signifies its connection with the *solar plexus chakra* where our *'gut sense'* is located, while the white petals converging on the centre signify the influences, perspectives and *ideas that come together* and are *'digested'* there. A *mandala*-like pattern is visible in the arrangement of the tiny florets that form the centre, symbolising a *balance of feelings and thoughts*.

The multiple white petals represent the many different *inspirations and ideas* available to us. Shasta Daisy flower essence can help us to bring these ideas together and find a *holistic perspective*. Although the centre of the daisy is made up of *hundreds of little florets*, they merge to form one entity – a perfect, *whole*, single flower.

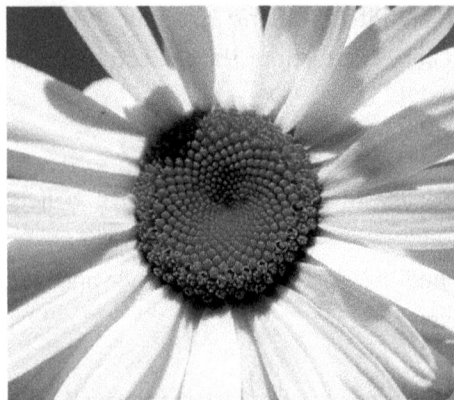

The Shasta Daisy state of mind

When your brain is cluttered with information and your mind is overloaded with ideas you can't bring together, consider using Shasta Daisy flower essence. At this moment in history, although we constantly collect new information, instead of feeling more informed we often just feel overwhelmed. The mind becomes cluttered and congested with ideas and thoughts that seem to be unconnected and without a common theme. You may know a lot but be unable to put your knowledge together so that it makes sense.

Consider Shasta Daisy when you are studying and need to draw comparisons between different subjects, when you are busy with many different tasks and need to know how one task can help to get another done, and when you are learning new ideas and tasks and need to understand how your previous experience relates to them.

Benefits of taking Shasta Daisy

Shasta Daisy flower essence helps us achieve a better balance between emotion and intellect, allowing us to see the bigger picture while attending to detail. We become better at integrating ideas and making meaningful associations between them. Kaminski and Katz (1996) tell us that Shasta Daisy helps develop our archetypal or holistic consciousness, 'stimulating great forces of intelligence and insight into life experience.'

Possible physical imbalances

A mind constantly cluttered and congested with ideas and thoughts needs to decongest itself and eliminate its 'psychic waste.' 'Waste' resulting from excessive cerebral ('above the shoulders') activity can eventually be processed and eliminated through physical means – catarrhal expressions such as sinus congestion, hay fever and head colds, or headaches and even structural neck and cranial problems.

Common uses

For the collector/hoarder of bits of information; when you just can't see the big picture; for those who are overly cerebral, with a head full of disjointed ideas; to help get a better 'feel' for things; to help integrate our feeling side with our thoughts; to help package and promote your knowledge; to develop a more holistic view

Complementary &/or similar flower essences

Cotton, Crab Apple, Crowea, Dill, Elm, Filaree, Fuchsia, Harvest Brodiaea, Hibbertia, Hound's Tongue, Iris, Lemon, Madia, Nasturtium, Pansy, Passionflower, Paw Paw, Rabbitbrush, White Chestnut

Supporting the changes

- Develop a more meditative/mindful approach to life. Meditation, yoga and tai chi will help you to do this.
- Develop lateral thinking through mental exercises – try connecting seemingly unrelated subjects or words in unusual ways. Be prepared to be silly!
- Be selective about the sorts of things you commit to memory. Don't try to remember details that a computer or diary will store for you.
- Meditate on a mandala.

She Oak

Casuarina glauca (Reddish / Aus)

Positive state

Fertility/creativity
Hormonal/emotional balance (Ian White)

Negative state

Frustrated creative expression
Hormonal dysfunction/emotional imbalance

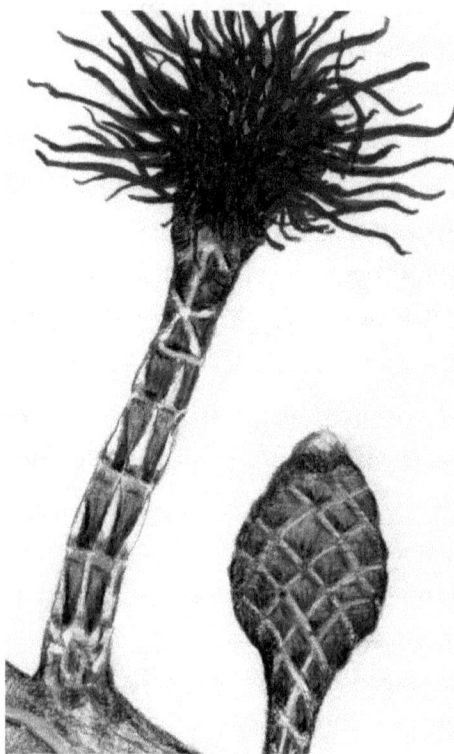

She Oak's male and female flowers are found on the same tree, as with many Casuarina species, although Ian White chose to use only the *female flower* to produce this Australian Bush Flower Essence. She Oak grows in marshy ground, along slow streams or beside the backwaters of tidal rivers and has also been referred to as the Swamp Oak.

The fact that it grows close to water emphasises the She Oak's relationship with the *water element* which is said to govern our *emotions/ passions* on a metaphysical level. Another strong aspect of the plant signature is the similarity in shape and size of the female cone to human *ovaries*. The female flowers appear as globular heads and the styles which hang out to catch pollen resemble the shape of *human fallopian tubes* that receive eggs released from the ovaries (White 2008).

The She Oak personality

Ian White (2008) recommends She Oak flower essence for women who are having difficulty conceiving where there is no clear physical reason. Infertility can be heartbreaking and sometimes seems like an insoluble problem, but She Oak acts on emotional patterns that may be inhibiting fertility. Such unconscious blocks may revolve around feelings of inadequacy or doubt about the possibility of conception and gestation. Many of the women who have responded well to She Oak have been over-concerned about how they will cope with gestation, delivery and child-rearing from a variety of perspectives, including practical or financial issues.

Benefits of taking She Oak

As a therapist, I have found that She Oak flower essence is useful in the area of hormone balance in general, especially for women, and is most effective when prescribed in conjunction with other relevant natural medicines. Hormone imbalance has a close relationship with emotional states, so it is reasonable to expect that when appropriately selected for individual emotional needs, flower essences such as She Oak will generally assist in re-establishing the hormonal balance that plays a role in fertility.

Many different flower essences can play a significant role in helping women conceive. It is important to remember that issues around fertility can be complex and that the partner's involvement must also be considered.

Possible physical imbalances

She Oak flower essence has helped many women with general hormonal imbalance before or during menstruation, particularly when fluid retention is an issue. It is often prescribed in conjunction with other appropriate natural female remedies.

Common uses

For hormonal imbalance; to enhance creativity in all its forms; to increase fertility (always speak with a qualified health practitioner); to embrace your femininity

Complementary &/or similar flower essences

Aloe Vera, Basil, Billy Goat Plum, Calla Lily, Crab Apple, Easter Lily, Fairy Lantern, Hibiscus, Indian Paintbrush, Manzanita, Mariposa Lily, Pomegranate, Quince, Sticky Monkeyflower, Watermelon

Supporting the changes

- Study the feminine energies as portrayed in mythology, the work of Carl Jung or the yin principle in Traditional Chinese Medicine. Learn to acknowledge and respect feminine energy for its strength, wisdom and intuitive power.
- Love and respect your body, especially those aspects that express your gender.
- Find creative outlets for your passion!

Shooting Star

Dodecatheon hendersonii   (Violet-pink / FES)

Positive state

Feeling 'at home' on Earth and in one's body
Feeling part of the warmth of the human family (FES)

Negative state

Not at home in one's family or on Earth (FES)
'Profound feeling of alienation' (FES); disengaged in relationships

Shooting Star's name, as with so many plants, gives insight into its healing qualities. We sometimes use the phrase 'shooting star' to describe someone who appears as if from nowhere, has a profound impact on the lives of others, then disappears from view. They may arrive in the spotlight with a 'bang' but never really *commit and settle* into ordinary, everyday life. The classic beneficiary of Shooting Star flower essence is an *unsettled soul*. They often have *traumatic births* involving arrested labour and then a quick delivery (Kaminski and Katz 1996) after they get over their reluctance to be born! They resist the *transition* from the warmth of the womb into the cold material reality of life, like a deep sea diver who delays his ascent and then suffers the bends because he has to surface too quickly. These babies often suffer from colic – as if they cannot comfortably 'digest' what comes to them from their new environment.

The merged *pink and violet* colours of the flower are an important aspect of the plant's signature – violet represents the *crown chakra* and pink represents the *heart chakra*. Their merging symbolises integration of the *spirit/purpose* and *heart/body/feeling* aspects of the Self. Shooting Star flower essence helps you confirm your *commitment to being here* and heightens your *sense of belonging*.

The Shooting Star personality

In my experience as a therapist, clients who benefit from taking Shooting Star flower essence often tell me that they have never really felt at home in the family. They feel that they are 'different' on some level and don't truly belong. As one client eloquently related to me, 'I'm in the world but I'm not of it!' As parents they may also feel 'on the outer' and not fully part of the family they have created with their partner. This sense of 'being on the outside looking in' is often deeply ingrained.

For some, this feeling originates in the experience of a traumatic transition into life because of birth complications which leave them feeling that they have never properly adjusted to being here. It seems they have not properly undergone their 'rite of passage.' At some level they have lost connection with the feeling of support and love that was there in the womb. Shooting Star flower essence can help you reconnect with that loving support, here and now.

Benefits of taking Shooting Star

Shooting Star flower essence helps us to accept the Earth as our home and make a deep, 'heartfelt' connection with life, so that we feel we really belong in our body, our family and on this planet (Kaminski and Katz 1996). This connection is felt as a new warmth and harmony experienced with loved ones, family and others on the journey.

Possible physical imbalances

Shooting Star helps us 'connect' and feel more comfortable in our bodies. This awareness helps us to better understand what our body needs in terms of nutrition and exercise, and how to respond to environmental stresses. If we are more in tune with our body's needs, we can make better choices about diet and lifestyle.

Common uses

Feeling disconnected and alienated; feeling as though you don't fit in; not grounded or involved; feeling disembodied; after rapid and/or complicated or traumatic birth; to be comfortable in your body; to feel part of the (human) family; to speak from the heart and be heard and understood; to feel the warmth of humankind

Complementary &/or similar flower essences

Angelica, Arnica, Calendula, Californian Poppy, Cayenne, Corn, Cosmos, Forget-Me-Not, Lotus, Mallow, Manzanita, Mariposa Lily, Nicotiana, Red Lily, Rosemary, Sweet Pea, Tall Yellow Top, Violet, Water Violet, Wild Rose

Supporting the changes

- Professional psychotherapy which involves properly supervised regression therapy may be useful.
- Engage in grounding activities such as gardening or pottery, or physical exercise such as bike-riding or bushwalking to get the blood flowing, making you aware of your body and giving you a sense that it belongs to you.
- Join a group that is dedicated to something you feel passionate about, such as conservation of the environment – your home on Earth.
- Make heart-connections with the world.

Silver Princess

Eucalyptus caesia   (Red / Aus)

Positive state

Dynamically motivated
Clear sense of purpose/direction

Negative state

Lacking drive; ambivalent
'Aimless' (Ian White)

Silver Princess's budding flowers are covered by a small hard cap that fits tightly. This dry, protective lid is thrown off by the *expanding* stamens of the flower as it blooms (White 2008).

There is rich symbolism here: the old hat no longer fits. A *new role* in life is *emerging* and you are ready to tread a path in which guidance from your *higher Self* is becoming clearer. A protective membrane of naivety is shed painlessly as the essential Self, strengthened by experience, embarks on the next stage of its journey.

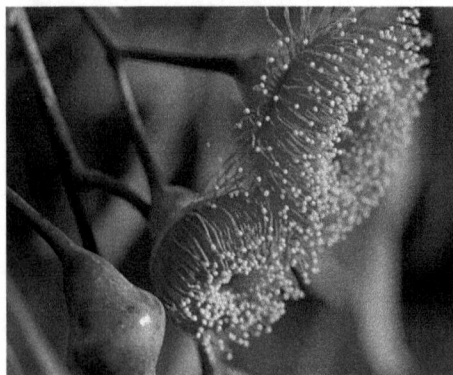

Each of the many stamens which provide much of the flower's beauty is distinctive and *stands out from the crowd*. This aspect of the plant's signature relates to the quality of certainty in one's *direction and purpose* that does not get lost in the blur and activity of life.

Eucalypts are grown for their beauty but they also help to stabilise soil and drain swampy land. Ian White (2008) reminds us that they have an ability to adapt to a 'harsh environment with extremes of temperature and rainfall, bushfires and poor soil.' Their growth is not inhibited and they manage to *find their place in life* in spite of the restrictions and demands imposed on them by their habitat. Silver Princess flower essence helps you to be *vitally adaptable*, so that you can create a *niche* for yourself even in the competitive and fast-paced world we live in.

The Silver Princess state of mind

When we sense that our lives are not on the right path but we are unclear about what direction to take, Silver Princess flower essence can be helpful. Without direction or a clear purpose we lack the motivation and energy needed to explore

THE **ESSENTIAL** FLOWER ESSENCE BOOK

new directions in life. We may recognise our needs but become passive and resigned to leaving them unmet as we wander aimlessly through life, apathetic and withdrawn.

Benefits of taking Silver Princess

Always consider Silver Princess flower essence during significant life transitions such as the astrological 'Saturn Return' which first occurs at around twenty-seven to twenty-eight years of age, or use it to support the opportunity for 're-visioning' your life at midlife. It is especially useful if you have achieved a goal only to be plagued by the question, 'Is that all there is?' Silver Princess allows a greater sense of purpose and meaning to re-emerge.

Possible physical imbalances

What usually accompanies the unbalanced Silver Princess state of mind is a lack of physical energy and motivation. Part of a positive response to the flower essence is an increase in energy and purpose.

Common uses

Lack of direction; lack of motivation (and energy); for resignation; to get back on the right life path; for clarifying direction; to develop a sense of purpose; for drive and motivation

Complementary &/or similar flower essences

Aloe Vera, Blackberry, Borage, Bottlebrush, Californian Pitcher Plant, Cayenne, Chrysanthemum, Clematis, Deerbrush, Forget-Me-Not, Hornbeam, Iris, Madia, Pomegranate, Red Lily, Shasta Daisy, Tansy, Walnut, Wild Oat, Wild Rose

Supporting the changes

- Grounding activities such as physical exercise, gardening and other types of earthy work are useful.
- Explore a more emotional and intuitive approach to your life.
- Try to be more down-to-earth and listen to others who have this capacity.
- 'If the hat fits wear it!'

Snapdragon

Antirrhinum majus (Yellow / FES)

Positive state

Articulate and dynamic verbal communication (FES)
Balanced libido and creative expression

Negative state

Frustrated/tense/'snappy' verbal communication
Misdirected psychic drive or desire

The Snapdragon flower has a shape like a mouth and this is part of the plant's signature. The healing qualities of Snapdragon flower essence relate to the *vocal cords*, lips, *jaw*, facial tissue and muscles and all aspects of *verbal communication*. The texture of the flower is soft and flaccid and the 'mouth' seems to lack definition. Looking at its photograph, my clients have commented that the flower looks *'wishy-washy'* and ask, 'What is the flower trying to say?' These responses show insight into the capacity of Snapdragon flower essence to help us become *clearer and more direct* in our verbal communication rather than just *'jawing on'*.

In the wild, plants are usually *pinkish purple*, often with *yellow* tips, and this signifies its connection with the *heart chakra* and the *solar plexus chakra* and a capacity for *genuine, heartfelt expression* and balanced Self-assertion, rather than 'snappiness.'

The Snapdragon state of mind

When we have difficulty articulating how we feel, especially when we are discouraged from acknowledging our emotions, emotional energy may become misdirected, for example through an inappropriate sexual persona, verbal aggression or excessive tension in the jaw (Kaminski and Katz 1996). A very repressive upbringing, often associated with a strict, religious atmosphere, can result in emotional inhibition and distorted or repressed sexual expression. Snapdragon flower essence helps us balance our psychic drives and desires, allowing their appropriate expression in life.

If we fall into the habit of talking too much about superficial things in order to compensate for not talking about how we genuinely feel, others may tune out. Snapdragon flower essence helps us to get away from the idea that if we talk enough others might eventually get the point. Dynamic and direct, but non-aggressive, oral communication is enabled with Snapdragon flower essence.

Benefits of taking Snapdragon

When appropriately prescribed, Snapdragon flower essence can aid all aspects of effective communication, subtly aligning the emotional and mental bodies and supporting the integrity of the physical structures involved in communication.

Snapdragon helps us to access and integrate the powerful creative forces of the lower and intrapersonal chakras to give potency and clarity to our spoken words.

Possible physical imbalances

People who have benefited from taking Snapdragon flower essence often suffer from problems related to the jaw. Tension held in the jaw often leads to tooth-grinding in sleep or creates other conditions that may require (expensive) dental work.

Common uses

For verbal aggression; for 'jawing on' aimlessly; for TMJ and teeth grinding issues; for misdirected libido; for healthy expression of basic drives; for dynamic communication; to articulate your essence

Complementary &/or similar flower essences

Angelsword, Calendula, Californian Pitcher Plant, Calla Lily, Cayenne, Cosmos, Deerbrush, Lotus, Mullein, Quince, Scarlet Monkeyflower, Sticky Monkeyflower, Tiger Lily, Trillium, Trumpet Vine, Yerba Santa

Supporting the changes

- Relaxation techniques and activities that aid the release of tension in the facial area are therapeutic.
- Public speaking classes will help you refine your articulation.
- Grounding activities such as gardening, vigorous physical exercise or making pottery can help you engage your lower chakras.

Squash (Zucchini)
Cucurbit species   (Yellow / FES-res)

Positive state

Security with Self and sexual identity
Positive masculine (yang) expression

Negative state

Gender identity insecurity
Unassertive; repressed masculine side

Squash has both *male and female* flowers and the key quality associated with this flower essence is *balance* between the masculine and feminine principles. It can help to ease a *gender identity insecurity* (Calla Lily flower essence should also be considered). In the case of Zucchini and its signature, the vegetable bears a resemblance to the *male sex organ* and the flower essence's greatest value is in its positive influence on the expression of healthy and balanced *masculine energy*. The *yellow* colour of the flower relates it to the *solar plexus chakra* which governs *individual expression and healthy assertiveness* in the world.

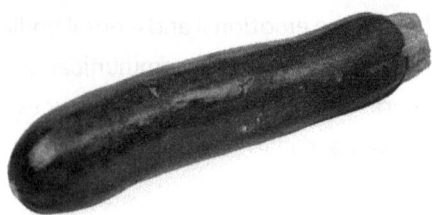

The Squash personality

Squash flower essence can help to stabilise overly dominant masculine or yang energy or to free this energy up if it has been repressed. An overly masculine/yang personality often displays itself in the form of aggressive behaviour and a desire to dominate others, whereas in the person with a repressed masculine side the ability to stand up for self or be assertive and directive is lacking. Squash flower essence can help both men and women to access their positive masculine qualities to assert themselves and take action for the good of all.

The essence is also useful for members of either sex who are confused about their gender identity and unsure of what it means to be 'male' or 'female,' especially in relationships. Whether masculinity has been 'pumped up' or repressed, Squash flower essence can help people to express their masculine potential with warmth and confidence.

Benefits of taking Squash

Squash flower essence can help to restore the balance of yin/feminine and yang/masculine energy and free us from being totally reliant on a rational and analytical, 'left-brain' approach to life at the expense of feeling and intuition. When the head completely rules the heart we suffer a loss of spontaneity and enJOYment in life. Squash facilitates a more confident and spontaneous approach where we refrain from rationalising (away) our feelings and allow our 'right-brain,' intuitive side to hold equal sway.

Possible physical imbalances

There is a potential for hormonal imbalance in persons requiring Squash flower essence. In keeping with its emphasis on bringing masculine energy into balance, it should be considered in health problems associated with the reproductive organs in all sexes.

Common uses

For the insensitive male; for confused sexual identity; to develop positive masculinity or yang forces; for confident self-expression; for warmth, spontaneity and outgoingness

Complementary &/or similar flower essences

Borage, Buttercup, Calendula, Calla Lily, Golden Rod, Larch, Mountain Pride, Mullein, Pomegranate, Quince, St John's Wort, Snapdragon, Sunflower, Tiger Lily, Violet, Watermelon

Supporting the changes

- Study the concepts of anima and animus, yin and yang, feminine and masculine energies.
- Look out for workshops and reading material etc that aims to help you develop your intuition and achieve a more contemplative approach to life.
- If you rebel or conform, make sure it's an action rather than a reaction.

Star of Bethlehem
Ornithogalum umbellatum   (White / Bach)

Positive state

Subtle anatomy dimensions re-aligned for healing
Release of shock and trauma

Negative state

Disturbed/shaken at a physical and subtle body level
Effects of present and past shock and trauma

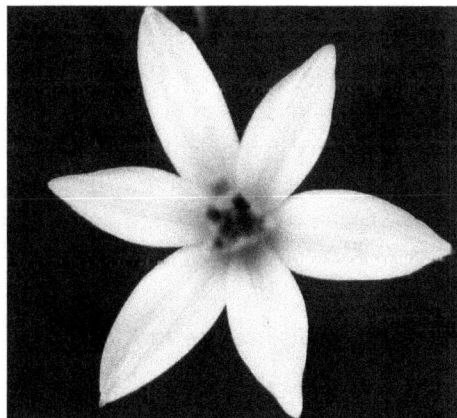

Star of Bethlehem's flowers have a *star-like* corolla of six petals that make two triangles, one pointing up and the other down. This configuration symbolises the merging of heaven and Earth, *body and soul*. When the soul is engaged with the body, *physical healing is divinely-directed*.

The flowers open only when the sun is shining, and this aspect of the plant's signature relates to the essence's capacity to allow us to respond selectively to the most *beneficial and life-energising* aspects of our environment. The *intense white* of the flower is another symbol of its *protective and purifying* qualities. In the process of protective visualisation, people often surround themselves with *'white light'* that creates a safe space for *emotional healing.*

The Star of Bethlehem state of mind

When we are thrown into disarray by some shock – bad news, an accident, general anaesthetic (when the etheric and physical bodies become temporarily dislocated), physical or emotional violence, childbirth or other prolonged stress, even where these occurred many years ago, Star of Bethlehem flower essence helps to restore inner calm.

When we don't have the opportunity to recover fully from shock or trauma, the hurt remains like a festering sore or sensitive scar that can cause further emotional pain. We learn to live in a defensive state, constantly guarding this vulnerable area. Like an athlete carrying an injury and only playing their game to a fraction of their capacity, when we carry an emotional injury we can't fully experience the spontaneity and joy of life.

Benefits of taking Star of Bethlehem

After traumatic experiences, the subtle levels at which our thoughts and emotions arise are disturbed and shaken out of harmony. Star of Bethlehem flower essence helps guide the body-mind back into alignment so that healing can take place in a smoother, more profound and permanent way. It assists in healing recent trauma and also helps recovery from old emotional and mental wounds. It helps to dissipate shock and its effects, whether immediate or delayed, and soothes the sorrows of those who decline to accept consolation even from friends or family.

Under the soul's reconnecting influence, the body becomes healthy again and can be a true temple for the spirit once more.

Possible physical imbalances

For the after-effects of physical trauma – accidental injury, dental or medical procedures – Star of Bethlehem flower essence (especially in conjunction with Arnica) will always provide solace and steer healing and recovery in the right direction. It is especially useful to realign the subtle bodies after their (necessary) disorientation and displacement due to general anaesthetic.

Common uses

For any shock/trauma; for unresolved past emotional trauma; for 'dislocation' of the subtle bodies; to remove obstacles to the healing process

Complementary &/or similar flower essences

Aloe Vera, Arnica, Crowea, Echinacea, Fringed Violet, Glassy Hyacinth, Golden Ear Drops, Nectarine, St John's Wort, Self-Heal, Rescue Remedy, Waratah, YES formula

Supporting the changes

- Professional medical and/or psychotherapeutic guidance is often appropriate for people who need Star of Bethlehem.
- Always give yourself time to recover in a nurturing environment after experiencing a shock of any kind. Often we don't give ourselves enough space or time to acknowledge how deeply something has affected us.
- Learn methods of self-protection such as visualising protective white light around you, especially in the area of the solar plexus.
- Learn to sense and recognise places and situations in which you don't feel secure, so that you can anticipate or avoid them.

Star Thistle
Centaurea solstitialis   (Yellow / FES)

Positive state

Inner sense of abundance
Generous, inclusive and trusting (FES)

Negative state

Poverty-consciousness
'Stingy', ungenerous; 'fear of lack' (FES)

On battlefields long ago, soldiers planted *caltrops* – metal balls with four spikes – to damage the feet of the enemy and the hooves of their horses. The word *caltrop* comes from *trapa*, the Latin word for thistle, and in particular some species of Star Thistle. The *prickly nature* of this roadside plant points to its usefulness as a flower essence for those who, consciously or unconsciously, seem to send out the warning: *'Tread carefully around me!'*

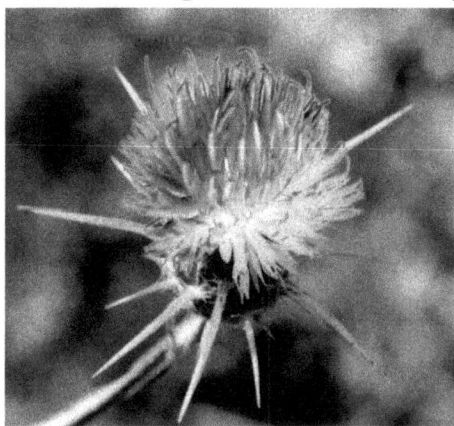

Star Thistle has been specified in herbalism as an antipyretic – an agent that helps reduce fever and inflammation – and the flower essence can help us resolve deep-seated, *painful and inflamed* emotional responses to hardship or rejection earlier in our lives. Like artichokes, the young leaves of the Star Thistle are edible, and the young, *tender* stems make a *generous* contribution to salads. The flower essence helps us to heal and revert to the *softer, emotionally open nature* we had before experiences caused us to lose our *trust* in the world.

The Star Thistle personality

On an emotional level, the unbalanced Star Thistle person sends out a message to others to 'keep away'; we need Star Thistle flower essence when we have become a little too 'prickly'! When we become too emotionally self-protective to give of ourselves, we lose our emotional generosity, and our responses are ruled by a sense of emotional poverty.

Benefits of taking Star Thistle

Star Thistle flower essence helps us to release emotional defences and blockages resulting from painful life experiences. It can re-awaken us to the innate sense of abundance of the soul and free us to respond more openly and unconditionally in our lives and relationships once again. 'Give, and it will be given to you.' (Luke 6:38)

Possible physical imbalances

Because of internal guarding and defensiveness, some who could benefit from Star Thistle flower essence may develop problems such as constipation and/or nervous tension as a result of an inability to 'let go.'

Common uses

For fear of lack; for poverty consciousness; to be less 'stingy'; to trust others with your feelings; to access your generous streak; to give and receive with ease; for a greater sense of abundance

Complementary &/or similar flower essences

Baby Blue Eyes, Bleeding Heart, Chicory, Chrysanthemum, Dogwood, Flannel Flower, Hibiscus, Holly, Oregon Grape, Tiger Lily, Trillium, Willow

Supporting the changes

- Incorporate some spiritual perspectives in your life beyond the materialistic view.
- 'Open up' your pelvic region through yoga, tai chi and/or exercise.
- Buy the next round of drinks!

Sticky Monkeyflower

Mimulus aurantiacus   (Orange / FES)

Positive state

Able to express deep and intimate feelings (FES)
Feeling comfortable and nurtured in intimacy

Negative state

'Repressed sexual feelings' (FES)
Unreceptive to warmth and pleasure of intimacy

Sticky Monkeyflower's *orange* flower expresses its connection with the *sacral chakra*, which relates to issues of *intimacy* with ourselves and others, especially in sexual relationships.

When looking at the flower from above, its *boundaries* seem ill-defined and *nebulous*, as though dissolving at the edges the way the white of an egg spreads when its fragile shell is *shattered*. Sticky Monkeyflower essence is useful for those whose *emotional boundaries* have been abused or invaded and who, as a result, have set up *protective barriers* against *intimate contact*, which feels threatening or overwhelming to them.

The Sticky Monkeyflower personality

Intimate relationships require us to be secure enough in ourselves to be able to risk making ourselves vulnerable to another. Fear of intimacy can disguise itself in many ways. Often it takes the form of retreat into a cerebral or intellectual approach in which we are able to talk very calmly and objectively about sex and sexuality but find it difficult to 'give in' and lose ourself in the experience of physical sensuality. Another approach is to speak coarsely about sex and degrade the experience as a cover for insecurity, or engage in superficial, 'heartless' sexual encounters without becoming emotionally available (Kaminski and Katz 1996).

Benefits of taking Sticky Monkeyflower

Sticky Monkeyflower is part of the Mimulus family and essences made from these flowers assist in dealing with fear of fully experiencing intense emotions. It has a particular emphasis on helping people deal with the intensity of emotion associated with intimate relations.

Sticky Monkeyflower essence can help us be more receptive to experiencing intimacy and not allow our fears to inhibit the pleasure it can bring. Great joy and harmony can be gained through sexual communion but an equally strong alienation can be felt if there is an absence of real warmth and connection. Without intimacy, sex can be a cold and barren experience – 'so near and yet so far.'

Current portrayals in marketing and the media compound the problem (Kaminski and Katz 1996), presenting the body and sexuality as a 'package' separate from the whole person. This can create a self-protective reaction, especially among women, causing them either to harden themselves or to withdraw from intimate contact.

Sticky Monkeyflower plays a role in creating a better relationship between body and soul and a more balanced integration of human warmth and sexual intimacy. It can bring a sense of inner security that allows us to embrace and appreciate intimate relations without fear of losing the Self.

Possible physical imbalances

Some of my clients who have benefited from taking Sticky Monkeyflower essence have experienced problems relating to the reproductive organs and the menstrual cycle in particular.

Common uses

For fear of sex; for discomfort about intimacy; for repressed feelings around sexuality; to help be more receptive to pleasurable sexual feelings; to enjoy the warmth and closeness of intimacy; to help express deep feelings of love; to trust others on an intimate level; to allow yourself to feel vulnerable

Complementary &/or similar flower essences

Baby Blue Eyes, Basil, Billy Goat Plum, Calendula, Crab Apple, Dogwood, Easter Lily, Echinacea, Flannel Flower, Fringed Violet, Fuchsia, Hibiscus, Mallow, all the Monkeyflowers, Oregon Grape, Quince, St John's Wort, Star of Bethlehem, Star Thistle, Star Tulip, YES formula

Supporting the changes

- If traumatic experiences have made you vulnerable and insecure it would be wise to seek professional counselling/therapy.
- Gentle bodywork, massage, tai chi and yoga provide ways of becoming more comfortable in your body, fully sensing it, and ultimately processing ingrained inhibitions.
- Create your own refuge or sanctuary – this may be an actual room or personal shrine or it may be an internal space, created through meditation and relaxation techniques or creative visualisation.

THE **ESSENTIAL** FLOWER ESSENCE BOOK

Sturt Desert Pea

Clianthus formosus (Red and black / Aus)

Positive state

Recovery – emotional pain processed
Past burdens released; receptive to NOW

Negative state

Deep hurt and sadness (Ian White)
Guilt and regret; repressed grief

Sturt Desert Pea is a spectacular native plant with a *powerful presence*. The *rich*, glossy *scarlet* flower with a *black centre* signifies its usefulness as a flower essence for those who have a deep sense of *dark sadness* mixed with *fiery rage*. Those who can benefit from taking Sturt Desert Pea flower essence have deep, unresolved *sadness and hurt* and, like wounded animals, they can be dangerous to themselves and others.

Sturt Desert Pea seeds 'have been known to flower after forty years ... germination often does not take place until the seeds have been subjected to a great force like fire or boiling water' (White 2008). These aspects of the plant's signature reflect the way emotional hurts can be stored for long periods and held in the psyche until they become dislodged through a *cathartic release*.

The Sturt Desert Pea personality

Aboriginal legends based on the Sturt Desert Pea are numerous and Ian White, creator of this essence, writes that they all concern grief, sadness and loss. Aboriginal tribes knew it as the flower of blood. For many First Nations people today the flower still provides a symbol of their ancestors' blood, spilled over the years since invasion and colonisation. With the essence's help, healing of a painful past can proceed, easing the grief that keeps us stuck and unable to experience the joy of the moment.

Benefits of taking Sturt Desert Pea

Ian White believes that Sturt Desert Pea and Waratah are the most powerful of all the essences he has produced. Sturt Desert Pea is capable of healing deep pain and sorrow while Waratah can guide you through your darkest hour, bringing courage, strength and faith. Sturt Desert Pea can help you let go of long-harboured emotional pain by exploring its origins and expressing and diffusing the associated feelings. A heavy weight that has burdened you for a long time is released. You feel re-energised, grounded in the present, and motivated to make things happen.

Possible physical imbalances

In Traditional Chinese Medicine the emotion of grief is associated with the lungs. When health has been affected by grief (even from years before), especially when lung afflictions are present, you would be wise to consider Sturt Desert Pea flower essence. Psychoneuroimmunology studies show how deep-seated and unresolved emotional pain becomes implicated in a wide range of illnesses.

Common uses

For loss or when grieving; for long term sadness/sorrow; to express and diffuse emotional pain; to heal old emotional wounds; to let go of the burdens of the past; to re-commit to NOW and become motivated; to renew trust and optimism about the future

Complementary &/or similar flower essences

Arnica, Baby Blue Eyes, Black Eyed Susan, Bleeding Heart, Borage, Dogwood, Echinacea, Fringed Violet, Fuchsia, Gentian, Golden Ear Drops, Holly, Honeysuckle, Mariposa Lily, Star of Bethlehem, Yerba Santa, Walnut, Waratah, Wild Rose, Willow, YES formula

Supporting the changes

- Consider professional grief counselling or investigate regression therapy.
- Explore the concept of karma.
- Meditation, yoga or any technique that acts to help transform pent-up emotions is beneficial.

Sunflower
Helianthus annuus   (Yellow / FES)

Positive state
Aligned with your inner (higher) authority
Upstanding, honourable and 'your own person'

Negative state
Poor relation to authority and/or father
Self-inflation or self-effacement (FES)

Sunflower is impossible to miss! It stands up to four metres tall and *projects itself* to the world without reserve. It is outrageous and non-conforming, *strong and upstanding*. Most of all it is itself. *Being yourself*, standing up for yourself and not conforming to anyone else's standards or expectations is the quality conveyed by this plant.

The whole plant including the seeds is rich in mineral *silica*, which is extremely important to the *structural* components of the body. Silica is known as 'nature's sculptor' because it 'shapes' crude elements – calcium and magnesium – into appropriate structural forms in the body, such as bones, nails and hair. Silica is vital for the integrity of the spine and other bones and joints; a human without silica is a human without 'spine.' Sunflower essence helps bring *confidence* to people who are very self-effacing and fearful of displaying their *true worth*. It allows them to '*show some spine*' and stand up and be counted, just like the outstanding Sunflower. It helps both men and women to develop and display their *positive masculine qualities*.

Another salient aspect of the Sunflower's signature is the way the golden-yellow flowers, composed of small tubular florets arranged compactly on a flat disk, look like the *sun*. In many cultures the sun has traditionally been associated with the *Father*, the masculine principle and *spiritual knowledge, authority and leadership*.

The Sunflower personality

Sunflower is recommended for those who are self-effacing to the point where they hold back from expressing their full potential, or by contrast, for those who behave in an egotistical or haughty manner (Kaminski and Katz 1996). In both cases there is often a sense of having something to prove to the father (or father-figure) or the world! Both situations share the same underlying theme – low self-esteem and a need for recognition, approval and acceptance. Some more reserved individuals are just very unsure of their real truth or, on the flip side, other more outgoing individuals think they do know it (all) but are, in reality, subservient to external influences 'hard wired' in them from a young age – this often leads to 'intrapsychic conflict that results from the introjected voice or voices of significant others' (Harte, 2019).

Sunflower people often take an ambitious course in life in order to prove something to society, their family or father. Eventually they may burn out, become disillusioned or suffer physical setbacks and this causes them to question their motives. As a therapist, I have found that some women in the negative Sunflower state may resent their menstrual cycle, believing that it prevents them from functioning at their optimum in their career; they may suffer from intense pre-menstrual tension as part of this struggle.

Benefits of taking Sunflower

Sunflower essence helps us to sort out our priorities in life. For example, it can assist men to bond with their young children and enjoy the immediate reward and emotional nourishment of this relationship, as opposed to a more elusive or temporary recognition derived from their career.

Sunflower can assist healing and reconciliation with the father, or our idea of who he is and what he demands of us (Kaminski and Katz 1996). If Sunflower is an important flower essence for you, your relationship with your father-figure may hold the key to many of your personal issues, especially around your relationship with authority.

Sunflower helps us radiate warmth of soul, truly shining in life. Then the only authority and expectations we need to live up to are those associated with our own values and principles. Spiritual direction/guidance and leadership are found within and there is less need to seek it outside ourselves.

Possible physical imbalances

The height and upright posture of the plant points to its relationship with the spine. A number of my clients have reported, as an aside, an improvement in their back problems when taking Sunflower essence. Bodywork practitioners and psychologists agree that posture can reflect the 'stance' we take in life. Are we using our backbone, are we standing up for ourselves or are we 'spineless' in the face of life's challenges?

Common uses

For low self-esteem; for difficulties with authority; for an inflated ego; for those with something to prove (to their dad!); to answer only to your highest good; to know what you stand for; for a healthy masculine/feminine balance; to 'shine' warmly, genuinely and confidently in the world

Complementary &/or similar flower essences

Baby Blue Eyes, Buttercup, Californian Poppy, Calla Lily, Chrysanthemum, Elm, Goldenrod, Hibbertia, Mullein, Pretty Face, Quince, Sagebrush, Saguaro, Tiger Lily

Supporting the changes

- Study the Jungian concepts of anima (feminine) and animus (masculine). Nurture your feminine side.
- Consider doing some public speaking or other personal development activities.
- Spend more time with your kids or your father if possible.
- Don't take yourself too seriously! Learn to laugh at yourself.

Sweet Chestnut

Castanea sativa   (Yellow female & green male / Bach)

Positive state

Courage and faith
Irrepressible resilience

Negative state

Total despair
'Dark night of the soul'

The Sweet Chestnut tree grows to a huge size and has a *powerful, self-reliant* quality, embodying great and *enduring strength*. These trees can live for over a *thousand years*, and even very old trees are capable of producing *new growth*. The *deeply furrowed* bark is reminiscent of the skin of an old, *wise* person who has *been through it all* and still stands strong and vital. The blossoming tree reminds us of our potential for *irrepressible resilience* and *innate ability to recover* from life's most extreme tests of emotional endurance.

The Sweet Chestnut state of mind

When life has tested the limits of our endurance, Sweet Chestnut flower essence can help us climb out of the depths of despair into a new, enlightened era. It can help us change our 'no pain, no gain' philosophy and come to the realisation that life doesn't have to be so hard.

Sweet Chestnut can help us when we experience despair and despondency associated with midlife, menopause, deep-seated emotional trauma or after any long, arduous, demanding and stressful period in life. Such a dark night of the soul can make or break us. We can either submit to misery or forge ahead in a new and better way – 'what doesn't kill us makes us stronger!'

Benefits of taking Sweet Chestnut

When we hit rock bottom the only way out is up. Sweet Chestnut flower essence can bring a return of hope, with a sense that the end of torment is near and we can arise like a phoenix from the ashes. Sweet Chestnut helps restore our dignity, strength and self-assurance – qualities displayed abundantly by this tree that can live for a thousand years.

Possible physical imbalances

Sweet Chestnut flower essence can assist at crisis points when we have carried an illness for a long time. It can be used in terminal illness or for those on the threshold of death to help achieve a more peaceful and serene disposition (consider also Angel's Trumpet flower essence). The deep despair associated with the physically incapacitating aftermath of spinal injuries and strokes may also call for Sweet Chestnut.

Common uses

For 'the straw that breaks the camel's back'; for total despair and hopelessness; for the symbolic deaths in our lives – and the rebirths; for courage and faith; to surrender; for peace of mind after prolonged anguish

Complementary &/or similar flower essences

Angelica, Angel's Trumpet, Arnica, Borage, Chaparral, Echinacea, Gorse, Mustard, Nectarine, Rescue Remedy, Scotch Broom, Sturt Desert Pea, Waratah, Willow

Supporting the changes

- Seek professional counselling and guidance and look for emotional support from friends and family.
- Vocational reassessment may be essential and timely. Seek professional guidance.
- It is essential to establish a healthy, nourishing diet and lifestyle.
- Remember that things can only get better.

Sweet Pea

Lathyrus latifolius   (Pink / FES)

Positive state

Sense of 'social connectedness' (FES) and belonging
Feeling comfortable and 'at home'

Negative state

Feeling disenfranchised
Wandering, 'seeking one's place in life' (FES)

Sweet Pea flower essence is made from flowers of the *pink* variety of the plant. This colour is a sign of its strong connection with the *heart chakra* and the qualities of *emotional attachment* (or *detachment* in the negative state) and *receptiveness* to one's surroundings. The heart chakra governs the thymus gland which plays a pivotal role in our *natural immunity*, allowing us to be *nourished by our surroundings* and to ward off what is not beneficial.

Numerous seeds are *enclosed together* in each Sweet Pea pod. This growth pattern relates to the flower essence's capacity to help us to live in close proximity with each other, a feature of *crowded city living*. The saying 'like peas in a pod' is appropriate here as Sweet Pea essence helps people adjust to living in group situations such as cities where *congested living conditions* can cause antisocial behaviour. Often a way of surviving such harsh conditions is for people to disconnect and allow the mind to disassociate from what's happening around them. Unfortunately, they then feel isolated and that they don't really belong.

I was once consulted by an extended family that had been through two marriage break ups, the suicide of a teenager and numerous changes in place of accommodation; they were currently living in a modest house with *little room to move*. Before they came to me as clients, I visited their home on an unrelated matter. I came to the open front door and from there I could see: two teenage children watching television; the mother in the kitchen (in full view of the front door); a toddler playing with her toys on the other side of the small living room; and a fourth child playing a computer game. It seemed like an eternity before anyone responded to my presence. One by one they came out of their inner worlds and became aware of someone different in their space. Each family member had 'split off' and become detached as a way of surviving recent emotional trauma and dealing with new and oppressive living conditions. When the family consulted me at my clinic, I was able to prescribe Sweet Pea flower essence for each member of the family. It helped family members to feel more comfortable to come out of their separate and isolated 'head spaces' and be emotionally nourished by engaging in more *heart-warming* activity with other members. Kaminski and Katz (1996) describe how 'by acknowledging and experiencing [the] pain which has numbed the Self, the soul can begin to heal, and find its true connection to the Earth and *to other human beings*.'

The Sweet Pea personality

If we don't feel nurtured by our surroundings, we begin to feel alienated. Sometimes this sense of not belonging has no apparent cause, as for example when someone moves into a 'dream home' built to their exact specifications only to find that they don't feel at home in their new neighbourhood. Sweet Pea flower essence can help people to open their hearts so that they can appreciate their surroundings, be nourished by them, and develop a greater sense of belonging.

Adults who as children grew up in a family that moved residences a lot, for instance, can often benefit from taking Sweet Pea, which can enable them to develop a sense of 'home' and belonging in their community, something they may never have developed in the past.

Benefits of taking Sweet Pea

Sweet Pea flower essence helps us to 'feel at home' or at least get a sense of where home is. Sweet Pea has a positive effect on our heart energy, reviving our sense of place on Earth (Kaminski and Katz 1996). At a deep level, it can help us commit to life, right here, right now. Sweet Pea flower essence also helps pets adjust to new surroundings after moving house. It helps them as it does us to be open and receptive to the nurturing already available in our surroundings and allows us to develop a sense of belonging and community.

Possible physical imbalances

If we don't feel truly nurtured by our environment, we can easily develop allergies and intolerances to it. A number of clients who have responded well to Sweet Pea flower essence also found that their environmental allergies improved. Allergies and intolerances reflect much about the state of our overall natural immunity and its interaction with our immediate environment.

Common uses

For congested living conditions; for feeling like an alien; to adapt to a new home; to be open to the positives in one's environment; to find where your heart belongs; to socially connect with your community; to experience heartfelt presence and home comfort where you are, right here, right now!

Complementary &/or similar flower essences

Baby Blue Eyes, Californian Poppy, Corn, Dill, Foxglove, Honeysuckle, Mallow, Nicotiana, Quaking Grass, Shooting Star, Silver Princess, Star Tulip, Tall Yellow Top, Water Violet, Wild Oat, YES formula

Supporting the changes

- Engage in grounding activities such gardening, pottery or any outdoor physical exercise.
- Join a local club or sports team and engage in community work.
- Explore all the options available to you in your local community.
- Bloom where you are planted!

Tall Yellow Top

Senecio magnificus   (Yellow / Aus)

Positive state

Heart and head reconnect
Home is where the heart is – I belong

Negative state

Alienation and loneliness (Ian White)
Unsure where home is

Tall Yellow Top is a *tall* perennial with yellow flowers that are *borne aloft*, as its common name suggests. The *yellow* reminds us of the plant's relationship to the *solar plexus chakra* and the expression of individuality. When the intellect holds sway, our heart and feelings become deprived and a sense of *alienation and disconnection* can develop. Tall Yellow Top flower essence allows the pendulum to swing back towards a *felt sense* for who and where we are – this provides a greater sense of *belonging* (see also Sweet Pea flower essence). Each flowerhead is composed of many small, daisy-like flowers that give the impression of a single large flower, suggesting *self-containment*. This is a useful human quality but when it pervades our life and relationships we become *isolated*.

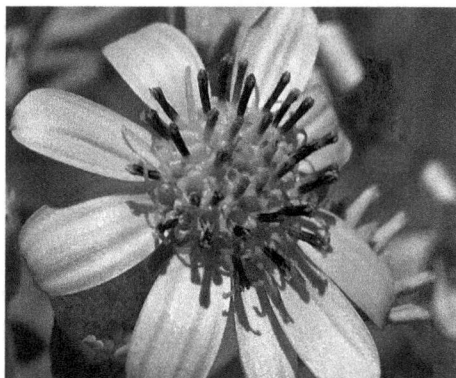

Tall Yellow Top is a *Senecio*, which belongs to the Daisy family, one of the largest and most widespread in the world. As part of this huge extended family, Tall Yellow Top flower essence helps us re-connect and *re-acquaint* ourselves with our family, workplace and networks and once again start to feel a *sense of belonging*.

The Tall Yellow Top personality

If we have spent much of our life drifting or have had jobs and roles with which we coped well intellectually but had no real connection, we can benefit from Tall Yellow Top flower essence. In the unbalanced state, Tall Yellow Top people are restless and this may keep them on the move to such an extent that they become alienated from family, friends and home country, with ensuing loneliness and longing. The sense of alienation may also result from experiences of abandonment in childhood (White 2008). I have had people tell me that they feel they don't belong anywhere – at work, at home or even on this planet! Tall Yellow Top flower essence can help restore a sense that we are home, part of something bigger, giving us a true sense of belonging.

One client who was single and in his late twenties had deliberately chosen to live as far away as possible from his family. He was very intelligent and had proved a capable worker in a number of jobs but suffered from bouts of depression. He thought the main problem was his uncertainty about whether he should settle down where he was and make a definite commitment to living there. Tall Yellow Top helped him become clearer about where he belonged – which turned out to be exactly where he was – and he was able to develop closer, more meaningful relationships with those around him. Even his communication with his family became more relaxed, enjoyable and regular and he felt closer to them although the physical distance between them remained the same.

Benefits of taking Tall Yellow Top

Ian White (2008) tells us that Tall Yellow Top flower essence 'helps to reconnect the head and the heart' so that we can feel at home wherever we are – with our family, in the workplace and in our homeland. It helps us establish and put down roots, open our hearts to others and develop a desire to participate in our community.

Possible physical imbalances

People who respond well to Tall Yellow Top may tend to take a very 'cerebral' approach to life. As a consequence they are prone to 'above the shoulder' health issues such as headache/migraine, neck/cervical problems, sinus problems and also a tendency to anxiety and depression. Tall Yellow Top helps reconnect heart to head and I often tell clients that many headaches are the result of the head struggling to go the way of the heart. In Traditional Chinese Medicine, sinus congestion is regarded as resulting from 'the heart trying to get into the head.'

Common uses

For loneliness; for a deep sense of alienation; to reconnect the heart with the head; to accept yourself and commit to life; to stop 'drifting' and drop anchor; to feel you really belong; to finally come home to Self

Complementary &/or similar flower essences

Angelica, Baby Blue Eyes, Californian Poppy, Forget-Me-Not, Golden Yarrow, Lotus, Nicotiana, Saguaro, Shooting Star, Silver Princess, Sweet Pea, Water Violet, Wild Oat, Wild Rose

Supporting the changes

- Counselling, psychotherapy and other professional guidance may help you find

and accept your true Self.
- Heart-focused meditation will assist you as long as it is practised in moderation and is balanced by grounding activities.
- Try to spend more time with those who respect you and your personal space.
- Engage in activities that are emotionally stimulating – follow your passions!

Tansy

Tanacetum vulgare (Yellow / FES)

Positive state

Decisive, committed and motivated
Self-directed, purposeful (FES)

Negative state

Indolent; prone to procrastination
'Habits undermine or subvert real intentions of Self' (FES)

Tansy is *resistant* to frost and cold and the strong-smelling flower *lasts* a long time. Patches of Tansy can *survive* for decades in the same location. Herbalists claim that the common name Tansy is a corruption of the Greek word for immortality, *athanasia*. As a flower essence, Tansy can help us develop a stronger, more *enduring commitment* to our aspirations and goals, even if we have repressed these aspirations early in life as OUR WAY of navigating/surviving difficult circumstances. It reminds us that the ability to endure manifests in different ways – some helpful, some not.

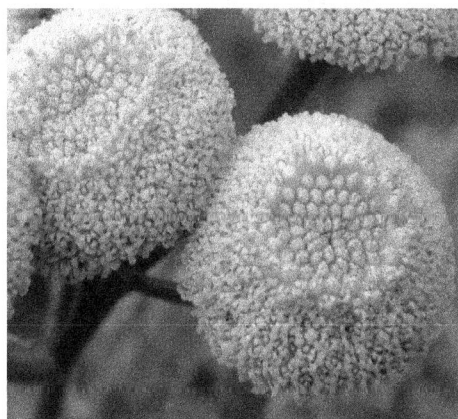

For example, a child who grows up in a chaotic, unstable home may cope silently, *suppressing* their *instinctive reactions* as a way of keeping the peace at the price of their own *inner drive and vitality*. Although it is a member of the Daisy family, Tansy flowers have no petals and this 'contractive' aspect of the plant's signature points to its usefulness as a flower essence for those whose 'outward' *growth has been repressed* or those who have a tendency to *retreat* or withdraw.

The Tansy personality

When we are lethargic, unmotivated and directionless, Tansy flower essence helps us to develop our true potential, to be self-directed and self-driven. When procrastination rules our responses, we can free up the vitality within us and decisively pursue our goals. As a therapist I sometimes hear clients say: 'After talking to you I feel motivated to make changes in my lifestyle or habits. However, knowing me, I'll lose the plot in a week or so and fall back into my old ways.' If this sounds like you, Tansy can help you to maintain your motivation and stay determined and goal-oriented.

I have found in practice that some people who have benefited from Tansy flower essence grew up feeling they had to 'hold their tongue,' often 'walking on eggshells' for fear of stirring things up or getting into trouble in a chaotic or very repressive home environment. Unfortunately, they can easily fall into the trap of becoming that outwardly 'happy go lucky' person who swallows their true feelings, literally developing eating disorders, with weight issues often being a real challenge.

Benefits of taking Tansy

Tansy flower essence helps stimulate greater self-awareness through a more meditative approach to life, allowing us to realise our strengths and become more purposeful and forthright, especially in getting our needs met. We are better able to focus on what we really desire and far less likely to fall back into old habits that undermine or subvert our personal goals.

Possible physical imbalances

Some clients in my practice who have responded well to Tansy flower essence have had a history of mildly underactive thyroid with related weight gain. The thyroid governs many metabolic processes in the body and if underactive, can bring about a feeling of sluggishness and lethargy. The throat chakra, which influences the thyroid, very much relates to how effectively we are able to communicate our needs and how well the world responds to them.

Common uses

For lack of motivation; for complacency and procrastination; for inability to make change and break undermining habits; for lethargy; to bring increased motivational energy; for a sense of purpose; to speak up for our SELF; for decisiveness and clear goals; for self- directed and sustained ACTION!

Complementary &/or similar flower essences

Blackberry, Cayenne, Deerbrush, Forget-Me-Not, Hornbeam, Iris, Lady's Slipper, Macrocarpa, Madia, Morning Glory, Pansy, Scleranthus, Self-Heal, Silver Princess, Wild Potato Bush, Wild Oat, Wild Rose

Supporting the changes

- Take part in non-confrontational assertiveness courses.

- Attend to lifestyle and diet and include more movement and exercise in your week. See a health professional for guidance.
- Take time to identify your current goals and set out a program that will help you to reach them.
- Don't just sit there – get moving and speak up!

Tiger Lily

Lilium humboldtii   (Orange with brown spots / FES)

Positive state

Capacity for cooperation – enhanced feminine/receptive energy (FES)
Win/win mentality – living in harmony

Negative state

'Overly aggressive; excessive yang forces' (FES)
Power struggles; 'separatist tendencies' (FES)

The *orange and brown* colours of the Tiger Lily flower relate strongly to the qualities of the *sacral chakra*. The *warm receptivity* associated with the sacral chakra is expressed through the colour orange; a sense of *abundance* of Earth energy and resources through the colour brown. These are the positive qualities enhanced by the flower essence. Together they instil a sense of *cooperation and harmony*.

The Tiger Lily personality

The nickname 'Tiger' is sometimes given to people who compete ferociously against those they identify with – usually siblings, friends and peers. In the unbalanced state, Tiger Lily people may be avoided by others because of their aggression or hostility; they see themselves as separate from others and strive against them rather than working for the good of the family, company or team (Kaminski and Katz 1996). This kind of fractiousness is often most marked during adolescence when teenagers attempt to develop autonomy as adults. It may also surface in midlife (especially at menopause) during reassessment or redefining of social roles, especially in terms of inner balance between masculine and feminine energies.

I once treated an eight-year-old boy who was continually sick with colds, tummy aches, allergies etc. In the olden days they would have called it 'failure to thrive.' His twin brother, on the other hand, was five or six inches taller and was healthy, with a totally different demeanour. Over a month or so of taking flower essences (including Sunflower) aimed at increasing self-confidence, along with some homoeopathic remedies to support immune function, the 'sickly' twin's health improved significantly. He also became much more self-assured and confident. This changed the dynamic between the twins quite dramatically – now the bigger boy became more aggressive towards his brother (who seemed pretty unfussed by it) and also towards the rest of the family. I prescribed Tiger Lily to help this previously 'top dog' twin adjust to his previously weaker brother's newfound confidence. Within a few days he had settled down and was much more cooperative – he seemed more secure and was able to adapt to the change in his now 'thriving' twin!

Benefits of taking Tiger Lily

Tiger Lily flower essence helps us to receive others warmly in a spirit of cooperation in situations of potential stress, for example when families or groups of refugees must share crowded living conditions. It can also help us develop a greater appreciation for the positive aspects of our life circumstances.

Tiger Lily helps to balance the masculine (yang) and feminine (yin) forces, especially when the masculine is dominant at the expense of the feminine (Kaminski and Katz 1996). This often manifests as aggressive tendencies that arise out of a sense of competition for resources and a perceived need to dominate in order to 'win out' in the struggle to survive. Tiger Lily can help to mellow the competitive masculine side by enhancing the feminine side and allowing it to come to the fore in social situations.

Possible physical imbalances

According to Traditional Chinese Medicine, a body with excessive yang energy is more prone to illnesses involving heat and congestion. 'Hot flushes' can be thought of as a yang response which occurs as part of a rebalancing of feminine/ masculine, yin/yang and female/male hormones that occurs during menopause. As a therapist I have found that Tiger Lily flower essence can often be helpful for women who experience this temporary 'excess yang' effect, allowing them to negotiate menopause more comfortably on many levels.

Common uses

For subtle power struggles; for sibling rivalry; for fear of lack or missing out; for an aggressive personality; to balance overly yang forces; to be more warm and receptive; for cooperation; to trust in abundance; to develop a true win/win attitude

Complementary &/or similar flower essences

Calendula, Calla Lily, Chicory, Chrysanthemum, Dogwood, Flannel Flower, Impatiens, Mariposa Lily, Oregon Grape, Pomegranate, Quince, Snapdragon, Star Thistle, Sunflower, Trillium, Vervain, Willow

Supporting the changes

- Explore the concepts of yin and yang and anima and animus.
- Develop a more meditative approach to life through practices such as tai chi and yoga and/or exercise your competitive spirit among consenting adults in a sport of your choice.
- Practise active listening, also called 'accurate receiving' and 'listening with the heart.'
- Remember that everyone can be a winner!

Trillium

Trillium chloropetalum   (Maroon / FES)

Positive state

Secure sense of personal welfare (FES); motivated by altruism
'Selfless service' (FES)

Negative state

Greed, lust, ambition for power (FES)
Self-service

Trillium flower's *purple-red* (maroon) colour and *phallic* appearance as it emerges from the ground points to its role in working with *crude power* that must be transformed and refined before it can be used to benefit the world. The colour purple is symbolic of our *higher (spiritual) self* and its capacity to *transform* (refine) our *basic urges, desires and passions* (red) in accordance with a *higher* or more *altruistic purpose*. The symbolism in this plant reflects its potential for helping us to re-channel *primal energy* in the service of humanity rather than in *self-gratification*.

The Trillium personality

When the base chakra (which relates to survival) is over-energised, we may suffer from an inordinately aggressive and competitive attitude so that accumulating power, status and material gain becomes our main motivation (Kaminski and Katz 1996). The survival instinct may be distorted so that it takes the form of excessive concern or obsession about material security and personal welfare. It may also drive a hedonistic approach to life as our erotic desires and sensuality are also intrinsic to the base chakra.

Benefits of taking Trillium

Trillium flower essence can transform an obsession with material security into an understanding and awareness of others' material and emotional needs. When we work together for the common good, we can achieve infinitely more than when we work alone. Kaminski and Katz (1996) speak of how 'Trillium encourages [us] to shift [our] awareness to a transpersonal level' so that our lonely and defensive stance in life can shift towards a more generous attitude. As we open ourselves up to give, we also create space to be able to receive.

Possible physical imbalances

Adrenal fatigue and male sexual issues are areas where energy imbalances of this kind have the potential to emerge on a physical level.

Common uses

For greed and over-indulgence; for sex addiction; for blind ambition; to enable us to trust life; to appreciate others' achievements; to enjoy working in a team; for satisfaction through altruism; to thrive through selfless service (to a cause)

Complementary &/or similar flower essences

Baby Blue Eyes, Basil, Chicory, Chrysanthemum, Hibbertia, Holly, Impatiens, Lotus, Quaking Grass, Quince, Snapdragon, Star Thistle, Sunflower, Tiger Lily, Vine

Supporting the changes

- Investigate the concept that there are no losers, only winners. Explore the idea of karma.
- Join a sports team or group working for charitable, community-based causes you admire.
- Take pleasure in someone else's good fortune!

Trumpet Vine
Campsis tagliabuana   (Orange-red / FES)
Positive state
Warm, dynamic communication
Eloquent and vibrant speech

Negative state
'Lack of vitality or soul force in expression' (FES)
Monotone and lacklustre speech

Like a 'flower essence manual for dummies,' Trumpet Vine provides an introduction to the doctrine of plant signatures. Named and shaped like a *trumpet* that *projects outward* as it *unfolds from within*, this flower leaves us in no doubt that that its qualities relate to *'blowing your own trumpet.'*

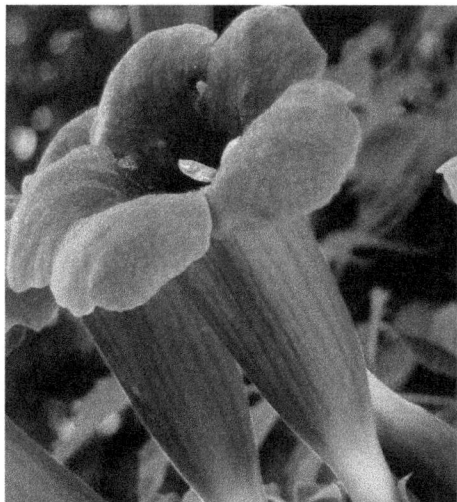

The flower essence helps us to speak our truth, fuelled by personal *passion*. The *warm, intimate* qualities of the colour *orange* (*sacral chakra*) are combined with the *passionate and stimulating* energy of *red* (*base chakra*) and both are conveyed in vibrational form through the flower essence to help us *communicate* a more vital self to the world.

Trumpet Vine flower essence helps to free the *dynamic* forces of our *lower chakras* to generate and vitalise our *speech*. It can add *emotional depth, passion and warmth* to verbal expression, which may otherwise be *flat, dry and bland*.

The Trumpet Vine personality

Our speech may be technically correct but if we lack the power and passion to invest it with interest or meaning we may bore those who listen to us or lose their attention. In the unbalanced state, some Trumpet Vine people may be concerned about sounding dull or clumsy and refuse to speak out, while others courageously endeavour to improve their skills (as one of my clients did by joining a public speaking group).

Trumpet Vine flower essence is also useful for children with speech problems such as stammering.

Benefits of taking Trumpet Vine

Trumpet Vine flower essence helps us to draw energies up from the lower chakras so that they can be integrated and articulated via the throat chakra. These centres – especially the sacral chakra – provide energy for expressing our mental creativity and for grounding our plans and ideas. 'As the soul learns to project and express itself' (Kaminski and Katz 1996) via the voice, our capacity to share our unique qualities with others grows, and we become more confident and less concerned about how others may judge us.

Possible physical imbalances

In my practice, I have found that a number of people who benefited from taking Trumpet Vine flower essence also had a history of throat problems (the area associated with the throat chakra and communication) such as frequent sore throats or recurring tonsillitis.

Common uses

For devitalised expression; for speech problems; for monotone vocalism; to add colour to your expression; for more dynamic projection of the Self; to learn how to 'blow your own trumpet'; to captivate your audience and really be heard!

Complementary &/or similar flower essences

Angel's Trumpet, Buttercup, Calendula, Cosmos, Deerbrush, Iris, Larch, Mallow, Morning Glory, Mullein, Nasturtium, Snapdragon, Sunflower, Yerba Santa

Supporting the changes

- Investigate personal growth courses, especially those addressing assertiveness and communication skills.
- Become involved in activities such as psychodrama, eurhythmy, singing, public speaking and performing, dance or other artistic outlets that encourage the expression of creative energies.
- Take part in courses that encourage the development of your presentation skills.
- Practise voice projection, exploring your full vocal range.
- Join a choir!

Vervain

Verbena officinalis   (Pink-mauve / Bach)

Positive state

Relaxed and accepting of others' paths in life
Natural enthusiasm for life

Negative state

Trying to convert others to your way of thinking
Over-identification with a cause

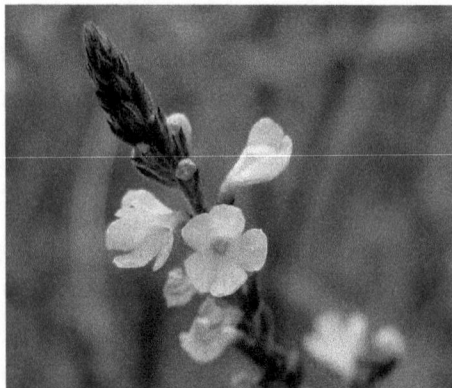

Vervain has tough and erect branches that are *spear-like*, aspiring to greater height and *spiritual penetration* – like the spires of a church or cathedral. Each branch grows individually towards the heavens while remaining *joined at the root*. (This reminds us that we are basically united and yet, at the same time, also have aspirations as individuals.) Traditionally the plant has adorned places of worship as a symbol of spiritual connection to the heavens and our *search for universal truth.*

Vervain flower essence teaches the lesson that you don't have to kill yourself in the process of attaining your goals or *'die for the cause'*! Vervain's vigorous growth supports a flower that is modest and unspectacular (Barnard 1988). The *calming mauve* or *pink* colour of the flower relates to the *heart chakra* and our ability to *let go* of *overzealous and unyielding attachment to an ideal.* When we approach our goals calmly, we often achieve them more fully than when we *try too hard.*

The Vervain personality

Vervain flower essence moderates the desire to convert everyone else to our way of thinking, even when we mean well. Attachment to a cause is frightening in its extreme form and accounts for many atrocities that have occurred in the name of religion or politics. In the negative Vervain state we try to force an idea on others because we fervently believe it to be right (as happens with fundamentalism). However, no ideology, however exalted, is adequate to the whole of human experience and all ideas have to pass through the distorting filter of our own personal and cultural limitations. This is the insight that is lost to those in need of Vervain flower essence.

Benefits of taking Vervain

Vervain helps us to understand that it is possible to inspire others to reach their own unique path without having to convert them to our beliefs. It allows us to pursue our quest to awaken and spiritually unite with the divine in others without imposing ourselves on them.

Vervain flower essence helps us become more secure in our beliefs and grounds them in our inner experience. We become better able to see the truths in other life paths and understand that differing life experiences may lead us to different conclusions. In the positive state, Vervain people do not lose their enthusiasm and perseverance – they continue to fight for justice in the world but their view is no longer narrow and insular and they do not claim to have all the answers.

Possible physical imbalances

Nervous and muscular tension is a very common result of an overzealous approach to life. Our inability to relax because our 'cause' will not allow it can predispose us to many health problems, particularly sleep difficulties. Eventually a tense, 'type A' personality approach to life can easily lead to heart problems.

Common uses

For over-enthusiastic health practitioners; for 'bible-bashers'; for fanatics and fundamentalists; for the over-zealous; for 'try-hard' personalities; for the martyr for a cause; for those who invade the personal space of others ('for their own good'!!); to help learn to ride with rather than override others; to remind us that we often teach best what we need to learn ourselves; to resist wanting to heal everybody; to allow people to come to their own conclusions through personal experience (or inner work as in Buddhism); to relax and to live and let live

Complementary &/or similar flower essences

Beech, Bleeding Heart, Calendula, Californian Poppy, Canyon Dudleya, Dandelion, Hibbertia, Impatiens, Larkspur, Lavender, Lotus, Quaking Grass, Rock Water, Zinnia

Supporting the changes

- Relax and take a holiday from your cause.
- Try to find some passive and introverted activities that you enjoy.
- Engage in exercise such as walking, gardening, swimming that relaxes as well as gets your mind off the 'cause.'
- Meditate on it!

Vine

Vitis vinifera   (Green / Bach)

Positive state

Unconditional, compassionate and cooperative
Accommodating of different ways/opinions

Negative state

Wilful, domineering
Only one way – my way!

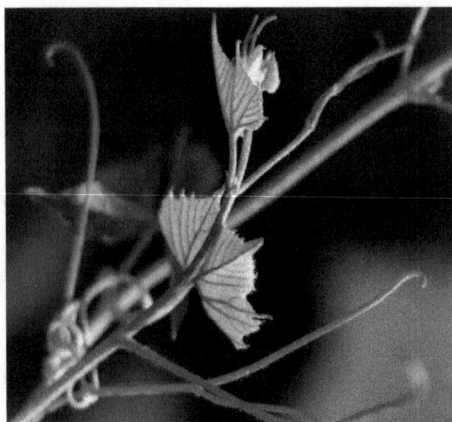

The grapevine is a *climber* that can live for *several hundred years*. It is one of humankind's oldest plant companions, mentioned in the Bible as having survived the Great Flood, after which Noah planted a vineyard. Its flowers are small, *green* and bud-like and appear in branched *clusters* like the grapes that follow. Green relates to the *heart chakra* and the capacity for *unconditional love*, *compassion* and the ability to *set others*

free.

The heart chakra also assists in developing *group consciousness* and the clustered growth of the Vine flower signifies the essence's capacity to foster *growing and working together in harmony.*

Julian and Martine Barnard (1988) describe how the vine will 'reach out and grip whatever is nearby, twisting the tendrils to fasten and hold.'

This *forceful overpowering* of others is seen in the negative state addressed by Vine flower essence. Five petals join to form a small cap that is *forced off* as the stamens mature and grow. This aspect of the signature can be interpreted as another illustration of a Vine person's sheer *willpower.*

The Vine personality

In the negative state, Vine people only know one way – their way – and they often have the strength of will to get it (unless they 'lock horns' with another Vine person!) They are strong, assertive, decisive and self-sufficient, and because they have been successful in the past, they believe they can continue to impose their will on everyone else. In their desire for power, they sometimes use others as stepping stones to increase their own stature, just as the plant uses the branches of its host to pull itself up.

In order to reach wholeness and balance, we need to recognise our genuine need of others – they are not just a means to an end. However, we cannot draw those we care about to us by will alone, nor would this bring us peace of mind ultimately. Vine flower essence can help us to allow our heart to open and its warmth to be felt by those around, as symbolised by the blossoming of the Vine plant's green flowers.

Benefits of taking Vine

In the positive Vine state, we are capable of heart-felt compassion which, when combined with a strong will and commitment, makes us formidable exponents of kindness and consideration. We are natural leaders, and when our heart transforms the desire to dominate into a desire to cooperate, we become inspirational, supportive, dependable and flexible enough to respond to the needs of others as well as our own.

Possible physical imbalances

Flexibility is a key issue for Vine people. The fact that mind and body are two sides of the same coin means that many who respond well to Vine flower essence tend to experience some form of physical rigidity, especially as they get older. They may experience symptoms ranging from simple tension to general stiffness, to movement-limiting arthritis. 'Hardening' of the blood vessels can also occur which potentially leads to heart problems and circulatory complaints.

Common uses

For people who use expressions like 'I'm the boss! Do it because I say so!'; 'Let me steer!'; 'It's my way or the highway!'; for the petty tyrant; for those who are stuck in their own ways; to change 'rigid' aspects of our character; to use your drive for the good of all; to help loosen up and let it be!

Complementary &/or similar flower essences

Beech, Dandelion, Impatiens, Larkspur, Lotus, Mallow, Nicotiana, Oregon Grape, Quaking Grass, Quince, Star Tulip, Sunflower, Tiger Lily, Trillium, Vervain

Supporting the changes

- Any form of relaxation practice will help you learn to 'let go' physically and mentally.
- Engage in regular stretching exercises or practices such as yoga to improve and maintain flexibility (and also 'let go').
- Join a team where someone else is leader or captain!
- Let someone else run the show!

Violet

Viola odorata   (Violet / FES)

Positive state

Modestly self-assured
'Sharing with others while remaining true to oneself' (FES)

Negative state

Shy and sensitive (FES)
Reluctant to share thoughts and opinions

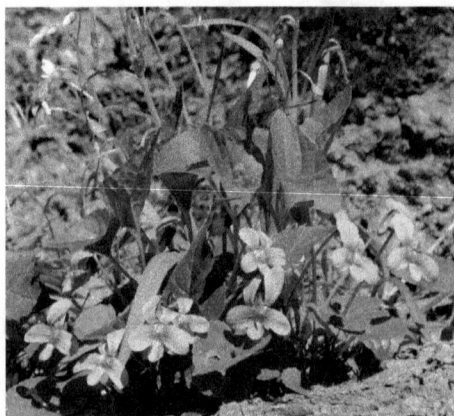

Violets have been admired for thousands of years and used for medicinal purposes for just as long. They grow and *creep close to the ground* beneath taller plants that provide shade and *protection*.

The Violet plant is *extremely sensitive* and its *vulnerable* constitution is easily affected by pollution or *parasites*. This is why it prefers to grow in partially shaded, sloping sites in meadows and woods.

Violets have an *attractive* perfume that *draws attention*. People who can benefit from taking Violet flower essence are *'shrinking violets'* who are *dying* to be noticed but are often too *shy* to speak up, so their insights do not receive the *acknowledgement* they deserve.

Traditional use has given the Violet herb a reputation for having beneficial effects in the treatment of cancer. While this has not yet been tested scientifically, it is interesting to note that some psychotherapists perceive a connection between unlived potential or repressed emotion and the development of cancer. Just like the plant that prefers to live in shade, parts of the self are never expressed in the light of day, and *unfulfilled* longings or *repressed* memories may *'eat away'* at an individual on a deep level. Psychoneuroimmunological research has confirmed that this can lead to serious immune dysfunction. (I am definitely not suggesting that Violet flower essence is a cure for cancer but I am suggesting that it is worth exploring the relationship between mental or emotional states and the manifestation of physical conditions because of the mind/body connection.) Violet flower essence can enable a person to find *creative expression* for aspects of the Self, especially when they have remained unexpressed because of shyness/timidity.

The Violet personality

Violet people are often shy and sensitive but want to be noticed and appreciated for their acute perception. Unfortunately however, this very sensitivity works against them in this respect because they 'shrink away' from speaking up in public. Kaminski and Katz (1996) inform us that Violet flower essence is helpful for those who are reticent and 'fear that their sense of Self will be lost or submerged' in group situations, despite a strong desire to join in and share valuable insights and perceptions.

Another group of people who find Violet flower essence very helpful are those who find their niche and become very confident in a certain area – whether 'out there' in the arts world or at home parenting – but who become timid and insecure as soon as they move outside their comfort zone. Violet flower essence can help these people develop better subtle boundaries so that they feel more comfortable and secure when 'venturing out' into other areas of life so that 'their beautiful soul nature may be shared with the world' (Kaminski and Katz 1996).

Benefits of taking Violet

Violet flower essence gently supports and assists us to feel safe and secure when speaking up in public, while remaining true to our sensitive, perceptive and open nature. Validation and appreciation follows naturally.

Possible physical imbalances

Sensitivity on subtle levels often expresses itself on a physical level. Just like the Violet plant itself you may need to be aware of reactions to foods and also environmental sensitivities, especially geopathic stresses.

Common uses

For over-sensitivity; for shyness in groups; for those easily overlooked; for those 'dying to be heard' but lacking confidence; to develop inner security; to establish better (subtle) boundaries; for more self-promoting confidence; to be heard in the crowd; for a modest but captivating presence

Complementary &/or similar flower essences

Almond, Angelica, Angelsword, Black Eyed Susan, Buttercup, Fairy Lantern, Fringed Violet, Fuchsia, Garlic, Golden Yarrow (and all the Yarrows), Mallow, Mimulus (and all the 'Monkeyflowers'), Red Grevillea, St John's Wort, Wallflower, YES formula

Supporting the changes

- Violet people benefit from taking refuge on a regular basis in their private 'sanctuary,' whatever that may be, in order to safeguard their sensitive and delicate natures. The sense of sanctuary can also be created internally through prayer, meditation and relaxation techniques or through creative visualisation. Visualising white light around the self is a common protective practice.
- A balanced approach to diet and lifestyle is extremely important for sensitive individuals. Occasional gentle cleansing programs such as herbal and fresh juice days are extremely beneficial.
- Never forget that what you have to say is very valuable, because you notice what a lot of other people don't!

Wallflower
Erysimum capitatum   (Orange / FES-res)

Positive state
Desire to participate
Socially self-assured and outgoing

Negative state
Tendency to retreat to the sidelines
Shyness (particularly with the opposite sex)

Young women who are *relegated to the sidelines at social functions* have often been called 'wallflowers,' being shy and unsure of the correct social etiquette. Wallflowers often stand alone on mountain slopes, with their showy bright yellow glow appearing as little splashes scattered about, here and there. Once again, the plant's common name (and its growth description) gives insight into the type of person who might benefit from taking the flower essence. *Romantic associations* have often been made with the Wallflower and at one stage it became a symbol for *adversity in love*. In my practice, I have found that Wallflower essence has, on a number of occasions, helped female clients to overcome *shyness* with the opposite sex.

The flower's predominantly *orange* colour signifies its influence on the *sacral chakra*, which is associated with *warmth and intimacy* in relationship. Wallflower helps us to feel more comfortable in sharing and expressing the *warm-hearted* aspects of our being. The orange-yellow, mustard-coloured flowers (like Mustard Bach Flower essence) also fills the Wallflower essence with a quality that can inspire a more hopeful and brighter outlook.

The Wallflower personality

Wallflower people may want to protest that they're 'not just a pretty face!' and seek recognition for the depth of their character but this often remains unvoiced because of their shyness and timidity. Their sensitive nature can easily leave them feeling overwhelmed and even violated in social situations; retreating from the social arena too often becomes their preferred option, sometimes leading to depression.

Benefits of taking Wallflower

Wallflower essence encourages involvement in self-assured social exchange, rather than retreat from social situations through shyness. It helps us to 'stand up and stand out' without the need for excessive makeup, sexually alluring clothes or other veneers. At the same time it helps to strengthen our dynamic boundaries, enhancing the integrity of the sacral chakra so that we keep our 'core' composure and don't absorb harmful energies even in volatile social situations.

Wallflower helps us to achieve a natural balance between expenditure and conservation of energy in social situations so that our warmth and dynamism can shine through.

Possible physical imbalances

As a therapist, I have found that people who respond well to Wallflower essence often match the old saying, 'cold hands, warm heart,' and for some of these clients there was even an improvement in physical circulation to the extremities, with less over-sensitivity to cold.

Common uses

For 'wallflowers'; for shyness with the opposite sex; for over-sensitivity and exhaustion in social situations; for dynamic self-assurance; for social confidence; to support joyful participation

Complementary &/or similar flower essences

Angelica, Angelsword, Buttercup, Calla Lily, Cayenne, Corn, Fairy Lantern, Forget-Me-Not, Garlic, Golden Yarrow (and all the Yarrows), Golden Rod, Hibiscus, Larch, Mallow, Mimulus, Oregon Grape, Pretty Face, Quaking Grass, Rosemary, St John's Wort, Shooting Star, Sticky Monkeyflower, Sweet Pea, Violet, Water Violet, YES formula

Supporting the changes

- Learn techniques that strengthen your aura and help you to feel more secure in social situations. White light visualisations, chakra meditations that focus on the solar plexus, prayers and affirmations may be useful.
- Read about the lives of quiet achievers.
- Consider doing some assertiveness training courses.
- Maintain regular, enjoyable social activities – don't just retreat.
- Join in the fun!

Walnut

Juglans regia   (Green / Bach)

Positive state

Able to steer one's own course
Coping and adapting to change

Negative state

Deflected from one's path by the influence of others
Overwhelmed by change/major transitions

When a Walnut shell is cracked open, the inner nut resembles a brain. This aspect of the plant's signature reminds us of Walnut flower essence's ability to stimulate the mental body and help us to make intellectual (*brain-driven*) rather than emotional (*heart-driven*) decisions when required. This is necessary at certain stages of development and *change* (often coinciding with outer change in our lives), when some of our *emotional attachments* no longer serve our higher good. At transitional times in our lives we often need

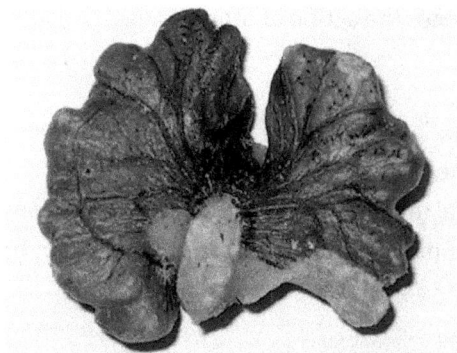

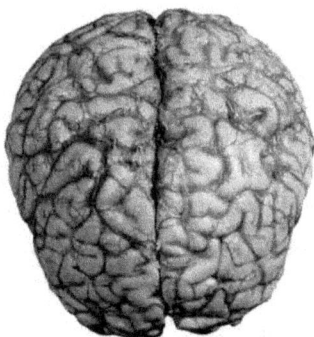

to *re-commit* to our *soul purpose* and not be distracted from our true path in life.

The leaves of the Walnut tree have a pungent, acrid scent, which deters other plants, animals and insects from coming too close. This aspect of the plant's signature symbolises how Walnut flower essence helps to create a *protected psychological space* that allows us to negotiate internal changes and *rites of passage* necessary for new growth, without distractions. (It is interesting to note that the scent is at its strongest when the new growth is occurring and leaf buds are just breaking open.) The green colour of the flower reminds us of its close affinity with the heart chakra and the qualities of natural immunity, 'personal space', protection and natural resistance to pathogens.

The Walnut state of mind

When we are easily influenced by others to the point that it obscures our true path in life, Walnut flower essence can be of assistance. During times of major transition such as teething, first separation from parents, puberty, leaving school, first job, moving house, loss of a loved one, midlife or menopause, we are more vulnerable to external influences and more likely to fall back on old patterns and attachments that may no longer serve our higher good. At times of change and upheaval we cling to our connections with individuals, groups or routines that feel safe and familiar. While part of us may long for what we know, even if it is 'the devil we know', another part knows that change is inevitable and necessary. Dr Bach called this remedy 'the link breaker', as it breaks emotional ties and habits that no longer serve the whole Self.

Benefits of taking Walnut

Walnut flower essence helps you conjure the inner resolve needed to realise your ideals and ambitions despite adversity or criticism and without needy dependence on another. It frees you from old ties and previous ways of thinking that no longer serve your true purpose.

In its capacity to positively influence the heart chakra, Walnut helps to strengthen natural immunity on all levels, including our ability to adapt to change. For this reason, it often complements and enhances the action of other flower essences.

Possible physical imbalances

Oversensitivity to outside influences applies to the physical environment also. In its capacity to positively influence the heart chakra and its associated thymus gland, Walnut helps improve natural immunity against recurring infections in childhood after exposure to new environments such as creche, kindergarten or school.

Common uses

As the 'link breaker'; for adjusting to separation; for the loss of a loved one; for over-attachment to family, friends, peer group; to improve natural immunity on all levels; to be less under the influence of others; to adapt to change; to help you let go of what no longer serves your greater good

Complementary &/or similar flower essences

Almond, Angel's Trumpet, Bleeding Heart, Boab, Bottlebrush, Canyon Dudleya, Centaury, Honeysuckle, Onion, Pink Yarrow, Red Grevillea, Sagebrush, St John's Wort, YES formula

Supporting the changes

- Call in a third party who remains emotionally objective when you need to resolve conflicts and problems.
- Use creative visualisation to protect the heart and solar plexus chakras with white light. Meditate by yourself.
- Write down the pros and cons of a situation. This allows you to objectively appraise the direction you need to take.
- Move on!

Waratah

Telopea speciosissima   (Red / Aus)

Positive state

'Enhancement of survival skills' (Ian White)
Active and composed in a crisis

Negative state

Hopelessness and utter despair (Ian White)
In crisis and unable to respond

W aratah's majestic, *rich red* flower symbolises its connection to *instinctual survival* energies associated with the *base chakra*. The *Telopea* genus belongs to one of the oldest plant groups in the world, having survived a multitude of crises during sixty million years since its emergence on the ancient continent of Gondwana (White 2008). No wonder Waratah flower essence is used to help *stir* our survival instincts when we are facing a *life crisis*.

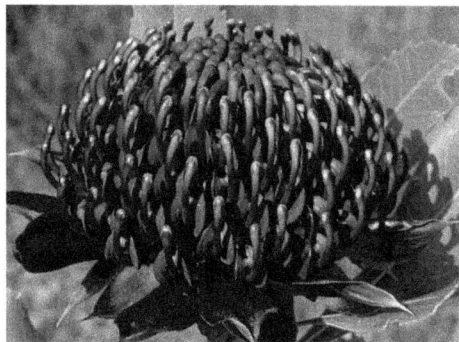

The many small flowers grow together in a *tightly integrated* head, *securely enclosed* in protective petal-like bracts, which reminds us (as does a similar formation in the Garlic and Red Clover flower) how the essence can help us to *'hold ourselves together'* in times of crisis. The look and feel of the red bloom, which can be up to thirty centimetres across, suggests *strength and integrity*. The Waratah flower is very important in Aboriginal culture, folklore and legends which tell the stories of individuals who survive crises, *ordeals and life challenges*, becoming stronger through the development of *courage, faith and endurance*.

The Waratah state of mind

Waratah flower essence is worth considering when we are in deep despair but it is also very helpful when we are just stuck in some way. When apprehension and hesitancy rule our thoughts, we feel trapped and a state of resignation and reluctance prevents us from moving forward. Progress and personal growth seem to cease, whether temporarily or in the long term. Sometimes we just need a little nudge in the right direction and at other times we need a more forceful push. The subtle but powerful action of this flower essence can be helpful in either circumstance.

Benefits of taking Waratah

Ian White, who first produced this flower essence, writes that in times of crisis, Waratah will sharpen the memory of previous survival skills (White 2008). (This also occurs in many animals when threatened by bushfire, for instance. They will instinctively move to safer ground.) The analogy I use for this remedy is driving a car on an unsealed country road; as the car drifts onto the gravel edge, an inexperienced and panic-stricken driver applies the brakes with disastrous consequences and the car careers out of control. A driver with defensive driving training and experience, on the other hand, knows that it is necessary to accelerate in order to get out of trouble and regain control in these circumstances.

Waratah flower essence can help us overcome the fear that prevents us from accelerating through and out of difficult situations. It helps us to regain composure by enhancing our innate survival skills, strengthening inner resolve and self-determination to move in the right direction.

Possible physical imbalances

I have noticed that a number of clients who have responded well to Waratah also experienced some improvement in postural issues, reporting improvement in lower back problems and ability to keep the spine in a more comfortable and upright position. Some similarities to Sunflower essence were noticed in this regard.

Common uses

For the 'dark night of the soul'; for hopelessness; for feeling stuck and unable to respond to crisis; for being 'frozen with fear'; to enhance (instinctual) survival skills; for faith and hope; for courage and strength; to help one adapt; to persevere beyond one's normal limit; to come through to the other side; to regain composure and peace of mind

Complementary &/or similar flower essences

Angelica, Arnica, Borage, Cayenne, Chaparral, Cherry Plum, Echinacea, Garlic, Gorse, Indian Pink, Nectarine, St John's Wort, Self-Heal, Sweet Chestnut, Red Clover, Rock Rose, Scotch Broom, Star of Bethlehem, YES formula

Supporting the changes

- Take part in regular, vigorous exercise or other activity that helps to develop your physical and mental endurance.
- Consider a program of bodywork therapy.
- Set yourself realistic goals. You may need to set short-term goals to achieve major aspirations. Then you can rebuild your life from the foundations up.
- Take a few calculated risks!

Watermelon

Citrullus vulgaris   (Greenish-yellow / FES-res)

Positive state

Nurturing the growth of the creative 'seed'
Creatively expressive

Negative state

Retarded development of creative potential
Creatively unexpressive

The Watermelon state of mind

In the negative state, Watermelon people are generally reluctant to share creative ideas or let others know about their talents for fear of criticism and/or judgment. They may be closet musicians or artists who never exhibit or novelists who keep their manuscripts buried in their dreams.

Benefits of taking Watermelon

Watermelon flower essence helps us to nurture and confidently display our 'baby' to the world – whatever form our creative output takes. There are obvious benefits for taking Watermelon during physical pregnancy. It helps a mother to accept the physical and emotional changes that occur and bond with her unborn baby, then care for it confidently once it is born. It is also very useful for those who are about to present a completed creative project to the world, whether in the workplace or as part of academic study/research. One of my clients had 'almost' completed writing her PhD thesis (it had been in the 'almost' category for the last year!) but just couldn't quite 'get it over the line' to present her findings and release it publicly. For her it would be the biggest achievement in her life and as she said: 'I am exposing a big part of myself that has gone into it, to the world.' She returned to see me after taking Watermelon flower essence for a month to let me know that she had successfully completed the thesis: 'It's finally out there!' For those on the verge of creative revelation, the flower essence will provide encouragement and support. In this instance, my client was offering something that meant a lot to her for the scrutiny of others. When we feel apprehensive or doubtful in the face of others' evaluation, Watermelon flower essence instils greater self-confidence and allows us to enjoy the whole creative process.

In the same way that it can help parents to bond with their unborn child, it can also make us more confident and proud about our creative abilities and able to stand up for our ideas and creations. And just as society recognises, acknowledges and protects an individual's creative work through intellectual property rights, copyright and patents, Watermelon encourages us to recognise and appreciate our own creations on an individual level.

Possible physical imbalances

If there is uncertainty or lack of confidence when planning to have a child, Watermelon flower essence is a great support for both partners – before conception, during pregnancy and after the child is born.

Common uses

For difficulties adjusting to pregnancy; for confidence in conceiving; to assist bonding with your unborn baby; for confidence in your 'creations'; to nurture your creative 'baby'; to pursue your creative dreams to their ultimate manifestation; to put 'it' out there!

Complementary &/or similar flower essences

Blackberry, Bleeding Heart, Bottlebrush, Buttercup, Californian Poppy, Cayenne, Chrysanthemum, Fairy Lantern, Forget-Me-Not, Indian Paintbrush, Iris, Larch, Madia, Manzanita, Mariposa Lily, Pomegranate, Quince, Violet, Wild Oat

Supporting the changes

- Follow your creative pursuits and dreams with determination.
- Explore the needs of your 'inner child'. Rediscover your creative 'baby' and nurture its growth.
- Find a creative outlet and take some responsible risks.
- If you've got it, flaunt it!

Water Violet
Hottonia palustris   (Pale mauve with yellow centre / Bach)

Positive state
Humble and engaging
Independent but able to collaborate

Negative state
Aloof and self-absorbed
Alone and unapproachable

Water Violets are *graceful* plants with feathery leaves that float on the surface of waterlogged ditches, ponds and lakes.

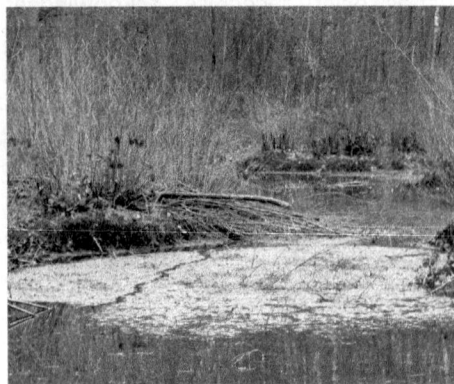

Access to the plant is limited because it *lives in water* which provides *protection* and support. People in the negative Water Violet state are also often *hard to reach* on a personal/intimate level. Their *emotionally guarded* disposition usually protects a very *sensitive* nature in which the *water element* (emotion) is strong.

The plant lives in hidden habitats of still waters and undisturbed springs. Because of its need to grow in *seclusion* the plant has always been comparatively rare and this rarity has increased as a consequence of development, pollution and drainage of wetlands (Barnard 1988). The primrose-like blooms are pale *lilac*, which relates it to the *crown chakra* (altruism and higher purpose) with a *yellow* centre, which shows its connection to the *solar plexus chakra* (sense of unique Selfhood). The sensitivity and *self-reliance* of personality types associated with the flower essences of aquatic plants such as Water Violet and Lotus can bring to mind the idea that they are *'old souls.'* However, while they may indeed have a more elevated perspective than the mere mortals around them, in the negative state this can tip over into arrogance and/or aloofness. No one wants to listen to a know-it-all or 'holier than thou' attitude, so their potential for valuable contribution may be lost.

The Water Violet personality

Just as the plant is unapproachable in its watery habitat, Water Violet people in the negative state can be unapproachable and aloof. All of us are drawn to seclusion and privacy to some extent – some people believe that one of the reasons we are here is to experience our spirits as separate entities in physical bodies. Most of the time we seek a balance between involvement and non-involvement, association and dissociation, committed and uncommitted relationships. When our lives are biased towards insularity and detachment and we begin to feel a certain heartlessness, Water Violet flower essence can help.

Water Violet people may have a nature that is highly spiritual and delicate, of which they are proud and protective. Artistic talents may have brought material rewards that assure their independence, so their desire to be alone is easily satisfied. But this may be cold comfort to the heart, which longs to merge with others and feel a sense of belonging, recognising that at an emotional level, others' needs and concerns are also ours.

Benefits of taking Water Violet

Water Violet flower essence can help to soften the impact of personal exchange on our hearts, much as water acts as a buffer between the plant and its connection to the Earth, leaving the delicate spirit pure and intact.

Water Violet flower essence allows you to maintain your innate humility, love and wisdom, renewing its appeal and making it accessible to others. You can continue to enjoy your own company but without the need to isolate yourself.

Possible physical imbalances

Water Violet people like to keep everything, including illness, 'close to their chest.' Even when they are sick they are not likely to ask for help.

When the heart centre is starved of relational nourishment because of an emotionally insular life, one is more predisposed to physical heart problems.

Common uses

For the aloof loner; for those too proud to ask for help; for those with a 'stiff upper lip'; for spiritual arrogance; to feel more comfortable getting involved; to have fun joining in; to 'feel the love'!

Complementary &/or similar flower essences

Golden Yarrow, Hibbertia, Impatiens, Larkspur, Lavender, Lotus, Mallow, Manzanita, Mariposa Lily, Shooting Star, Sweet Pea, Tall Yellow Top, Violet, Wallflower, YES formula

Supporting the changes

- Take a few risks with your independence – join a group, team or association that you know treats its members with respect. You may enjoy the interaction.
- Try socialising a bit more.
- Fall in love!

Wedding Bush
Ricinocarpus pinifolius   (White / Aus)

Positive state
Trusting and decisive
'Commitment to relationships … as goal or life purpose' (Ian White)

Negative state
Doubting and undecided
Lacking commitment (Ian White)

Wedding Bush is a shrub that grows up to two metres high in sandy soils in Queensland and New South Wales. Its many flowers are white and unisexual and were once used by brides in the outback, an association that has given the plant its common name (White 2008). The *white* colour of the flower links the plant to the *crown chakra*, which sheds *light on the subject* bringing mental clarity and helping us to get a deeper sense of meaning and *purpose*. This flower essence helps us understand the *nature of relationships and partnerships* and how well they relate (or not) to this purpose.

The unisexuality of the flowers points to the essence's usefulness for encouraging single-mindedness and decisiveness in being true to yourself – *commitment* follows.

The Wedding Bush state of mind

Those who have trouble making commitments, whether to relationships, jobs, projects, family or their own plans are displaying the negative Wedding Bush state of mind. It is not uncommon for men to fall into a pattern of going from one relationship to another, ending each one before any real commitment can be made, after the initial physical attraction wears thin and before deeper affection can begin to grow.

Apart from the emotional havoc this causes for others, it is ultimately a lonely and unsatisfying path for the commitment-phobe too. Wedding Bush flower essence can help bring self-insight to the situation so that it is possible to form and sustain deeper relationships that demand commitment.

Benefits of taking Wedding Bush

Wedding Bush flower essence assists us when we are considering going into a partnership – personal, social or business – or questioning whether to remain in one, by allowing us to become clear about whether the partnership is appropriate for us. If the answer is yes, we can feel more comfortable to make a deeper commitment to the growth and development of the relationship. This sense of 'rightness' is important when the initial enthusiasm, infatuation or attraction begins to fade.

Possible physical imbalances

Wedding Bush flower essence helps us commit – whether to a relationship or to a positive change in diet or lifestyle – so that we can build a new pattern into our lives. Wedding Bush flower essence will help you to discern whether or not the commitment you are considering is part of your higher purpose.

Common uses

For doubt about relationships or business partnerships; when unsure how others fit into your scheme of things; to understand another's place in your life direction; for purpose and commitment; to confidently sense a connection

Complementary &/or similar flower essences

Blackberry, Californian Poppy, Forget-Me-Not; Foxglove, Iris, Larkspur, Lavender, Mullein, Pomegranate, Quaking Grass, Saguaro, Scleranthus, Silver Princess, Tansy, Tiger Lily, Walnut, Wild Oat, Wild Rose

Supporting the changes

- Step back from a situation and meditate on it.
- Try to take an altruistic view of your situation and its potential development.
- Consult a good and impartial friend who can give you an honest opinion.
- Commit to something!

White Chestnut

Aesculus hippocastanum
(White with pink, red or yellow centre / Bach)

Positive state

Mentally calm, meditative
Dynamic stillness of mind

Negative state

Full of worry, tormenting thoughts
Cluttered, 'busy' mind

White Chestnut, better known as Horse Chestnut, is a strong, tall and erect tree, with *many branches* which spread until they almost touch the ground in what can seem a *top-heavy* way. People who respond well to White Chestnut flower essence may say things like: 'I feel *heavy headed*. My mind is never still; my *thoughts go round and round relentlessly.*' The spreading growth of the White Chestnut tree is also a key to the essence's ability to help *disperse unwanted thoughts*, leaving the *mind at peace*.

The talented graphic designer who created the cover for the first edition of my book, *The Bach Flowers Today*, was originally going to put images of a number of flowers on the cover, including White Chestnut. When I looked at the final draft, however, White Chestnut was not present. I asked him why he hadn't used it and he said, 'It was *too busy*; there was too much happening in it.' How interesting that, despite knowing nothing about the Bach Flowers, he identified the *cluttered* and busy characteristics of the negative White Chestnut mental state so accurately.

The bright, white flowers with vivid pink, red and yellow centres are produced in panicles scattered among the leaves. If you step back and view the flowering tree as a whole, it is very beautiful. White Chestnut flower essence helps us to step back from unwanted thoughts so that we can observe without resistance and *let them go*. This allows the mind to settle into a state of peace like that experienced during *meditation*.

The *red, yellow and pink* flowers signify the plant's ability to help us call on the energies of the *base, sacral, solar plexus and heart chakras*, reconnecting us with the body and emotions at times when we are 'stuck' in the more cerebral upper chakras. In this way a harmonious and peaceful balance between body and mind can be achieved once more.

The White Chestnut state of mind

When our minds are so cluttered with thoughts that we're unable to concentrate, we become easily distracted. We may worry obsessively about the past or something coming up in the future. Our thoughts run uncontrolled, going over conversations we have had or imagining arguments with people we haven't even met. We are preoccupied by recurring thoughts that prevent sleep or concentration and these may persist to the point of headache – we crave mental calm.

Too much work or simply becoming disconnected from our feelings may propel us into the negative White Chestnut state. Unwanted thoughts harass, torment and eventually exhaust us and we feel like their victim.

Benefits of taking White Chestnut

White Chestnut flower essence helps to ease the relentless round of thoughts that destroy our peace when the mind goes into a spin, chasing its own tail. This flower essence can release the mind from its addiction to constant thought, bringing new calm and clarity. We are then more able to respond to the moment in a spontaneous manner, achieving an open and dynamic stillness of mind.

Possible physical imbalances

When we remain in a state of mental tension, pain in the head, neck and shoulders often develops. A mind constantly 'congested' with thoughts will ultimately 'decongest' through physical expressions such as headache/migraine, sinus discharge and/or recurring head colds.

Common uses

For insomnia due to an active mind; for constant worry; for persistent unwanted thoughts; to help very 'cerebral' people 'get out of their heads'; for inability to concentrate; to help unwind and switch off mentally; to help one feel and not just think; for that elusive peace of mind

Complementary &/or similar flower essences

Californian Poppy, Chaparral, Cosmos, Crab Apple, Crowea, Filaree, Harvest Brodiaea, Hibbertia, Hound's Tongue, Iris, Lavender, Lotus, Madia, Mountain Pennyroyal, Nasturtium, Paw Paw, Rabbitbrush, Shasta Daisy, Zinnia

Supporting the changes

- Learn meditation and relaxation techniques.
- Physical activity or manual work can help bring balance to mental activity by getting us 'out of our heads.' Try going for a walk every day.
- Yoga, tai chi and other physical disciplines are relaxing and mentally calming.
- Learn to ask, 'What am I feeling right now?'

Wild Oat

Bromus ramosus   (White / Bach)

Positive state

Knowing one's part in the play of life
Sensing one's vocation

Negative state

'All dressed up with nowhere to go'
Directionless

Wild Oat is a grass that is commonly found in pastures, damp woods and thickets and by roadsides. It can be distinguished from the cultivated oat *Avena sativa* by its hairy stems. To prepare the flower essence, the greenish flowers are gathered in late summer and potentised using the sun method. The *green* of the flower shows its relation to the *heart chakra*. Wild Oat flower essence helps to marry the *ambition* in our nature with what is *most attractive* to our heart, allowing us to *follow our calling*. It helps us *stay true* to our heart (often despite what our head thinks) and follow its wisdom in understanding our true and most *fulfilling path*.

The plant itself is found growing *scattered* about 'on hedge banks and on the edge of woodland,' never seeming to form a communal patch like other grasses (Barnard 1988). This reflects both negative and positive aspects of the Wild Oat state. When unbalanced, there is difficulty in forming community and individuals may live *in limbo*, unable to maintain connections. In the positive state, however, you are able to find your own *niche* wherever you are and no matter what is happening around you.

The Wild Oat state of mind

Wild Oat flower essence acts as a vocational guide for the soul when we are unsure which of many directions to take in life. (Scleranthus on the other hand is more useful on an everyday level when there is a need to choose between a couple of immediate options.)

In the negative state, Wild Oat people are always searching for the perfect job or way of life. They change careers, lifestyles, skills and countries but never feel they have found their niche or that they really belong. Frequently, they leave a trail of unfinished projects and abandoned intentions behind them and feel unfulfilled or deeply dissatisfied.

Benefits of taking White Oat

The only real and lasting sense of belonging must be found within. Wild Oat flower essence helps us to make the committed connection to the world which is a prerequisite for clarity about our direction. We must be truly involved in life to see what role we can best play, and in this way share the prize of achieving a common purpose.

When we lose our bearings, Wild Oat can help put us back on track towards self-realisation and fulfilment.

Possible physical imbalances

Job dissatisfaction is often accompanied by a range of associated illnesses, some of them specific and some more vague. In this situation, the stress experienced is not only from external causes but is brought about by lack of internal direction and motivation. Whatever the cause, however, stress is stress – and it is always detrimental to health, especially the health of our immune system.

Common uses

For the 'Jack of all trades and master of none'; for the drifter; for midlife and/ or vocational crisis; for some types of adolescent apathy; for those desiring a change of direction; to help prioritise or redefine your future direction; to help reinvent yourself; to help you hear your calling

Complementary &/or similar flower essences

Angelica, Angelsword, Bottle Brush; Californian Poppy, Forget-Me-Not, Foxglove, Iris, Onion, Pomegranate, Sagebrush, Saguaro, Scleranthus, Shasta Daisy, Shooting Star, Silver Princess, Walnut

Supporting the changes

- Look for vocational counselling and other measures to enhance self-knowledge.
- Join in team or group activity that involves working towards a common goal.
- Remember, you must often lose sight of the shore before you can see a new horizon.

Wild Rose

Rosa canina   (Pink / Bach)

Positive state

Enthusiastic and involved
Renewed interest and passion for life

Negative state

Withdrawn resignation
Disinterested and dispirited

Wild Rose shrubs are common in woodlands and hedges throughout Europe. The white or pink, fragrant flowers bloom prodigiously in midsummer, followed by red rosehips that ripen in early winter. Many aspects of the Wild Rose signature relate it to the *heart chakra* – the *pink* of the flowers and their *heart-shaped* petals being the most outstanding. This flower has always 'spoken' to the hearts of artists and poets because of its *sweet scent and beauty*. Just as the condition of the heart chakra relates to our capacity for *delight and enjoyment* of physical life, so the *open* flowers and heart-shaped petals of Wild Rose display receptiveness to the sun and the dance of life.

It is interesting to note that the below-ground *root system* of the Wild Rose is almost the same size as the plant's growth above the ground. In the positive state, Wild Rose people are extremely *well-grounded* and are not easily uprooted or swayed from their life course. Wild Rose flower essence helps us to hold firm and remain *committed* through the struggles and joys of life.

The Wild Rose personality

In the negative state, Wild Rose people withdraw from full participation in life. They become resigned to being an effect rather than a cause and often find themselves stuck in a way of life designed around everyone else's needs. Apathetic detachment is their habitual response.

It is time to consider Wild Rose when we lack motivation and begin to think, 'What's the use? There's no future for me, no point in trying.' We may have encountered setbacks or experienced an illness that lasted longer than expected, and as a result we are dispirited and resigned to the notion that things will never get better. A teenager may think, 'Oh my God, it's all too hard. Too many responsibilities, too much to think about!' The negative state may also arise from a more global perspective when we begin to feel that there's no future in a world with so many insoluble problems to sort out (note also Scotch Broom).

There is also another Wild Rose type who is involved, busy and well-organised.

THE **ESSENTIAL** FLOWER ESSENCE BOOK

They are well-grounded, practical 'doers' but after a bit of delving we discover that underneath their 'busy' persona they have lost their enthusiasm. They have raised the white flag and surrendered to the struggle of life and the only thing that keeps them going is the fear that if they stop, they will 'drop their bundle.' Of course this is in fact very unlikely but their underlying fear of 'death through withdrawal from keeping active in life' is ever present. Wild Rose flower essence can help these people internally renegotiate their priorities and discover a new energy and passion for life.

Benefits of taking Wild Rose

When we are dispirited and discouraged, Wild Rose flower essence helps us to restore our passionate involvement in life. Like other members of the Rose family, these plants have a very strong and hardy root system that is deeply grounded and entrenched in the Earth. Wild Rose flower essence can be our teacher, restoring our inner joy, vitality and enthusiasm and helping us put our heart back into living.

Possible physical imbalances

Over a period of time, 'disconnection' from the heart chakra – a sort of 'disembodying' or partial retreat from life – means the etheric (fluid) body contracts to a degree. This then can result in physical circulatory symptoms such as cold extremities and decreased cerebral blood-flow. This in turn can lead to brain fag and vagueness. I have also found in practice that a history of low blood pressure has been quite common in those who respond well to Wild Rose flower essence.

Common uses

For chronic apathy; for those withdrawn from life; for lack of interest in one's surroundings; for loss of motivation; to help become grounded in the present; to truly commit yourself; to restore your enthusiasm and passion; to get back onto the dancefloor of life

Complementary &/or similar flower essences

Blackberry, Cayenne, Clematis, Coffee, Forget-Me-Not, Foxglove, Gentian, Gorse, Honeysuckle, Hound's Tongue, Iris, Larkspur, Morning Glory, Peppermint, Rosemary, Scotch Broom, Silver Princess, Wedding Bush, Wild Oat, Zinnia

Supporting the changes

- Vigorous physical exercise is far more useful than prolonged meditation while in the negative Wild Rose state. Develop a daily routine and avoid oversleeping.
- Bodywork and other somatic therapies are useful.
- Find out what excites your passion and lust for life!
- Recommit!

Willow

Salix alba var. vitellina (Green/yellow / Bach)

Positive state

Self-determination
Emotional resilience

Negative state

Victim mentality ('poor me')
Wallowing in resentment

Willow grows best beside rivers, creeks and in close proximity to water. The qualities of the *water element*, which represents *emotion*, are strongly associated with the Willow tree. Unexpressed, suppressed and internalised emotion creates *resentment*, the key word for Willow flower essence. Water is also cleansing and Willow helps *cleanse* our system of emotions that have become toxic. Willow helps us to assimilate painful experiences, preventing us from becoming stuck in the past, *wallowing* in *pain, sadness or grief*. We learn to understand ourselves more deeply and use the wisdom gained to facilitate change in our lives. This is truly *'moving on'* – very different from denial of past pain. Willow helps us to learn *resilience*, so that we can delve into our history and use the insights we gain to create a better and more joyous future without feeling victimised by the past.

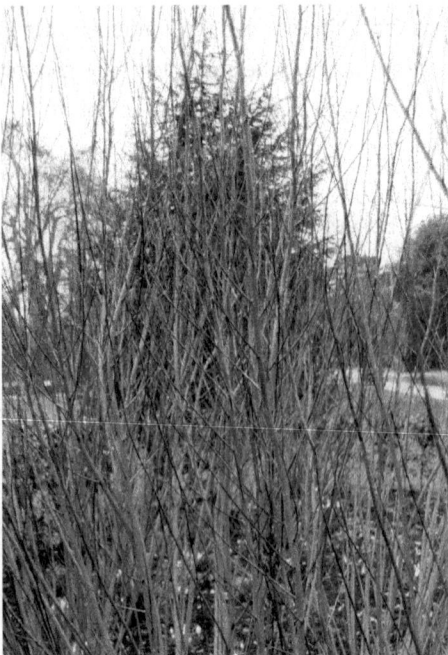

As a child I found refuge beneath the overhanging branches of a Willow tree that grew beside a creek near our house, especially when I was feeling 'hard done by' because I was in trouble with my parents! And maybe that was when I inadvertently began to practise meditation. Willow flower essence reawakens in us our ability to *accept, then release sadness to experience more joy.*

The smooth twigs are very *flexible* (*fluid* in movement) and make great whips! Their *resilience* means that they *do not break easily, even under duress* and are excellent for making baskets and light, moveable enclosures. Traditionally, trees used for this purpose are pollarded

– that is, the branches are cut back to the stump each year to force vigorous, *resilient* young shoots to *grow*.

Willow flower essence helps to foster resilience after *hurts and setbacks* so that we don't get stuck in resentment and feelings of victimisation. Another aspect of the plant's signature is its capacity to take root easily, even from a small cutting. Pieces of branch will *strike roots without difficulty*, and if you drive a cut Willow pole into the ground it will take root and become a tree. Julian and Martine Barnard (1988) marvel at how 'Willow has such a will to grow!' Even the tree's preferred habitat, wet ground by a river, would cause many other species to rot or be overgrown by other plants.

In addition, the *bright golden yellow* of this species' bare stems in the winter landscape symbolise the way our minds can be uplifted by the power of positive thinking. Willow flower essence can bring brightness and flexibility to our *mental attitude* when it has become too rigid and fixed.

The Willow state of mind

'Why does this always happen to me? Why do I always get a raw deal? I do the right thing, and look what happens – I miss out again! It's no wonder I've got an attitude problem when life treats me like dirt. I never asked to be born anyway!' These feelings are characteristic of the victim mentality of the negative Willow state, and they can create a negative reality for us. On days when you wake up in a bad mood, you are more likely to stub a toe getting out of bed. If you leave home in a foul temper, you are more likely to encounter hostility on the road and from your colleagues at work. If you are glum you will put a damper on everything around you, and what goes around comes around!

Benefits of taking Willow

Societal attitudes can sometimes create a victim mentality by fostering the notion that we have no part to play in our own health and wellbeing. Willow flower essence can help raise our awareness of our own role in maintaining good health and managing illness when it does occur. Taking responsibility (and Willow flower essence!) can empower us to make better decisions based on a realistic but positive mental outlook. Rather than feeling like a victim, we learn about the powers of self-determination. Willow flower essence can help us to rediscover a positive outlook and take responsibility for creating a better reality in our lives.

Possible physical imbalances

Willow can help us face physical illness with a more positive and proactive attitude, feeling less of a victim to it. Psychoneuroimmunology research supports the understanding that a positive attitude can play a significant role in prevention of illness, and in recovery if illness occurs.

Common uses

For feelings of bitterness and resentment; for 'attitude' problems; for those who play the 'blame game'; for those who have difficulty taking responsibility for anything that happens in their lives; to help release pain, hurt and sadness; to help mental flexibility, resilience and adaptability; to help maintain a positive attitude

Complementary &/or similar flower essences

Borage, Chicory, Dogwood, Garlic, Golden Ear Drops, Gorse, Hibbertia, Hound's Tongue, Holly, Hornbeam, Iris, Mountain Pennyroyal, Scotch Broom, Self-Heal, Star Thistle; Yerba Santa, Zinnia

Supporting the changes

- Think about ways in which you might create your own reality through your thoughts, beliefs and attitudes.
- Think about whether or not you have some responsibility for some of the things that have happened to you. This may allow you to see a problem coming next time around, so that you have a chance to change the outcome for the better.
- Keep your body as supple as possible through yoga, tai chi etc – some of the benefits will flow back to your mind.
- If some of your unhappiness is your own fault, the upside is that you also have the power to make yourself happy!
- Take a deep breath, let it go, get over it and spring back up (a dozen times a day)!

Yarrow
Achillea millefolium (White / FES)

Positive state
Luminous and secure auric field (FES)
Healed, dynamically shielded and protected

Negative state
Depleted and vulnerable auric field
'Overly absorbent of negative influences; psychic toxicity' (FES)

Yarrow gets its botanical name, *Achillea*, from the ancient Greek warrior Achilles, whose wounds were said to have been healed by this herb. Soldiers throughout the centuries have carried it among their provisions as they march into battle and it has been used both internally and externally for its styptic qualities in helping to stem bleeding. Yarrow flower essence *stems bleeding* on an energetic or subtle level by

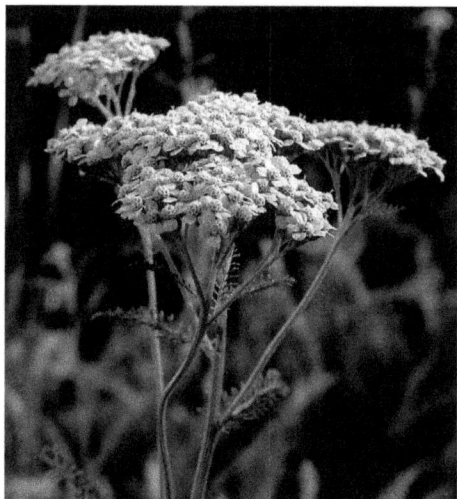

helping to seal, *protect and stabilise the life force*. There are a number of species of Yarrow that are made into flower essences and all of them *protect against negativity* of different kinds in the environment (Kaminski and Katz 1996).

All Yarrow flowers are recognised for their finely-detailed geometric patterns, interwoven to form *strong, enduring* structures (FES).

Achillea millefolium has a white flower, which points to its capacity to help us surround ourselves with a shield of *'white auric light.'* This acts like an energetic *buffer* between us and the environment – *energetic boundaries* become better defined and our *personal space* becomes more *secure*. In this way Yarrow provides protection against radiation, geopathic stress and general negativity in the physical environment (see also *YES formula*, which includes Yarrow).

The Yarrow state of mind

Yarrow is used as a flower essence to stem 'bleeding' on a subtle level (Kaminski and Katz 1996) in those who are oversensitive or highly susceptible to negativity in their environment. Yarrow helps to seal and protect the subtle body boundaries of the aura just as in herbal form it acts as a styptic and helps to seal and protect physical boundaries.

Benefits of taking Yarrow

Yarrow flower essence is a great protector against negativity in the physical environment, especially in the form of radiation, allergens, pollution and other problems relating to crowded city living. (Pink Yarrow flower essence, on the other hand, protects against negativity in the emotional environment.) Yarrow can help us to reinforce the shield of white light we place around ourselves when we want protection on a psychic as well as physical plane.

Possible physical imbalances

Those who respond well to Yarrow flower essence may have a history of health problems relating to compromised natural immunity such as repeated cold and flu infections, sensitivities and/or allergic reactions to the environment or chronic immune dysfunction. Yarrow flower essence (and YES formula) can often provide a starting point for addressing these immunity issues.

Common uses

For oversensitivity and reactivity to the environment; to protect against negativity in the physical environment; to improve the integrity of your auric field; to enhance your natural immunity on all levels; to strengthen your psychic shield

Complementary &/or similar flower essences

Angelica, Angelsword, Arnica, Aspen, Canyon Dudleya, Echinacea, Fringed Violet, Garlic, Golden Yarrow, Indian Pink, Mountain Pennyroyal, Pink Yarrow, Red Clover, St John's Wort, Star of Bethlehem, Walnut, Waratah, YES formula

Supporting the changes

- Visualise white light around you or develop other methods of dynamic self-protection such as meditation or protective rituals.
- Maintain a balanced lifestyle, especially when it comes to getting enough sleep and keep yourself grounded with activities such as gardening, pottery and outdoor exercise in open spaces full of greenery.
- Make sure your diet is rich in nutrients for the nervous system, especially Vitamin B.
- Create a haven where you can regularly take time out to regroup – your room, your study, your shed, YOUR SPACE!

YES formula
Yarrow Environmental Solution

(FES flower essences of *Achillea millefolium* (+ var. *rubra*), *Achillea filipendulina*, *Arnica mollis* and *Echinacea purpurea*, with Yarrow and Echinacea tinctures in a sea-salt water base)

Positive state

Enhanced integrity of the life-force (FES)
Dynamic natural immunity

Negative state

'Disturbance of life-force and vitality by noxious radiation, pollution or other geopathic stress; residual effects of past exposure' (FES)

Yarrow Environmental Solution (YES) is a unique and powerful blend of flower essences and plant tinctures in a sea-salt water base to help strengthen and protect against *toxic environmental influences*. It is like a personal body guard!

YES formula includes three different types of Yarrow (white, pink and golden), along with two allies from the same plant family – Echinacea and Arnica (see also description of specific YES ingredients elsewhere in this book). It was originally developed by the Flower Essence Society in response to practitioner requests after the Chernobyl nuclear disaster in 1986. Kaminski and Katz (1996) inform us that YES 'directly counteracts the destructive effects of radiation on the human energy field.' All the herbs used in the formula have a reputation for enhancing *natural immune response*. When combined, their *synergistic effect* amplifies their ability to strengthen *natural immunity on all levels*.

The sea-salt base of the formula further enhances the effectiveness of this remedy. Unpolluted ocean water contains minerals in similar proportions to that of human blood. Indigenous diets are typically high in these mineral salts (sometimes called 'tissue salts') which help maintain a healthy immune system.

As well as causing immediate physical damage, *geopathic stressors* such as *radiation* attack our *etheric energy system*. To protect the *integrity of the vital force*, vibrational medicines such as flower essences and homeopathic remedies are required, and YES formula is designed specifically for this purpose.

Benefits of taking YES formula

The purpose of YES formula is to strengthen and protect against toxic environmental influences, geopathic stress and other hazards of modern life. These include the effects of radiation from x-rays, televisions, computer monitors, cellphones, electromagnetic fields, radiation treatments and cosmic radiation to which we are exposed during high-altitude flights. Many practitioners use it as a baseline remedy and ongoing stabiliser when addressing fundamental health issues endemic to the modern world.

Some specific indications for use:

- As a general tonic and protection against technological and environmental challenges.
- Before, during and after exposure to any type of radiation from x-rays, medical treatments, computer equipment, televisions, household appliances (including microwave ovens), signal towers etc.
- When subjected to geopathic stress and strong electromagnetic fields.
- To strengthen the immune system, particularly in those who are prone to allergies and chemical sensitivities.
- During or after times of extremes stress, especially when left feeling shattered or 'disembodied.'
- For health practitioners/therapists, especially those helping clients that have experienced significant trauma.

YES formula acts as a strong energetic shield to help protect against 'environmental challenges to wellbeing and vitality; strengthening and protecting' (Patricia Kaminski, FES co-director).

Zinnia

Zinnia elegans (Red / FES)

Positive state

Levity and playfulness
Joyful, able to laugh and have fun (FES)

Negative state

Weighed down by life
Overly serious; joyless; 'lack of humour' (FES)

Zinnia bears single or double flowers in large, daisy-like heads. The plant, which is native to America and is very popular in Mexico, needs rich, fertile soil and blooms nearly all year round. The flower may be crimson, orange, *red*, *violet*, white or yellow and this *variety of vivid colours* reflects the way Zinnia flower essence can add *colour and brightness* to our lives. Zinnia flowers look *playful* – some say like a 'toy' flower – and they enhance any *festive* occasion. Zinnia flower essence creates better balance between the physical and emotional bodies, resulting in a better *sense of humour* so that our *inner child* can come out to play!

The Zinnia personality

We can benefit from Zinnia flower essence when life issues weigh us down and we find it difficult to enjoy ourselves, even during leisure time. It helps us contact our playful 'inner child' (Kaminski and Katz 1996) and rediscover our sense of humour, freeing us to not take ourselves so seriously. It can also help us to communicate better with children and join in their fun.

Zinnia can be extremely helpful for an older child (often the eldest in the family) who has become over-responsible for others in the family, and for overzealous parents and work managers who take themselves and everyone else too seriously. It can help us to release built-up tension, so that we can unwind and have some real fun. This can help to solve some very serious problems. Agitated and anxious, hypersensitive and depressed individuals have been helped by Zinnia flower essence.

Interestingly, Zinnia can also be very helpful in situations where an older pet has to come to terms with the arrival of a playful younger animal. Clients report things like, 'The old fella isn't so grumpy – he not only tolerates the pup now, he even plays with it!' He still lets the pup know who's boss when he needs to though!'

Benefits of taking Zinnia

Zinnia flower essence is useful when we get into the habit of taking life too seriously. It can help us let go and unwind, treating things in a more light-hearted manner, laughing at life (Kaminski and Katz 1996) and ourselves again. Zinnia teaches us that laughter is the best medicine!

Possible physical imbalances

The injection of more joy into one's life has a positive influence on the heart centre. This is turn benefits the associated thymus gland and in this way has helped to improve many 'Zinnia' clients' natural immunity. Psychoneuroimmunological research supports this observation. There is good evidence that Laughter Therapy (or Laughter Yoga) can benefit physical health and wellbeing.

Common uses

For lack of humour; for joylessness; for those who take themselves and everything else too seriously; to help 'lighten up'; to bring back the joy; to learn how to play again; to let the inner child come out to play!

Complementary &/or similar flower essences

Agrimony, Baby Blue Eyes, Borage, Calendula, Dandelion, Flannel Flower Garlic, Gentian, Golden Ear Drops, Harvest Brodiaea, Hibbertia, Hibiscus, Hound's Tongue, Iris, Larkspur, Mallow, Manzanita, Mountain Pennyroyal, Pansy, Quince, Scotch Broom, Willow

Supporting the changes

- Read about other people's positive philosophies on life.
- Play with your kids and/or join in other games and activities.
- Remember to take time out, stand back from your life and enjoy some happy day-dreaming.
- Think about what you used to do for fun and do it!
- School's out! Have some fun.

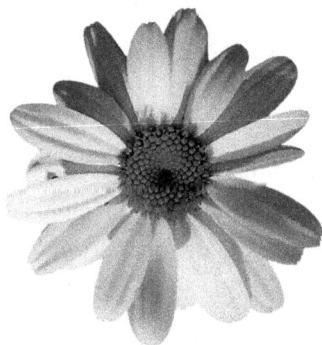

Supplementary flower essences

In the interests of offering a comprehensive guide, this section gives short summaries of a number of flower essences that are not covered in the first section and with which I have less experience prescribing as a therapist. (Successive editions will continue to add to this section, and some material currently included here will find its way into the section containing more detailed descriptions as more clinical experience is gathered.) Drawing on my experience thus far with these flower essences, I have endeavoured to describe succinctly the core theme or quality of each one so as to enable the reader to understand and use it to best effect. As with all the essences covered in this book, there is a vast body of extremely valuable information available through the flower essence organisations listed elsewhere in the book.

Once again I wish to draw attention to the original sources of information which provided me with a basic understanding of the flower essences, in some cases decades ago. All FES flower essence descriptions are based on information originally obtained directly from the FES Flower Essence Repertory researched and compiled by Patricia Kaminski and Richard Katz, and from FES brochures and the FES website. I have added my own findings and 'flavour' to the descriptions as a result of 40 years' experience and understanding gained from my work as a Naturopath/Homeopath. Similarly I formed my original understanding of the Australian Bush Flower Essences from the descriptions found in Ian White's book and other literature provided by the Australian Bush Flower organisation over the years. The same applies to literature and information provided by the late Steve Johnson, head of the Alaskan Flower Essence Project. Please refer to the Introduction section of this book for further detail about the original sources of information on the following flower essences.

Alpine Aster

Aster alpigenus (Pink-yellow / FES-RL)

Alpine Aster flower essence should be considered when we are fearful about anything beyond the physical realm or any form of altered consciousness – dream states, meditation, spirituality and mortality (FES). We may over-identify with materialism and the physical dimension and/or have a purely quantitative or left-brain-dominated approach to life. Alpine Aster helps us to be more comfortable in meditation. There can be a 'freeing of the spiritual body from the physical' (FES), enabling us to be more comfortable with our spiritual side. Alpine Aster flower essence can give us a greater sense of the unity of being that is shared by all forms of life, so that we can tap into the peaceful divinity which connects us all.

Alpine Lily

Lilium parvum (Red-orange / FES)

As with Chocolate Lily, Easter Lily, Evening Primrose, Fairy Lantern, Fawn Lily, Pomegranate, She Oak and Tiger Lily flower essences, 'Alpine Lily helps the feminine soul experience a more vibrant relationship to the female body' (FES). Negative impressions of the female body may be unconsciously absorbed from family and reinforced by today's culture (FES). Those who can benefit from Alpine Lily flower essence may experience a conscious or unconscious rejection of female physicality, whose functions are perceived as spiritually 'low' (FES). As a therapist, I find this response to be similar to the pattern found in the negative Manzanita state, where there is a rejection of the whole physical body based on a perception of its 'low' spiritual status. Alpine Lily can help women who identify with the self-sufficiency of the Virgo archetype but mistakenly assume that independence of this kind calls for a rejection of incarnated, bodily womanhood. It helps to integrate the feminine principle in a dynamic way, allowing women to live as splendidly complete human beings.

Black Cohosh

Cimicifuga racemosa   (White / FES)

Black Cohosh flower essence is useful when we are caught up in emotionally abusive relationships and/or abusive lifestyles involving addiction/dependency and violence (FES). We can easily become riddled with unexpressed and dark emotions that fester and become psychically toxic. Black Cohosh flower essence helps us conjure up the courage to recognise and confront our 'shadow' side, and become more enlightened so that we can recognise the part it plays in (recurring) abusive relationships, situations and lifestyles. It helps us cleanse ourselves of toxic emotions that are well and truly past their 'use-by' date.

Blazing Star

Mentzelia laevicaulis   (Yellow / FES-RL)

Blazing Star flower essence enhances the sun/fire soul forces when the water element predominates within (FES). It helps strengthen our willpower and courage and prevent us from 'going to water' under pressure. It fosters a radiant (sunny) vitality so that we can strike the right balance between the feminine/water/soul element (inwardly nurturing) and the masculine/fire/soul element (radiant warmth and strength). You can stand up and be counted, generate a warm presence and blaze forth in the world!

Bunchberry

Cornus canadensis (White / Alask)

Bunchberry helps us focus our mind's energy (Alask) by aligning the emotional, mental and spiritual bodies. It helps us 'get our (body/mind/spirit) act together' so that we can align with our higher purpose without distraction, even in demanding situations. Better concentration, persistence and patience – 'mental steadfastness' results (Alask) – as we now work toward our goals via the path of least resistance.

Californian Peony

Paeonia californica (Dark maroon / FES-RL)

Californian Peony flower essence is useful when we have an overly passive approach in life and lack 'get up and go.' We 'take a back seat,' unassertively choosing the devil we know in an attempt at 'risk-free' living. Californian Peony helps us rekindle the flame of passion, enabling us to experience pleasure and liveliness (as shown by the dark maroon signature relating to the *base chakra*). It can help us undergo our own 'mini-raising of the kundulini'! And it will foster 'charismatic' soul forces' (FES) that enhance our ability to attract the energy and resources we need for living (*sacral chakra*) – and share the resulting sense of abundance.

Californian Valerian

Valeriana capitata (White / FES-RL)

Californian Valerian flower essence helps to ease 'stress head'; it helps us breathe more easily in life; it helps lessen our expectation of more stress and trauma when this has been the pattern in the past (FES); it helps improve our sleep patterns, making it easier to let go, trust, and go to sleep; it eases anxiety and worries about the future (FES), by helping us to come to terms with and accept life experiences from the past so that they don't dictate our expectations of the future; Californian Valerian lets us get back in touch with inner peace and tranquillity (FES) and rediscover inner ease, while trusting and embracing what lies ahead.

Cassandra

Chamaedaphne calyculata (White / Alask)

Cassandra flower essence helps eliminate distracting thoughts and quiet the mind (Alask). It is useful when we are crying out for 'space' and 'time out' that will allow us to achieve calm and clarity in our thinking. This allows our focus to turn inward so that we can perceive life on a deeper level (Alask), gaining spiritual insight and a more meditative or mindful approach. Cassandra helps us experience stillness of mind, raising our awareness so as to attune better to our environment.

Cherry

Prunus avium (White / FES-RL)

Cherry flower essence should be considered when we feel bad about ourselves or down on ourselves – especially when a skin condition such as acne (FES) may be making matters worse. A traumatic adolescence or other past traumatic experiences can create toxic memories (FES) that continue to afflict the sense of who we are now. Cherry helps us heal so that we can begin to make light of our past experiences. We start to feel refreshed, 'born again,' more open, 'ripe for the picking' (cherry ripe!) and enthusiastically affirming of life. Cherry flower essence can help us to feel more youthful (FES), putting back the 'spring in our step.'

Chocolate Lily

Fritillaria biflora (Chocolate-brown / FES-RL)

Chocolate Lily flower essence is for those of us who lack awareness of the basic eliminatory functions of the body or have an aversion to them (FES). When we become disconnected from the base chakra and sacral chakra, physical and etheric blockage and congestion occurs within these lower chakras. As a therapist, I have found that Chocolate Lily is very useful as an adjunct to natural therapies when chronic menstrual and bowel health issues (not necessarily occurring at the same time) are part of a client's history. There can be a reawakening and embodiment (FES) of these lower chakras which leads to energetic and physical decongestion. It helps you to let go and leave unnecessary things 'behind.' Chocolate Lily helps the reproductive and eliminative systems to function more dynamically, tapping into a new energy flow. Then you become more able to 'listen to' and respond to all aspects of your body's needs.

Columbine

Aquilegia formosa (Red-orange with yellow / FES-RL)

Columbine flower essence adds spirit to your being, 'sparking you up' (the way a spark plug starts an engine up). The plant was so named because it typically blooms around the Christian feast of Pentecost, which commemorates a time when the Holy Spirit (often depicted as a dove or *columba*) descended in the form of 'tongues of fire' to inspire the faithful. In religious terms, the phrase 'speaking in tongues' is used to describe ecstatic speech in which the Holy Spirit is believed to speak through an individual. Columbine helps us to appreciate our unique talents and inner beauty (FES), regardless of how we differ from others, so that we can express ourselves better creatively in all areas of life. We become confident to take creative risks that can get us recognised 'in the crowd.' Columbine flower essence is particularly useful in developing our unique creative talents at midlife (FES) just when we might have become resigned to never expressing ourselves fully. It frees up the flow of creative energies from the lower chakras, especially the *sacral chakra*, as signified by the red-orange flowers, to be articulated to the world through the *throat chakra* (communication centre).

Comfrey

Symphytum officinale (Mauve / FES-res)

Comfrey flower essence is a nervous system tonic that helps restore nerve and brain tissue, especially after it has been damaged. It helps improve brain/nerve communication and coordination (including left-brain and right-brain balance) and helps utilise dormant, unused or atrophied portions of the brain. It can help heal the etheric body when its integrity has been damaged, whether recently or in the past (and even the distant past).

Compart-mental-isation is a key word and signature of the plant, which can be observed in the way the seed germinates. Comfrey flower essence aids in identifying and recognising certain aspects of our psyche that have, for whatever reason, including injury, been compartmentalised off from the whole. It allows us to heal/mend these aspects and facilitate their reintegration.

The analogy of a panel or grid used to harness solar power is useful here. If one or more of the individual cells on the grid is inactive or non-functioning it significantly affects the overall performance of the unit. But if all cells are functioning at their optimum, good energy results will be attained. Comfrey can help repair the nervous system at the cellular level, improving *synaptic communication* as a consequence of better bio-electrical or ethereal energy transmission. This has implications for all the subtle mechanisms in the human energy field.

Comfrey flower essence improves *connection between all aspects of the Self*, helping to better align the subtle bodies and aspects of our psyche – especially dormant and unused aspects – creating a well-*integrated* whole person. A more *'united'* Self can be achieved on all levels as a result of this gathering and re-uniting of subtle aspects. A greater sense of wholeness and a feeling that we 'have our act together' is experienced. The name Comfrey is derived from the Latin *conferva*, which means *'knitting together'* and its botanical name, *Symphytum*, means *'grown together.'* The herb has been used for centuries to help *reunite bone* after breaks and fractures, and for severe bruising trauma. It is interesting to note how Gurudas (1989) elaborates on this 'uniting' aspect. The *purple* of the comfrey flower signifies its connection with the *brow chakra* and its role in a gradual reawakening of the 'third eye.' The brow chakra 'oversees,' facilitates and harnesses the united energies of the chakras below for healing through the mind.

Corn Lily

Veratrum californicum (White with green centre / FES-res)

Corn Lily is a very good flower essence to consider during menopause, especially when there are negative thoughts about being 'over the hill' and 'all dried up' (FES). It also should be considered when there is depression associated with the physical ageing process, especially during midlife, or when we desperately try to deny our loss of physical youth and fertility. Corn Lily can help us age more gracefully, appreciating age as the 'getting of wisdom' (FES) and understanding that the lines, marks and changes in the body are the beautiful, honest and unadulterated result of a rich and full life experience. Corn Lily can help us celebrate midlife and view it as 'a glass half full' rather than 'a glass half empty'!

Daffodil

Narcissus Ajax (Yellow / FES-res)

The Daffodil flower's conical shape points towards its usefulness in helping us to be receptive to higher levels of being or our 'higher Self,' and this is underlined by its yellow colour which indicates its relationship with the higher octave of the *solar plexus chakra*. These two aspects of the flower's signature point to the essence's ability to foster a spiritualisation of the intellect as the mental body attunes better to the higher Self from which it receives direction. We are more able to comfortably negotiate 'personal growth spurts' that occur on more subtle levels, for example those experienced during psychotherapy. Much greater clarity and stillness of mind allows us to better understand what is happening within and how it shapes our perception of what is going on 'without.'

Evening Primrose

Oenothera hookeri   (Yellow / FES)

Those who can benefit most from Evening Primrose flower essence have a deep, core feeling of abandonment and/or rejection as a result of traumatic experiences while in the womb, during birth or in the early weeks of life. The trauma for the unborn child may be centred around anger/hostility received directly from a parent who may, even if only briefly, feel that they do not wish to have the child. Trauma may also occur as a result of a very difficult birth in which the mother becomes emotionally disconnected from the baby (heavy painkilling medication, for instance, may accentuate this 'disconnection') and the baby feels abandoned.

As a result of this kind of trauma occurring very early in life the underlying fear of rejection, if strong enough, often causes such a person to avoid commitment in relationships. They are also often guarded and emotionally cold in intimate relations with others.

Evening Primrose flower essence can help heal the deep emotional pain associated with feelings of rejection, especially those stemming from experiences that occur well before a capacity for cognitive recognition has developed. Healing of painful early emotions felt and absorbed from parents frees a person to 'open up' emotionally with others and feel safe enough to form deeper bonds and more committed relationships (FES).

Explorer's Gentian

Gentiana calycosa   (Blue / FES-RL)

As a therapist, I have found that Explorer's Gentian flower essence is a good midlife remedy for those who have lost interest, become disheartened and weary (FES) and have almost (but not quite) given up. Though they may have already achieved a great deal in their life, especially in the eyes of others, their sense of accomplishment is wearing thin. Explorer's Gentian helps people to reacquaint themselves with their life purpose (FES). As one client put it, 'If I'm still around I must be destined to do something useful!' Of course other situations besides midlife can bring about moments of re-evaluation – a severe financial setback or health crisis, for instance, can leave us searching for meaning. Explorer's Gentian gives us strength to recommit to our life purpose and destiny with new enthusiasm and recognise that there is more to 'explore.'

Fawn Lily

Erythronium purpurascens   (Yellow with purple / FES)

Those in need of Fawn Lily flower essence experience a need to withdraw (FES) to a safe haven that protects the delicate Self. There is a feeling of vulnerability and a lack of desire to face the world and its challenges. The sensitive Self wants to retreat but there is also an awareness that this brings a risk of becoming isolated. You also know that there are things of value that you need to disclose and share (FES) and a world that can benefit from them. Fawn Lily flower essence helps give you the strength to stick at it, to 'stay in the mix' and remain fully involved in life. You know in your heart that you have a lot to offer and Fawn Lily flower essence can help to make you feel secure as you become more and more creatively and socially involved, sharing your special gifts and talents with the world.

'Let Light and Love and Power restore [you to] the Plan on Earth' (from the 'Great Invocation' in *Esoteric Healing* by Bailey, 1984).

Fig

Ficus species   (Pink female & yellow male / FES-res)

Fig flower essence helps us gain deep insight (the flowers 'turn in on themselves' to become the fruit) allowing increased personal expression and the release of inhibiting influences and fears that have been hidden in the subconscious. It is very supportive when doing 'shadow' work as described in Jungian psychotherapy, for instance. It can help us to be more comfortable 'going inward' in Self-exploration in order to gain insight and creative inspiration. Our mind becomes a more 'fertile' terrain from which creative ideas can grow. As a result we can release disabling thought patterns (often developed in childhood) stored in the subconscious mind, allowing us to gain a better mental perspective, more clarity and thus more confidence.

Fireweed

Epilobium angustifolium   (Magenta / FES-RL)

Fireweed flower essence helps to cleanse old patterns so that new life energy can flow through you (FES). It can rekindle an 'old flame' or re-ignite a fiery passion that was extinguished before it had a chance to burn bright – perhaps one that you have always longed to express. Fireweed assists subtle body purification and recovery from past abuse, trauma or the metaphoric 'trials by fire' that are part of life's tribulations. Fireweed stands tall and radiant, quickly regrowing in areas where there has been forest fire or other major disruptive disturbances to the soil. Fireweed grew profusely in many parts of Europe after heavy bombing in World War II, and was especially visible around London. Fireweed flower essence helps us access regenerative, restorative and transformative energy from our environment, so that we can emerge like the phoenix from the ashes, revitalised and rejuvenated (FES).

Forget-Me-Not

Myosotis sylvatica   (Blue / FES)

Forget-Me-Not flower essence helps you remember what you are meant to be doing right now! It can help you to apply practically the ideals and purposes that your soul and its soulmates collaboratively designed for this life. Forget-Me-Not helps raise your awareness of deep (soul) connections in a 'down-to-Earth' way, with those you live with and those who are in the spiritual world (FES). As a therapist, I have found that this awareness usually manifests as a strong sense of direction/purpose in life, along with renewed energy and motivation for doing what is required to make aspirations real. Relationships are consolidated and deepened with those whose path aligns with your own and as a consequence you no longer feel so isolated or alone on your journey. You find yourself connecting with your loving heart rather than just your head, once you recognise your true 'soulmates.'

And finally, when a loved one has passed on, taking Forget-Me-Not flower essence can bring comfort by strengthening our sense of their enduring 'presence.'

Fringed Violet

Thysanotus tuberosus   (Purple/ AUS)

This little dynamo of a flower is entrancing from the very first glimpse. As Ian White says when he comes across a Fringed Violet flower in the bush: 'It stops you dead in your tracks! ... And even though it is quite small its OOMPH is quite amazing' (YouTube 2013).

From a few metres away, what I initially perceive as a purple haze surrounding the flower gradually transforms, as I move closer, into a well-defined, uniform fringe. This first impression of a purple aura around the flower conveys a powerful plant signature. As a flower essence, it is used to help heal and maintain the integrity of the human aura.

People may need Fringed Violet flower essence when they feel psychically unprotected and uneasy in the presence of someone who 'browbeats' them – a subtle example of intimidation through the third eye! Another person may have experienced emotional or physical abuse which has left them injured and vulnerable on a subtle energy level. Or it may be that someone is overly susceptible to the effects of disharmony within their environment in the form of the negative emotions of others or any kind of negative atmosphere. Fringed Violet helps you 'mend' and enhance the integrity of your aura, thus establishing dynamic boundaries to provide emotional and psychic strength and protection.

Glassy Hyacinth

Triteleia lilacina   (White / FES-RL)

Glassy Hyacinth is a close botanical 'cousin' of Star of Bethlehem. They both bring harmony and balance, centring and healing the mind, body and spirit after trauma. Glassy Hyacinth flower essence has the potential to bring peace and calm after major, cathartic crises (FES). With the help of this flower essence, when intense trauma brings a confrontation with our darkest demons and shadow side (FES) – the 'dark night of the soul' – we have an opportunity to transform and redeem these aspects at a soul level. It can help resurrect us (FES) from deep-seated trauma and from the unconscious and undermining influence of our personal demons. Glassy Hyacinth flower essence enables us to transcend trauma's associated emotional pain and suffering and stand triumphant in the light once more, just as this exquisite, white lily springs forth out of dark, volcanic rock.

Grapefruit

Citrus x paradisi   (White / FES-res)

Grapefruit flower essence helps to ease 'cerebral' tension, especially of the neck, scalp and face – it helps with general release of tension in the musculoskeletal system. Grapefruit helps clear and refresh your thinking, making you feel more awake and alive. As a therapist, I have been amazed at how often this flower essence has also helped clients suffering from pain/stiffness of the neck, often with associated lingering headache.

Green Cross Gentian

Frasera speciosa (Greenish-white with purple spots / FES-RL)

Like essences made from other members of the Gentian family, Green Cross Gentian addresses feelings of discouragement, especially in relation to our treatment of the 'green' Earth (FES). It helps us keep on track when we feel strongly about conservation and living 'green' and wish to set an example that others can aspire to. It secures our 'ability to carry the elemental "cross" of the world' (FES). Green Cross Gentian helps us to remain hopeful despite challenges and hardens our resolve to serve the world in the best way we can.

Hawthorn

Crataegus oxyacantha (White / FES-RL)

Hawthorn flower essence helps to moderate the force of the will when it is too strong (FES) and when the will is used to force others to believe (with you) that you are absolutely right. This puts pressure on heart energy, especially if you are frustrated in your attempts to bring others into line and are prone to becoming tense/angry/hostile – perhaps displaying the classical 'Type A' personality (FES). (It is worth noting that as a herb, Hawthorn is used to treat heart and circulation problems.)

Hawthorn flower essence allows 'positive assertive forces' (FES) to be exerted appropriately and for the good of all – under the influence of a balanced *heart chakra*. It helps you develop the courage to remain positive when your strong will is thwarted and avoid falling into hostile 'tantrum' reactions when you don't get your way.

As a therapist, I have found that clients who display the characteristics of the negative Hawthorn state often have a tendency to 'force the issue' because they have been thwarted in the past and feel let down in some way. Hawthorn helps to resolve deep feelings of loss, sorrow or grief which have affected the heart; when this resolution takes place, it becomes possible to let go of negative aspects of the past and feel more nurtured by positive past experiences. This creates an inner calm that brings with it our heart's content.

Hops

Humulus lupulus (Yellow-green / FES-res)

Hops flower essence helps to enhance balanced and coordinated spiritual and physical growth. This is especially useful in adolescence. It helps to ease social tensions by assisting teens to adjust better to rapid growth by facilitating a balanced maturation on all levels of being.

Hops flower essence provides a nervous system tonic (as does the herb); it helps you to create 'space and time' and balance for your Self in a fast-moving life – as therapeutic as a trip to the green open spaces of the countryside! The yellow-green of the flower signifies its relationship with the *solar plexus chakra* (yellow) and the *heart chakra* (green). Its calming influence on the *solar plexus* enables safe opening of the heart chakra and a more harmonious relationship between the two. A more meditative approach allows the nervous system to become nourished, balanced and rejuvenated. A better quality of health-inducing sleep is also a consequence.

Hyssop

Hyssopus officinalis (Blue / FES-RL)

Hyssop flower essence helps us to be more positive about the future by letting go of regrets about the past. Traditionally the herb has been used for respiratory ailments and the lungs are associated with grief in Traditional Chinese Medicine. Those who may benefit from Hyssop flower essence often experience guilt and self-reproach or shame and grief in relation to past experiences (FES) which may or may not involve abuse. Hyssop helps us to let go and forgive ourselves and others – to 'clean the slate' and move on with a buoyant heart and a more optimistic attitude.

Icelandic Poppy

Papaver nudicaule (Red / Alask)

Icelandic Poppy flower essence is very supportive of a balanced spiritual awakening (Alask); it supports the gentle unfolding of spiritual receptivity and facilitates insight so that we can find our truth within and feel more comfortable and less threatened about sharing it honestly with others. Icelandic poppy aids self-realisation and 'opening up' to the world, strengthening our charismatic capacity and ability to radiate spiritual energy in all areas of life.

Jacaranda

Jacaranda mimosifolia (Lavender-blue / Aus)

Jacaranda flower essence helps us when our energies have become scattered as we jump from one project to another (Aus). We start things but leave them unfinished to go off and start something else. We change our minds like the weather. Our enthusiasm, which often attracts others, is always genuine in the beginning but our friends and acquaintances soon feel let down or disappear out of our lives when they become aware of our lack of follow-through and commitment. Jacaranda flower essence helps us to remain centred, using our capacity for quick thinking and 'off the cuff' ideas in the service of productive and satisfactory outcomes.

Jasmine

Jasminum officinale (White, pink tinged / FES-res)

Jasmine flower essence helps release us from the restraints of a past that lingers beyond its 'use-by' date, so that we can appreciate the present and be nourished by it. It helps bring the heart back into the present and restores the ability to love when one has lost love in the past. As a therapist I have found that the qualities of Jasmine flower essence have many similarities to Honeysuckle – both flower essences often come up at the same time and seem equally appropriate.

Jasmine helps to release the 'emotional' past and enables expression of things that have been difficult to express till now. Often, the only expression possible is through production of respiratory catarrh or mucus. (It is not coincidental that many people have allergic-type catarrhal responses to the Jasmine plant It is triggering more than just catarrh!)   In Traditional Chinese Medicine, excessive production of mucus is seen as the body's expression of tenaciously-held emotions and upper respiratory/sinus congestion is perceived as the 'heart trying to get into the head.' Jasmine flower essence enables us to let go of the past and let in the heartfelt joy of the present.

Joshua Tree

Yucca brevifolia   (White to greenish-white / FES-RL)

Joshua Tree flower essence assists in reprogramming deep-seated, hereditary patterns, especially where there is a familial history of dependency or addiction (FES). In Australia, the Boab tree provides a flower essence that helps to transform generational karma and allow those afflicted by it to transform it and break free. In North America this role is filled by the Joshua Tree. This essence enables historical, cultural and familial patterns of dysfunctional behaviour (FES) and inherited illnesses to be addressed and changed for the better. A stronger and more autonomous YOU is the result. New insights into your family (and into the family and personal 'shadow side') and better understanding and empathy with struggles that have occurred over generations gives you a new-found *freedom of choice* in life. You can respect your origins and tolerate your connections while still clearly recognising your individuality (FES). Your family and its cultural and habitual behaviours can no longer control you as you regain autonomy.

Lady's Mantle

Alchemilla vulgaris (Yellow-green / FES-RL)

Lady's Mantle flower essence helps protect and nurture our relationship with the sacred feminine and Mother Earth, especially when a technical or clinical mental outlook dominates (FES). It can help reconnect women with their sensual and creative femininity so that the female reproductive system and cycle are no longer perceived as an inconvenient and uncomfortable nuisance. It can assist men in balancing their relationship with their mother, their inner child, and the feminine principle in themselves and others. Lady's Mantle promotes the release of long-held sadness and despair held in the *lower chakras* (especially the *sacral chakra*) and helps in their repair and healing so that we can feel truly 'Earthed' and grounded in the present. We become more dynamic, soulful and radiant once we are able to access and catalyse the energies of the Earth (FES).

Lady's Slipper

Cypripedium parviflorum (Yellow / FES)

The yellow colour of the Lady's Slipper flower relates to the *solar plexus chakra* and its influence on the way we 'go out' into the world and shine as individuals. Lady's Slipper flower essence helps us when the path we have chosen in life does not align with our inner truth or direction and we find ourselves engaging in disingenuous 'role play' that is exhausting to sustain. We all have a spiritual or higher purpose for being here – even though many of us are unaware of it – and this flower essence helps us integrate this meaning and purpose into our work and daily life (FES). The plant gets its name from the perceived resemblance of the flower to a slipper. It helps us to recognise and follow our true path (FES) in the world so that 'the shoe (or in this case, slipper) fits,' and we walk our true path, undistracted by peers or any external influence that does not align with our personal truth and inner authority.

Lavender Yarrow

Achillea borealis (Lavender / Alask)

As with all the members of the Yarrow family, Lavender Yarrow flower essence relates to psychic and energetic protection. More specifically it helps to strengthenand protect the *higher chakras* – healing and balancing the receptivity of the *crown chakra* so that it is not so susceptible to chaotic and overwhelming influxes of spiritual energy (Alask). This in turn allows an even, balanced and insulated flow of higher vibrational energy through the *heart chakra*. Energy depletion from scattered and dispelled energy through the upper chakras no longer occurs. A mindful, calm and centred conscious state results.

Lilac

Syringa vulgaris (Violet / FES-RL)

Lilac flower essence can help when the upper chakras are over-energised and the lower chakras cannot properly play their part in grounding our thinking and philosophies in the 'real world.' A lack of nurturing and/or having our basic emotional needs met in the past and during early childhood may have resulted in the lower chakras becoming 'anaesthetised' against the pain felt – FES describe it as 'soul amnesia' – so that we are unable to access these chakras' vital, playful and joyful energies (FES). Lilac can help us re-access this energetic input by generating a better 'memory' of the past – re-programming and re-visioning through 'neurological regeneration' (FES) (or changing established neural pathways in the brain, as it is described in Mindfulness/Meditation research these days). This facilitates increased vitality in the energy centres of the physical body, helping us to 'get out of our heads' so that obsessive spiritual idealism, for instance, can become grounded in practical reality, providing us with a real sense of purpose.

Love-Lies-Bleeding

Amaranthus caudatus (Red / FES)

Love-Lies-Bleeding flower essence helps us come to terms with our lot in life, not in a resigned way but with a compassionate and transpersonal understanding of our suffering and discomfort (FES). For example, rather than feeling isolated and alone in our struggle with pain, it enables us to sense how our burden is lightened when shared with our direct karmic connections and rest of the world (FES). When we are able to put physical pain and mental anguish in a broader perspective, this gives us access to an understanding that there is more to us than our pain. When we no longer identify with it completely, we can recognise our own and others' pain with compassion rather than be a slave to it.

To give an example from my own experience, I used to experience very painful migraines from my early teens through to my early twenties. One day I realised that after each migraine episode, although I did have a sore head (though no longer aching), I felt calmer, more relaxed and far less anxious! I became aware that the migraines were actually serving a purpose – they slowed me down so that I could recompose myself and start again calmly. Without them, the tense and anxious state that was my habitual pattern at the time might have become a life sentence, with very bad long term effects on my general health.

Love-Lies–Bleeding flower essence was one remedy that helped me come to realise the meaning behind my painful migraines. In finding meaning, I also came to a greater acceptance of the migraines and even the pain associated. I developed a different relationship with my pain which meant it had less impact on me. This was the beginning of what has become a lifelong study of different approaches to health and wellbeing that perceive illness, pain and suffering as always having a deeper meaning behind their more superficial and transient physical symptoms. In my case I began to look for ways of working with my anxious, stressed responses to life so that I could remain calm enough to avoid having a migraine intervene and do it for me! I learned relaxation techniques and began to meditate; I also began to use more flower essences and homeopathy and within a year the migraines had become a thing of the past.

Milkweed

Asclepias cordifolia   (Red-purple / FES)

Milkweed flower essence is useful when, as a result of previous deprivation (often experienced very early in life) we find it difficult to get the nurturing and sustenance we need. As a consequence we may become needy to the point where we are almost insatiable emotionally, or may look for comfort in food and/or over-eating, or develop a dependency on alcohol and drugs (FES). Lack of self-reliance, dependency on others for emotional nurturing and/or dependency on substances to numb emotional pain can become a strong pattern in our lives. Milkweed can put us back on the road to independence and help us to (re) build healthy ego strength (FES). It can help us to develop our ability to nurture ourselves and others, enriching our lives to the point where we can become self-sustaining.

Monkshood

Aconitum columbianum   (Purple / FES-RL)

Monkshood flower essence is useful when past shock and trauma consciously or unconsciously inhibits our behaviour in the present and creates anxieties about the future. (As a homeopathic remedy Aconite is also used to treat anxiety arising from shock and trauma.) A shocking experience or brush with death can have the effect of numbing or paralysing our spiritual forces to some degree, shutting down our responses to everyday experiences (FES). It is as if we are still in a state of 'spiritual shock or anaesthesia' which creates a sort of 'mental amnesia' although on a physical level we may seem to be functioning normally. Monkshood supports us when reaching into deeper levels of Self to heal and reconnect with our divine or spiritual nature. We start to feel more and more comfortable with integrating this nature into everyday activity at a broader social level (FES). We no longer need to bow our head under the monks' hood – on the contrary we can hold our head high!

Mountain Forget-Me-Not

Hackelia micrantha (Blue with yellow centre / FES-RL)

The flower essences of Mountain Forget-Me-Not and Forget-Me-Not have strong similarities (as you might expect). Here are some distinctions I have identified as a therapist. Mountain Forget-Me-Not essence is helpful for getting a better sense of overall purpose and direction in life, while Forget-Me-Not can help you gain a greater sense of commitment and purpose in everyday activities. Both can help you to be more receptive to the teachers, guides and relatives with whom you have an intimate spiritual connection on a karmic level (FES). Mountain Forget-Me-Not flower essence helps you to get a greater sense of your destiny, aligning you more closely with your soul's purpose (FES). In the negative Mountain Forget-Me-Not state, the feeling of alienation often goes deeper than in the negative Forget-Me-Not state. When we need Mountain Forget-Me-Not flower essence, it is as if we need to seek a higher vantage point (on the mountain!) to gain better perspective. From this more spiritual level, surrounded by soulmates familiar to our higher Self, we can remember our true intention 'down' here, which may have been forgotten.

Mountain Pride

Penstemon newberryi (Magenta / FES)

Mountain Pride plants perch on rocky ledges where they stand out like 'spot fires.' The flower essence helps us 'carry the flame' of our conviction despite fierce and confrontational headwinds. When we take a warrior-like stance, our spiritual light will not be extinguished! Sometimes we may withdraw, procrastinate or vacillate when faced with personal challenges, unable to step up and make a stand (FES). We become like 'a candle in the wind' as our spiritual flame flickers. Mountain Pride flower essence can help restore and/or maintain our pride in who we are and what we stand for. We can rely on ourselves to display courage and a balanced self-assertiveness (FES) when a situation calls us to stand up for our principles and convictions.

Mugwort

Artemisia douglasiana   (Yellow / FES)

Mugwort flower essence helps to ground us by bringing our dream and psychic states into balance with the rest of life, by integrating mind and spirit. Its yellow colour indicates its role in helping to balance the *solar plexus chakra*, calming 'hysteria and emotionality' (FES) by spiritualising the intellect. It allows us to integrate psychic and dream experiences into everyday activity in practical ways (FES) and helps us broaden our consciousness and general perception while keeping a firm grip on physical reality.

Mugwort flower essence is a must for anyone who keeps a dream diary and wishes to enhance their dream recollection and work practically with insights gained from their dreams.

Ocotillo

Fouquieria splendens   (Red / FES-RL)

Ocotillo has intensely red, flame-like flowers that project outwards in different directions from the tips of the stems and Ocotillo flower essence helps people who tend to project their feelings (and themselves) onto other people and situations. Subconscious or unexpressed feelings can lead to emotional over-reactivity and physical hyperactivity, and may erupt as uncontrolled anger and violence (FES). Some people in the negative Ocotillo state resort to alcohol and/or drugs to calm or deaden this fiery imbalance. Ocotillo flower essence helps to ground and give insight into and acceptance of emotions so that we don't feel victimised by them (FES). By 'owning' the fire element within, it becomes possible to integrate it properly. The heart chakra is nourished by and balanced with the fiery energies of the lower chakras, allowing us to radiate spiritual warmth and charisma.

Opium Poppy

Papaver commutatum   (Red and white / Alask)

Opium Poppy flower essence helps us strike the right 'balance between doing and being' (Alask); it helps us to live in the moment without losing sight of our longer term objectives; it really helps us to practise true mindfulness. It allows us to maintain an inner stillness, even in the midst of intense activity or the hustle and bustle of a busy life and helps us to keep perspective at all times, moving forward without wavering. This flower essence is a friend to all those on a quest for inner peace.

Orange

Citrus sinensis   (White / FES-res)

Orange flower essence helps us 'get our head around' intense emotions and come to terms with them. When a client comes to their first consultation in a highly emotional state, I often prescribe Orange flower essence, explaining that it will help them to access their 'inner counsellor' to help them 'get their head around' these overwhelming emotions. It helps to bring insight and clarity about rich, powerful emotions that rise to the surface and can be a good adjunct and support when undergoing any form of psychotherapy. Orange flower essence can facilitate a degree of self-realisation by assisting us to better understand the origins of powerful emotions. It can help us to release emotional tensions associated with strongly held views or opinions, enabling us to approach them in a more objective and less emotionally volatile manner. Communication is enhanced by warmth, not inflamed by emotion. A much better reception is had by all!

Pear

Pyrus communis   (White with violet-red / FES-res)

Pear flower essence helps us to use our brain as a tool without being dominated by it. Intellect becomes a genuine resource when we are able to acknowledge our emotional (feeling) nature – the brain can keep us rational while we explore how we feel and what we sense about a situation. It helps us to use the brain as a precision tool within the far expanses of the mind – it can therefore help us to 'think outside the square.' Pear flower essence might help discontented atheists to reconsider their position or persuade sceptics to broaden their phenomenological terms of reference, or even help some scientists to rethink their paradigm! If you are afraid that *changing* your mind is the same as *losing* your mind, this flower essence can help you to move out of your mental 'comfort zone' more easily and expend less mental energy on defending your belief system.

Back in the 1960s and 70s, hallucinatory drugs (especially LSD) were used to facilitate exploration beyond everyday realms of consciousness. Some users were terrified and even experienced psychotic episodes. Others, however, remained comfortable and never fully lost touch with reality during what was for them a peak spiritual experience which transformed their lives for the better. Pear flower essence can have the effect of keeping us grounded in this way while we seek understanding beyond our normal mental 'paradigms.' The flowers are white with violet-red anthers, signifying a connection between the spiritual aspirations of the *crown chakra* (white, violet) and the grounding effect of the *base chakra* (red). Pear flower essence can support and securely ground you when you venture into 'higher' realms of thought and experience, giving you confidence to venture into new mental territory rather than staying with 'the devil you know.'

Pennyroyal

Mentha pulegium   (Lavender / FES-res)

As a therapist, I have found that Pennyroyal flower essence has strong similarities with Mountain Pennyroyal. They both help us to protect ourselves from negative thought forms and patterns created by others in our immediate environment. Pennyroyal can aid gentle cleansing, inner purification and release of these negative 'mind fields' when they have become entrenched in our subtle anatomy. It can also work at this subtle level when the mind is dominated or obsessed by a specific pattern of thinking. Pennyroyal flower essence helps to protect against psychic malevolence.

Penstemon

Penstemon davidsonii   (Violet-blue / FES)

As with so many plants in the Penstemon family, *Penstemon davidsonii* displays an ability to endure, survive and thrive in spite of difficult and adverse habitats. As a flower essence, it helps us to overcome a tendency to feel sorry for ourselves and withdraw from confrontation and difficult circumstances. Penstemon enhances our 'intestinal fortitude' so that we can rise to the occasion and meet interpersonal difficulties and challenges 'head on' (FES). It helps us to become strong through adversity (FES), reminding us of the saying 'What doesn't kill you makes you stronger!' When the going gets tough, Penstemon flower essence helps the tough to get going and persevere beyond temporary setbacks.

Petunia

Petunia hybrid   (Purple / FES-res)

Petunia flower essence helps us to develop a more positive mental attitude that allows our behaviour to follow suit. Fixed attitudes can lead to fixed behaviours and habitual reactions. If these habitual behaviours and responses are antisocial and alienating, they can set up a self-reinforcing pattern that is very difficult to change. As a therapist, I have found Petunia flower essence to be particularly helpful for some children who seem to be locked into negative behaviour patterns and habits which are very difficult to break. Petunia essence's positive and expansive influence on the mental sphere can broaden and elevate our minds and attitudes. In my practice, I have also sent the essence home with some clients who wished to change long-standing unacceptable behaviours in their pets. Some success has been reported with the development of new and more socially acceptable habits – it seems you can teach an old dog new tricks!

Pink Monkeyflower

Mimulus lewisii (Pink / FES)

Like all Monkeyflower essences, Pink Monkeyflower helps people raise their awareness of certain intense emotions that they may fear and/or feel uncomfortable expressing. The Monkeyflowers enable people to 'sit with' these feelings and more fully experience and embrace them. They then become more comfortable to express these emotions, confident in their authenticity, and in Pink Monkeyflower's case, know that their responses come purely from the heart. The signature of the plant, in its colour and form, also informs us of its inner nature, with its strong connection with the heart centre.

Pink Monkeyflower can help a person overcome a self-denigrating sense of shame and unworthiness about the feelings they wish to express. The flower essence allows a person to display 'emotional transparency [and the] courage to take emotional risks with others' (Kaminski & Katz, FES Repertory, fesflowers.com)

This fear a person may have about their true, heartfelt feelings being exposed often stems from previous emotional abuse and humiliation as children and/or teenagers, when feelings were dismissed when at their most vulnerable. And highly sensitive people are always particularly vulnerable at all stages of life because of their sensitive nature that feels so deeply. Fortunately, with the help of Pink Monkeyflower to gently 'open' one's heart, an individual becomes more able to comfortably express what their heart truly feels and desires in their relationships and life. 'They begin to experience the love and the contact [and validation] which they so desperately need and want' (Kaminski & Katz, FES Repertory, fesflowers.com).

Poison Oak

Toxicodendron diversiloba   (Greenish-white / FES)

Once again we find a lot of meaning in a plant name. Poison Oak is a plant best known for its ability to cause allergic rashes and itching after contact. In the negative Poison Oak state, like the plant we become over-protective of our personal boundaries to the point where we overreact, rejecting friendly advances by others (FES). Aggressive or angry reactions to innocent overtures may disguise a strong 'fear of intimate contact' (FES). Poison Oak flower essence helps us to overcome our fears, releasing us from excessively self-protective behaviour and allowing us to be more emotionally open and receptive (FES). When it is appropriate and you are in the right company, with the help of this essence it becomes easier to drop your guard, relax and enjoy the benefits of being vulnerable and intimate.

Prickly Pear Cactus

Opuntia aciculata (Yellow / FES-res)

Prickly Pear Cactus flower essence helps us to avoid reacting in a 'prickly' manner when discussing sensitive issues so that we can engage in more objective discussion. It supports our ability to adapt better to our surroundings, and especially the people around us, like the plant which is able to survive in harsh environments. Emotional and social compatibility is enhanced so that we are able to communicate harmoniously with others, one-to-one and in groups. Prickly Pear Cactus flower essence helps us relax emotionally so we become more easygoing and amicable.

Purple Monkeyflower

Mimulus kelloggii (Purple / FES)

Purple Monkeyflower essence is useful for people who are intimidated by spiritual authority, religious convention or family and community culture (FES). They may fear the consequences of departing from 'the way' or straying outside a belief system they have been told is correct, true and 'normal.' This way of thinking may have helped them feel more secure and grounded until now, especially when some of their experiences and 'extra senses' scared them to the point of feeling they might be 'losing it.' While growing up, sometimes parents and others in authority reinforce this fear of having different ways of experiencing the world. One client (now in her 80s) explained to me how she, as a young child, had been close to death while in hospital suffering from pneumonia. After she recovered and was able to return home, she related to her mother that she had seen 'a tunnel of very bright light' when she was sick. Her mother quickly made her promise never to mention this again and told her that if she did, she would be 'put in a looney bin!' Only in her later years did this person come to feel comfortable to explore and trust some of her more spiritual experiences. Purple Monkeyflower helps us to trust our own spiritual experience and guidance (FES) and develop and follow our own conscience.

Quaking Grass

Briza maxima   (Green / FES)

Quaking Grass flower essence can help individuals to adapt better to working in groups (and living in families). It does this by fostering awareness of individual identity within the 'vision' or higher purpose of the group. I once worked with a client who described how, having joined a group because she felt attracted to its altruistic goals, she nevertheless developed a migraine by the end of every meeting because she found the behaviour of some members so upsetting. However, she was aware that she could be quite rigid and intolerant in imposing her 'standards' on other people, and she genuinely wanted to stay in the group to further its cause. I prescribed Quaking Grass flower essence, which helped her to become more flexible in her expectations of others while maintaining her own integrity. She became a very positive influence in the group (which has gone on to achieve significant results) and her meeting-related migraines stopped. 'Harmonious social consciousness is the special gift of the Quaking Grass flower' (FES).

Queen Anne's Lace

Daucus carota   (White / FES)

The cultivated carrots we eat have a reputation for providing nutrients that enhance vision, especially in the dark. As a flower essence, Queen Anne's Lace, the 'wild' carrot from which today's vegetable derives, is used to improve spiritual vision and insight (FES). It aids in the process of spiritual refinement, helping us to integrate the higher octaves and psychic faculties of the upper chakras with the lower chakras and our 'shadow' side. We could say that it helps to shed spiritual light on our primal nature, so that we are clearer and purer insofar as we know ourselves better and are less likely to project our own shadow onto others when giving advice or spiritual guidance. Queen Anne's Lace flower essence helps to ground us so that our psychic awareness is less likely to be contaminated or distorted by our own personal 'stuff' or 'emotional baggage.'

Red Larkspur

Delphinium nudicaule (Red / FES-RL)

    Red Larkspur flower essence is useful for natural leaders and inspirers who have temporarily lost their 'spark.' (By comparison, Larkspur flower essence is useful for reluctant leaders.) Red Larkspur is for those who accept their role as charismatic leaders but lack the energy and verve to carry out their work (FES). Their energy to inspire and motivate others has become exhausted and their usual exemplary physical energy (which also nourishes others) is depleted. Red Larkspur helps to recapture and harness the ability to radiate energy and influence and inspire others through positive leadership (FES). I have prescribed Red Larkspur with very positive results for a number of life coaches and personal trainers, for example, who were feeling unusually flat and depleted of energy.

Red Lily

Nelumbo nucifera (Red / Aus)

    Like Lotus flower essence, Red Lily helps bring the lower chakras into sync with the higher chakras. (Ian White reminds us in his book that Red Lily is in fact a lotus and as a therapist I find it almost interchangeable with Lotus for some clients.) Red Lily 'grounds' us securely in the present and helps us establish 'Earthly' foundations for our dreams and aspirations. In the negative state, the Red Lily personality is prone to daydreaming and 'splitting off' from the present, in a way that is sometimes unkindly referred to as 'airheaded.' As a result, their energies are scattered so that they are unable to focus on the task at hand. Red Lily flower essence is particularly useful for someone who is preparing to take responsibility and begin to 'walk the talk,' and not get off (their) track. It 'helps to balance the spiritual and earthly planes' (Ian White) by keeping us grounded and practical while we 'reach out and commune with spiritual realms.' At a deep level, it can help us reassert our commitment to being here and the evidence of this is a more dynamic presence in the world.

Red Penstemon

Penstemon rostriflorus (Red / FES-RL)

    Like Mountain Pride (*Penstemon newberryi*), Red Penstemon grows precariously from the sides of steep, rocky cliffs and has a similar form. However, Red Penstemon's environment is harsher, its shape is more distinct and its colour more vivid, 'like a red sword gleaming in the sun' (FES). All these aspects of its signature indicate how as a flower essence, it can enhance our vital force and physical expression. It can help us to be more physically adventurous and take more risks (FES), extending ourselves and growing as a person. It can help sportspersons to push their boundaries in order to reach new heights; it can help people at any age or stage to have the courage to engage in and enjoy adventurous physical activities. Red Penstemon flower essence instils the determination and tenacity that helps to overcome bodily restrictions, limitations and challenges (FES), enabling us to achieve all that is possible.

Redwood

Sequoia sempervirens (White/ FES-RL)

Redwood flower essence helps align all the subtle bodies, allowing the vital force to flow more freely through us. One of the tallest trees in the world, it helps us to 'stand tall' and become strong and 'upright' in our lives (FES). No room for 'yes'-people here! If we lack physical strength and vitality due to hereditary or other health issues, delayed or slow development or spinal or bone injuries and afflictions, Redwood can help us overcome limitations to reach our maximum physical and energetic potential (FES). As a therapist I have also found that it can play an important role in assisting the elderly to maintain a good level of vitality – Redwood trees can live for thousands of years! Regeneration and longevity are key words associated with the tree, and the essence can help humans to realise these potentials.

Rue

Ruta graveolens (Yellow / FES-RL)

In homeopathic form, Rue is prescribed for trauma and especially strain to ligaments and the periosteum. It helps to tone overworked elastic tissue and heals damaged protective tissue around bones and organs. In other words, it is used to tone and heal tissues responsible for elasticity and resilience. It is no surprise, then, to find that as a flower essence, Rue is used to promote the healing, cohesion and integrity of the subtle bodies and psychic forces (FES). It helps contain, consolidate, tone and cement 'scattered or confused psychic forces' (FES) so as to strengthen natural immunity at all levels, protecting the psyche and bringing mental clarity and discernment. It can help heal deep-seated past trauma and improve resilience of mind, body and spirit. In other words, it helps us rebound after trauma.

Sage

Salvia officinalis (Violet / FES)

Sage flower essence helps us to perceive and appreciate the wisdom, higher purpose and meaning behind events in our lives (FES). It helps us to appreciate the 'sage' within who has come into being as a consequence of our life's rich experience. This insight can be especially pertinent at midlife, enabling us to view our lives from the perspective of the higher Self. From this viewpoint, we no longer see life in general and our individual life in particular as ill-fated or lacking importance and meaning (FES), but rather the contrary.

Skullcap

Scutellaria lateriflora (Blue / FES-res)

Skullcap's common name refers to the shape of the flower which resembles a helmet with the visor raised. This aspect of the flower's signature conveys an opening up ('visor raised') to a clearer, more forward-reaching vision in life. (Many flower essences from the Mint family aid in mental clarity.)

Skullcap flower essence assists many of the uncomfortable cerebrally related symptoms that the herb does. It eases muscular tension and headaches caused by mental strain, relaxes the thinking process and allows a broader, more mindful vision. To misquote Monty Python, 'My brain doesn't hurt!'

Star Tulip

Calochortus toliei (White and purple / FES)

Star Tulip has the common name of 'Pussy's Ears.' We all recognise the way cats show their sensitivity, awareness and receptivity to their surroundings through their ear movements. Star Tulip flower essence helps us develop a more 'sensitive and receptive attunement' (FES) to others and our environment. Listening on all levels of our being is enhanced, from the ability to really hear what someone else is saying and get a sense of what they are feeling to 'inner listening ... to higher worlds' (FES). While taking Star Tulip flower essence, many of my clients report that they can meditate more easily and effectively, and gain better awareness and understanding of their dreams and generally become more aware, receptive and 'in sync' with the subtleties of what's happening around them. 'I've noticed things I've never noticed before, and I'm glad.'

Stinging Nettle

Urtica dioica (Green / FES-res)

Stinging Nettle flower essence helps repair emotional damage that occurs as a result of breakups in relationships, families and other groups. When emotional bonds are traumatically severed, Stinging Nettle can start the healing process after the initial shock. The green signature of the flowers relates to the heart chakra and signifies the plant's ability to heal issues of the heart and natural (emotional) immunity. Stinging Nettle restores the emotional integrity of personal boundaries that have been 'badly bruised' energetically. Like the Nettle plant, after emotional trauma we sometimes develop the self-protective habit of 'stinging' those who come too close. Stinging Nettle eases emotional tension and allows us to function and interact more comfortably on an intimate level with others.

Sundew

Drosera spatulata (White / Aus)

The signature of this plant is clear. Sundew's tiny white flowers are raised high above the solid red rosette of leaves that forms the base. The flower wavers in the breeze, barely connected to the base via a long thin stem, almost like a miniature balloon on a long string. The stem can be seen as representing a connection with the higher Self or crown chakra (the white flowers), while the red base signifies our 'earthing' or base chakra grounding in the reality of life. Sundew flower essence is useful when we are feeling vague, disconnected or split from the moment (White), or too often find ourselves daydreaming. Our ability to concentrate, focus and remain in the moment is lacking. Sundew helps fully ground us so that we can embrace each moment with passion. We can bring our basic instinctual urges and senses into consciousness and at the same time respect what we are doing by giving it the attention to detail and focus (White) that it deserves.

Tall Mountain Larkspur

Delphinium glaucum (Deep blue-purple / FES-RL)

All the Larkspur family essences have qualities that relate to embracing dynamic leadership qualities. Tall Mountain Larkspur has effects that focus on enabling receptivity to higher (spiritual) guidance (FES) and enhancing the capacity to influence people to align themselves with altruistic or spiritual aspirations. When you feel disconnected and lack trust in real inner guidance, this essence can help you to 'see and feel' a true higher calling to lead others (FES). Tall Mountain Larkspur can help leaders, whether of a small group or a big company, to get a real sense of what their group's motto or company's mission statement might be.

There are followers and there are leaders; there are politicians and there are true statesmen. Tall Mountain Larkspur essence helps you to access inner guidance so that you can act confidently, setting an example and inspiring others through your capacity for soul leadership that transcends ego and personality.

Thyme

Thymus vulgaris (Bluish-purple / FES-res)

As a therapist, I have found Thyme flower essence very useful for those who become too 'time urgent.' It seems to put time back 'on your side'! I have also found that Thyme tends to enhance the activity of other flower essences. I feel sure that one aspect of the way this works is that it helps to ensure that we actually make time for our flower essence doses rather than becoming so caught up in the rush that we forget or neglect to take them. When taking Thyme essence we get better at 'taking time' and not neglecting important things that should take priority in our lives. The day flows better, we utilise our time better and as a result we accomplish more without an uncomfortable and distracting sense of urgency and anxiety.

Turk's Cap

Malvaviscus arboreus (Yellow / FES-RL)

Turk's Cap flower essence helps us turn intense energy, passion and drive into direct and constructive action – in this way it is very 'grounding.' As a therapist I have found, for instance, that some male teenagers become better able to adapt and focus their newfound, testosterone-driven energy so that it's not such a source of frustration to them and aggravation to others. Turk's Cap helps them transform their energy so that it becomes a source of creative, constructive and fulfilling self-expression. The essence can, though, be equally applicable for all ages and both genders. Turk's Cap helps us refine our raw/instinctual passions, arising from overly yang energy, into calm, confident and creative self-expression.

Yellow Star Tulip

Calochortus monophyllus (Yellow / FES)

Yellow Star Tulip flower essence helps restore 'empathy' (FES) and enhances our sensitivity to the feelings of others when it has become dulled or numbed, especially when this happens because of desensitisation through overexposure to other people's suffering. This hardening may occur as a survival measure for social workers, therapists, counsellors, healers or those who have repeatedly been exposed to traumatic situations.

At the other end of the 'sensitivity' spectrum, Yellow Star Tulip essence can be useful for those starting out in healing, counselling or teaching careers and endeavouring to develop greater awareness of others' needs and refine their empathetic qualities (FES). Yellow Star Tulip helps develop our capacity for receptive and insightful presence, enabling us to really listen, hear and respond with our hearts to the hearts of others.

Yerba Santa

Eriodictyon californicum   (Violet / FES)

Yerba Santa flower essence assists the comfortable release of energy blockages and constriction in the chest area resulting from experiences of profound loss, such as separation from a parent or carer early in life. The effect of Yerba Santa flower essence can be compared to that of an electrical adaptor, in that it allows 'deeply repressed emotions [such as] internalized grief and melancholy' (FES), which may be felt physically in the region of the heart, to be released in a steady, gentle manner, without an intense and overwhelming 'surge.' In homeopathic and herbal form, Yerba Santa has traditionally been used to treat asthmatic and bronchial conditions; when energy becomes stagnant or blocked in the chest/heart area, there are physical effects which invariably render a person more vulnerable to lung congestion, asthma and even pneumonia. Yerba Santa flower essence helps to 'free up' the chest area so that it becomes possible to 'harmonise breathing with feeling ... and express a full range of human emotion' (FES). It works well when taken in conjunction with other flower essences whose action is potentially more cathartic, enabling emotions which have remained repressed over a long period to be processed in a gentle and manageable way.

Quick flower essence selection guide

Refer to the emotional/mental states or life situation/aspirations/stages in development listed below to find the best description of your **current feelings** or **current predicament**. Then look up the flowers recommended for those feelings or situations and choose one or more with the personality profile(s) that correspond most closely with yours.

Flower essences for the way you now feel – 'mood matching'

abandoned *(see also alone, rejected and unloved)*

Angelica, Baby Blue Eyes, Bleeding Heart, Bottlebrush, Chicory, Evening Primrose, Forget-Me-Not, Golden Ear Drops, Lilac, Mariposa Lily, Milkweed, Shooting Star, Sturt Desert Pea, Sweet Pea, Tall Yellow Top, Waratah

abused *(see also shocked and traumatised)*

Arnica, Baby Blue Eyes, Black Cohosh, Crowea, Dogwood, Echinacea, Evening Primrose, Glassy Hyacinth, Golden Ear Drops, Fringed Violet, Hibiscus, Joshua Tree, Lilac, Love-Lies-Bleeding, Mariposa Lily, Monkshood, Pretty Face, Purple Monkeyflower, Rue, Star of Bethlehem

afraid *(see also apprehensive, fearful and terrified)*

Angelica, Aspen, Cherry Plum, Garlic, Mimulus (and all the Monkeyflowers), Monkshood, Mountain Pride, Oregon Grape, Red Chestnut, Red Clover, Red Grevillea, Red Penstemon, Rock Rose, St John's Wort, Violet

aggressive *(see also hostile)*

Calendula, Cherry Plum, Flannel Flower, Hawthorn, Holly, Lilac, Impatiens, Larkspur, Mallow, Nicotiana, Oregon Grape, Poison Oak, Prickly Pear Cactus, Quince, Snapdragon, Squash (Zucchini), Star Thistle, Stinging Nettle, Sunflower, Tiger Lily, Trillium, Turk's Cap, Vervain, Vine, Zinnia

alienated *(see also lonely)*

Baby Blue Eyes, Evening Primrose, Fawn Lily, Forget-Me-Not, Heather, Impatiens, Lady's Slipper, Manzanita, Mariposa Lily, Mountain Forget-Me-Not, Nicotiana, Saguaro, Shooting Star, Silver Princess, Strut Desert Pea, Sweet Pea, Tall Yellow Top, Violet, Water Violet, Wild Oat, Wild Rose

alone *(see also abandoned, rejected and unloved)*

Angelica, Angelsword, Baby Blue Eyes, Echinacea, Evening Primrose, Fawn Lily, Forget-Me-Not, Honeysuckle, Lilac, Lotus, Mariposa Lily, Milkweed, Mountain Forget-Me-Not, Red Lily, Shooting Star, Sweet Pea, Tall Yellow Top, Violet, Water Violet

aloof

Fawn Lily, Hibbertia, Lilac, Lotus, Mallow, Nicotiana, Pear, Pink Monkeyflower, Red Lily, Rosemary, Sundew, Tall Yellow Top, Violet, Water Violet, Wild Rose

ambivalent *(see also indecisive)*

Angelsword, Calla Lily, Cayenne, Cerato, Clematis, Coffee, Easter, Foxglove, Iris, Jacaranda, Madia, Manzanita, Mullein, Onion, Paw Paw, Peppermint, Pomegranate, Red Lily, Rosemary, Saguaro, Scleranthus, Shasta Daisy, Silver Princess, Shooting Star, Sundew, Tansy, Violet, Wedding Bush, Wild Rose

angry/annoyed *(see also furious and irritable)*

Almond, Beech, Black Eyed Susan, Chamomile, Cherry Plum, Dogwood, Fuchsia, Hawthorn, Holly, Impatiens, Mulla Mulla, Indian Pink, Ocotillo, Orange, Poison Oak, Prickly Pear Cactus, Red Grevillea, Scarlet Monkeyflower, Snapdragon, Stinging Nettle, Tiger Lily, Turk's Cap, Willow

anxious *(also see nervous, tense, worried)*

Agrimony, Angelica, Aspen, Californian Valerian, Cassandra, Chamomile, Cherry Plum, Crowea, Dandelion, Elm, Filaree, Fuchsia, Garlic, Golden Yarrow, Hawthorn, Impatiens, Indian Pink, Kangaroo Paw, Larch, Lavender, Mallow, Mimulus, Nectarine, Oregon Grape, Passionflower, Red Chestnut, Rock Rose, St John's Wort, Thyme, Vervain, Violet, Wallflower, Waratah, White Chestnut, Zinnia

apathetic *(see also listless)*

Californian Pitcher Plant, California Peony, Clematis, Gorse, Explorer's Gentian, Hornbeam, Lemon, Madia, Peppermint, Red Larkspur, Red Lily, Red Penstemon, Redwood, Silver Princess, Sundew, Tansy, Wild Potato Bush, Wild Rose

apprehensive *(see also afraid, fearful and terrified)*

Alpine Aster, Angelica, Angelsword, Aspen, Cherry Plum, Crowea, Forget-Me-Not, Fringed Violet, Garlic, Golden Yarrow, Kangaroo Paw, Larch, Mallow, Mimulus, Mountain Pride, Oregon Grape, Purple Monkeyflower, Red Clover, Red Grevillea, Red Penstemon, Redwood, Rock Rose, St John's Wort, Violet, Waratah

awkward *(see also clumsy)*

Almond, Dogwood, Flannel Flower, Hibbertia, Kangaroo Paw, Mallow, Manzanita, Pink Monkeyflower, Pretty Face, Red Penstemon, Redwood, Shooting Star, Sticky Monkeyflower, Violet, Wild Potato Bush

bad tempered *(see angry/annoyed, irritable)*

Beech, Black Eyed Susan, Calendula, Chamomile, Cherry Plum, Crab Apple, Dogwood, Fuchsia, Holly, Impatiens, Indian Pink, Lotus, Mulla Mulla, Ocotillo, Oregon Grape, Poison Oak, Prickly Pear Cactus, Quince, Scarlet Monkeyflower, Snapdragon, Star Thistle, Tiger Lily, Vine, Willow

bewildered *(see also confused)*

Calla Lily, Cerato, Chestnut Bud, Clematis, Echinacea, Explorer's Gentian, Filaree, Forget-Me-Not, Green Cross Gentian, Lilac, Mountain Forget-Me-Not, Foxglove, Indian Pink, Iris, Jacaranda, Onion, Paw Paw, Queen Anne's Lace, Rabbitbrush, Red Lily, Rosemary, Rue, Scleranthus, Shasta Daisy, Silver Princess, Star of Bethlehem, Sundew, Walnut, Wild Oat

bitter *(see also resentment)*

Almond, Baby Blue Eyes, Chicory, Dogwood, Holly, Oregon Grape, Red Grevillea, Willow

blue *(see also gloomy, depressed and sad)*

Baby Blue Eyes, Black Cohosh, Bleeding Heart, Borage, Explorer's Gentian, Gentian, Glassy Hyacinth, Golden Ear Drops, Gorse, Harvest Brodiaea, Honeysuckle, Hound's Tongue, Hyssop, Iris, Love-Lies-Bleeding, Mustard, Pansy, Petunia, Red Larkspur, Scotch Broom, Sturt Desert Pea, Sweet Chestnut, Wallflower, Waratah, Wild Rose, Willow

burdened *(see also responsibility)*

Borage, Centaury, Chicory, Crowea, Elm, Hornbeam, Larkspur, Love-Lies-Bleeding, Oak, Paw Paw, Red Chestnut, Sturt Desert Pea, Wild Potato Bush, Willow, Zinnia

burnt out *(see also exhausted)*

Aloe Vera, Chaparral, Hornbeam, Indian Paintbrush, Macrocarpa, Morning Glory, Nasturtium, Nectarine, Olive, Peppermint

clumsy *(see also awkward)*

Almond, Dogwood, Flannel Flower, Kangaroo Paw, Mallow, Manzanita, Red Penstemon, Redwood, Sticky Monkeyflower, Violet, Wild Potato Bush

confused *(see also bewildered)*

Angelsword, Blackberry, Californian Poppy, Calla Lily, Cerato, Chestnut Bud, Clematis, Coffee, Corn, Cosmos, Dill, Elm, Filaree, Forget-Me-Not, Foxglove, Indian Pink, Iris, Jacaranda, Lemon, Madia, Mullein, Onion, Paw Paw, Pomegranate, Quince, Rabbitbrush, Red Lily, Rosemary, Scleranthus, Shasta Daisy, Silver Princess, Sundew, Wedding Bush, White Chestnut, Wild Oat

critical

Almond, Baby Blue Eyes, Beech, Calendula, Crab Apple, Dogwood, Filaree, Holly, Honeysuckle, Hound's Tongue, Impatiens, Lotus, Quince, Rock Water, Saguaro, Snapdragon, Vine, Willow

day-dreamy *(see also vague)*

Blackberry, Bunchberry, Cayenne, Clematis, Corn, Honeysuckle, Lotus, Madia, Morning Glory, Mugwort, Nicotiana, Peppermint, Red Lily, Rosemary, Shooting Star, Sundew, Tall Yellow Top, Wild Rose

deceived

Almond, Baby Blue Eyes, Bleeding Heart, Dogwood, Hibiscus, Holly, Mallow, Mariposa Lily, Oregon Grape

defensive

Black Eyed Susan, Calendula, Flannel Flower, Holly, Mallow, Oregon Grape, Poison Oak, Prickly Pear Cactus, Quince, Snapdragon, Star Thistle, Stinging Nettle, Tiger Lily, Trillium

depressed *(see also blue, gloomy and sad)*

Baby Blue Eyes, Black Cohosh, Bleeding Heart, Borage, Chrysanthemum, Explorer's Gentian, Gentian, Glassy Hyacinth, Golden Ear Drops, Gorse, Harvest Brodiaea, Honeysuckle, Hornbeam, Hound's Tongue, Hyssop, Iris, Love-Lies-Bleeding, Milkweed, Mustard, Pansy, Petunia, Red Larkspur, Scotch Broom, Sturt Desert Pea, Sweet Chestnut, Wallflower, Waratah, Wild Oat, Wild Rose, Willow

despair *(see also hopeless)*

Angelica, Forget-Me-Not, Gentian, Glassy Hyacinth, Gorse, Iris, Mustard,

Pansy, Scotch Broom, Silver Princess, Sturt Desert Pea, Sweet Chestnut, Waratah, Wild Oat, Wild Rose

desperate

Cherry Plum, Gorse, Nectarine, Orange, Rescue Remedy, Sweet Chestnut, Waratah

discouraged

Bleeding Heart, Borage, Bottlebrush, Elm, Explorer's Gentian, Foxglove, Gentian, Green Cross Gentian, Iris, Larch, Mountain Pride, Mustard, Pansy, Penstemon, Scotch Broom, Self-Heal, Silver Princess, Sturt Desert Pea, Tansy, Violet, Wallflower, Walnut, Wild Oat, Wild Rose, Willow

disingenuous

Agrimony, Almond, Angelsword, Calla Lily, Cerato, Chrysanthemum, Deerbrush, Fairy Lantern, Forget-Me-Not, Goldenrod, Hibbertia, Lady's Slipper, Mallow, Mountain Forget-Me-Not, Mountain Pride, Mullein, Northern Lady's Slipper, Pomegranate, Purple Monkeyflower, Red Grevillea, Sagebrush, Saguaro, Sunflower, Tall Yellow Top, Violet, Walnut, Wild Oat

disorientated

Cayenne, Clematis, Corn, Dill, Fringed Violet, Honeysuckle, Indian Pink, Lotus, Madia, Morning Glory, Nicotiana, Paw Paw, Peppermint, Rabbitbrush, Red Clover, Red Lily, Rescue Remedy, Rosemary, Shasta Daisy, Shooting Star, Silver Princess, Sundew, Sweet Pea, Tall Yellow Top, Walnut, Wild Oat, YES formula

distracted *(see also concentration and focus)*

Blackberry, Bunchberry, Californian Poppy, Canyon Dudleya, Cayenne, Clematis, Corn, Dill, Foxglove, Honeysuckle, Indian Pink, Jacaranda, Lemon, Madia, Morning Glory, Mountain Pennyroyal, Mugwort, Nicotiana, Paw Paw, Peppermint, Rabbitbrush, Red Lily, Rosemary, Shasta Daisy, Shooting Star, Sundew, Wild Oat, Wild Rose, YES formula

doubtful *(see also confidence)*

Angelsword, Aspen, Blazing Star, Buttercup, Californian Valerian, Calla Lily, Cerato, Centaury, Cosmos, Elm, Forget-Me-Not, Garlic, Gorse, Kangaroo Paw, Larch, Mimulus, Mountain Pride, Onion, Pansy, Penstemon, Pretty Face, St John's Wort, Scleranthus, Sunflower, Self-Heal, Tansy, Trumpet Vine, Violet, Wallflower, Wedding Bush

envious *(see also jealous)*

Boab, Bottlebrush, Buttercup, Chicory, Goldenrod, Holly, Pretty Face, Sunflower, Tiger Lily, Trillium, Walnut

erratic *(see also scattered)*

Blackberry, Bunchberry, Chamomile, Corn, Dill, Dogwood, Impatiens, Indian Pink, Jacaranda, Madia, Morning Glory, Paw Paw, Rabbitbrush, Scleranthus, Shasta Daisy, Silver Princess, Wild Oat, YES formula

exhausted *(see also fatigued and tired)*

Aloe Vera, Californian Peony, Cayenne, Coffee, Echinacea, Fireweed, Forget-Me-Not, Hornbeam, Lady's Slipper, Macrocarpa, Morning Glory, Nasturtium, Olive, Peppermint, Redwood, Larkspur, Wild Potato Bush, Wild Rose

fanatical

Angelsword, Californian Poppy, Canyon Dudleya, Dandelion, Green Cross Gentian, Hawthorn, Hibbertia, Impatiens, Lilac, Rock Water, Vervain, Vine

fatigued *(see also exhausted and tired)*

Aloe Vera, Californian Peony, Cayenne, Coffee, Fireweed, Forget-Me-Not, Hornbeam, Lady's Slipper, Lemon, Macrocarpa, Morning Glory, Nasturtium, Olive, Peppermint, Red Larkspur, Silver Princess, Wild Potato Bush, Wild Rose

fearful *(see also afraid, apprehensive and terrified)*

Angelica, Aspen, Blazing Star, Cherry Plum, Fawn Lily, Garlic, Larch, Mimulus (all Monkeyflowers), Monkshood, Mountain Pride, Oregon Grape, Red Chestnut, Red Clover, Red Grevillea, Red Penstemon, Rescue Remedy, Rock Rose, St John's Wort, Violet, Wallflower, Waratah

forgetful

Angelsword, Bunchberry, Cassandra, Chestnut Bud, Clematis, Coffee, Cosmos, Crowea, Forget-Me-Not, Harvest Brodiaea, Lemon, Madia, Mountain Forget-Me-Not, Nasturtium, Peppermint, Rabbitbrush, Rosemary, Shasta Daisy, Sundew, White Chestnut

frustrated

Almond, Blackberry, Boab, Bottlebrush, Californian Peony, Cayenne, Cosmos, Crowea, Impatiens, Indian Paintbrush, Iris, Joshua Tree, Red Grevillea, Silver Princess, Snapdragon, Tansy, Trumpet Vine, Turk's Cap, Wild Potato Bush

furious *(see also angry/annoyed)*

Almond, Black Eyed Susan, Chamomile, Cherry Plum, Dogwood, Fuchsia, Hawthorn, Holly, Impatiens, Indian Pink, Lotus, Ocotillo, Red Grevillea, Scarlet Monkeyflower, Snapdragon, Stinging Nettle, Tiger Lily, Willow

gloomy *(see also blue, depressed, joyless, sad)*

Baby Blue Eyes, Bleeding Heart, Borage, Explorer's Gentian, Gentian, Golden Ear Drops, Gorse, Harvest Brodiaea, Hibbertia, Hound's Tongue, Hyssop, Iris, Mustard, Pansy, Petunia, Scotch Broom, Sturt Desert Pea, Waratah, Wild Rose, Willow, Zinnia

greedy

Chrysanthemum, Chicory, Milkweed, Opium Poppy, Quaking Grass, Star Thistle, Sunflower, Tiger Lily, Trillium, Vine

grief *(see also heart-broken, sad, sorrow)*

Angel's Trumpet, Angelica, Bleeding Heart, Borage, Bottlebrush, Evening Primrose, Forget-Me-Not, Fuchsia, Gentian, Glassy Hyacinth, Golden Ear Drops, Honeysuckle, Hyssop, Love-Lies-Bleeding, Onion, Star of Bethlehem, Sturt Desert Pea, Walnut, Waratah, Wild Rose, Yerba Santa

guilt

Basil, Billy Goat Plum, Chestnut Bud, Crab Apple, Easter Lily, Hyssop, Larkspur, Mullein, Oak, Pine, Pomegranate, Sturt Desert Pea, Tansy

hate

Almond, Black Cohosh, Boab, Bottlebrush, Cherry Plum, Dogwood, Holly, Joshua Tree, Ocotillo, Oregon Grape, Red Grevillea, Willow

heart-broken *(see also broken-hearted, sad, sorrow)*

Bleeding Heart, Borage, Bottle Brush, Evening Primrose, Forget-Me-Not, Glassy Hyacinth, Golden Ear Drops, Hawthorn, Honeysuckle, Hyssop, Jasmine, Lilac, Love-Lies-Bleeding, Mallow, Mariposa Lily, Pink Monkeyflower, Rescue Remedy, Star of Bethlehem, Stinging Nettle, Sturt Desert Pea, Waratah, Wedding Bush, Wild Rose, Yerba Santa

helpless

Angelica, Cerato, Chestnut Bud, Fairy Lantern, Forget-Me-Not, Glassy Hyacinth, Iris, Hound's Tongue, Larch, Love-Lies-Bleeding, Mariposa Lily, Milkweed,

Mountain Forget-Me-Not, Mountain Pride, Penstemon, Red Grevillea, Rescue Remedy, Self-Heal, Sweet Chestnut, Wallflower, Waratah, Wild Rose

hesitant

Angelica, Angelsword, Angel's Trumpet, Blazing Star, Cerato, Coffee, Fairy Lantern, Fawn Lily, Forget-Me-Not, Larch, Mimulus, Mountain Forget-Me-Not, Mountain Pride, Mullein, Paw Paw, Pomegranate, Purple Monkeyflower, Red Grevillea, Red Penstemon, Scleranthus, Self-Heal, Shasta Daisy, Silver Princess, Tall Mountain Larkspur, Tansy, Violet, Wild Oat, Wedding Bush

hopeless

Baby Blue Eyes, Borage, Explorer's Gentian, Glassy Hyacinth, Gentian, Gorse, Honeysuckle, Iris, Mustard, Pansy, Petunia, Rescue Remedy, Scotch Broom, Sturt Desert Pea, Sweet Chestnut, Waratah, Wild Oat, Wild Rose

hostile *(see also aggressive and angry/annoyed)*

Baby Blue Eyes, Calendula, Flannel Flower, Hawthorn, Holly, Impatiens, Mallow, Ocotillo, Oregon Grape, Poison Oak, Prickly Pear Cactus, Quince, Saguaro, Snapdragon, Star Thistle, Stinging Nettle, Sunflower, Tiger Lily, Trillium, Turk's Cap, Vervain, Vine, Willow

hysterical

Bunchberry, Californian Valerian, Canyon Dudleya, Chamomile, Cherry Plum, Cosmos, Crowea, Daffodil, Fuchsia, Impatiens, Indian Pink, Lavender Yarrow, Monkshood, Mugwort, Nectarine, Orange, Purple Monkeyflower, Red Clover, Rock Rose, Rescue Remedy, Rue, Snapdragon, Star of Bethlehem.

impatient *(see also irritable)*

Baby Blue Eyes, Beech, Calendula, Californian Valerian, Chamomile, Cherry Plum, Cosmos, Crowea, Dandelion, Dogwood, Fuchsia, Hawthorn, Holly, Jacaranda, Impatiens, Indian Pink, Lotus, Orange, Quaking Grass, Quince, Snapdragon, Stinging Nettle, Tiger Lily, Water Violet

inadequate *(see also confidence and self-esteem)*

Blazing Star, Bottlebrush, Buttercup, Calla Lily, Cerato, Centaury, Cherry, Corn Lily, Elm, Cosmos, Evening Primrose, Fairy Lantern, Fawn Lily, Green Cross Gentian, Hyssop, Kangaroo Paw, Larch, Mountain Pride, Onion, Penstemon, Pine, Pretty Face, Red Grevillea, Red Larkspur, Red Penstemon, Redwood, Scleranthus, Sunflower, Self-Heal, Tansy, Trumpet Vine, Violet, Wallflower

indecisive

Angelsword, Bottlebrush, Bunchberry, Californian Poppy, Cayenne, Cerato, Clematis, Coffee, Foxglove, Iris, Jacaranda, Larch, Madia, Mullein, Onion, Paw Paw, Quince, Red Grevillea, Scleranthus, Shasta Daisy, Silver Princess, Sundew, Tansy, Walnut, Wedding Bush, Wild Oat, Wild Potato Bush

inflexible

Baby Blue Eyes, Bottlebrush, Dogwood, Kangaroo Paw, Hibbertia, Lilac, Lotus, Mallow, Morning Glory, Nicotiana, Oak, Quaking Grass, Quince, Rock Water, Vine, Walnut, Willow, Zinnia

influenced (too easily) *(see also boundaries)*

Angelsword, Blazing Star, Boab, Bottlebrush, Californian Poppy, Canyon Dudleya, Centaury, Cerato, Corn, Fringed Violet, Garlic, Goldenrod, Joshua Tree, Hyssop, Indian Pink, Larkspur, Mountain Pennyroyal, Pink Yarrow (and all the Yarrows), Red Clover, Red Grevillea, Rue, Walnut, YES formula

insecure *(see also protection and vulnerable)*

Agrimony, Angelica, Aspen, Blazing Star, Buttercup, Echinacea, Garlic, Golden Yarrow, Kangaroo Paw, Larch, Mallow, Mimulus, Monkshood, Mullein, Oregon Grape, Pink Monkeyflower, Pretty Face, Purple Monkeyflower, Red Clover, Rock Rose, St John's Wort, Self-Heal, Star Thistle, Sticky Monkeyflower, Sunflower, Violet, Wallflower, Waratah, YES formula

intolerant

Baby Blue Eyes, Beech, Bottlebrush, Calendula, Chamomile, Crab Apple, Hawthorn, Hibbertia, Impatiens, Indian Pink, Hibbertia, Holly, Lotus, Love-Lies-Bleeding, Quaking Grass, Quince, Rock Water, Saguaro, Snapdragon, Vine, Water Violet, Yellow Star Tulip

irritable *(see also angry/annoyed and impatient)*

Almond, Beech, Black Eyed Susan, Californian Poppy, Chamomile, Crab Apple, Crowea, Dogwood, Filaree, Fuchsia, Hawthorn, Holly, Impatiens, Indian Pink, Lavender, Ocotillo, Orange, Poison Oak, Prickly Pear Cactus, Scarlet Monkeyflower, Snapdragon, Stinging Nettle, Tiger Lily, Turk's Cap, Walnut, Willow, YES formula

jealous *(see also envious)*

Boab, Bottlebrush, Buttercup, Chicory, Goldenrod, Holly, Pretty Face, Sunflower, Tiger Lily, Trillium, Walnut

joyless *(see also blue, depressed, gloomy, sad)*

Baby Blue Eyes, Bleeding Heart, Borage, Crowea, Explorer's Gentian, Gentian, Golden Ear Drops, Gorse, Harvest Brodiaea, Hibbertia, Hornbeam, Hound's Tongue, Hyssop, Iris, Mustard, Pansy, Petunia, Scotch Broom, Silver Princess, Sturt Desert Pea, Waratah, Wild Oat, Wild Potato Bush, Wild Rose, Willow, Zinnia

lethargic *(see also apathetic, listless)*

Aloe Vera, Blackberry, Californian Peony, Californian Pitcher Plant, Cayenne, Clematis, Coffee, Explorer's Gentian, Foxglove, Hornbeam, Hound's Tongue, Indian Paintbrush, Iris, Lemon, Macrocarpa, Madia, Nasturtium, Olive, Pansy, Peppermint, Red Larkspur, Red Lily, Rosemary, Silver Princess, Sundew, Tansy, Wild Potato Bush, Wild Rose

listless *(see also apathetic, lethargic)*

Californian Peony, Californian Pitcher Plant, Cayenne, Clematis, Coffee, Explorer's Gentian, Foxglove, Hornbeam, Indian Paintbrush, Iris, Lemon, Macrocarpa, Olive, Pansy, Peppermint, Red Larkspur, Red Lily, Rosemary, Silver Princess, Sundew, Wild Potato Bush, Wild Oat, Wild Rose

lonely

Angelica, Baby Blue Eyes, Bleeding Heart, Evening Primrose, Fawn Lily, Forget-Me-Not, Heather, Honeysuckle, Lilac, Lotus, Love-Lies-Bleeding, Mallow, Mariposa Lily, Milkweed, Mountain Forget-Me-Not, Red Lily, Shooting Star, Sturt Desert Pea, Sweet Pea, Sweet Chestnut, Tall Yellow Top, Violet, Wallflower, Waratah, Water Violet

miserable *(see also joyless)*

Baby Blue Eyes, Bleeding Heart, Borage, Explorer's Gentian, Gentian, Gorse, Harvest Brodiaea, Hibbertia, Hound's Tongue, Hyssop, Iris, Mustard, Pansy, Petunia, Scotch Broom, Silver Princess, Sturt Desert Pea, Sweet Chestnut, Waratah, Wild Potato Bush, Wild Rose, Willow, Zinnia

misunderstood *(see also communication)*

Angelsword, Calendula, Columbine, Cosmos, Deerbrush, Goldenrod, Green Cross Gentian, Kangaroo Paw, Larch, Larkspur, Lemon, Lotus, Mallow, Mullein, Pink Monkeyflower, Quince, Red Lily, Saguaro, Shooting Star, Snapdragon, Sundew, Tall Yellow Top, Trumpet Vine, Violet, Water Violet

negative

Baby Blue Eyes, Beech, Blazing Star, Borage, Chicory, Corn Lily, Crowea, Explorer's Gentian, Gentian, Gorse, Holly, Honeysuckle, Hyssop, Larch, Lilac, Nectarine, Oregon Grape, Pansy, Petunia, Red Larkspur, Red Penstemon, Scotch Broom, Silver Princess, Snapdragon, Sturt Desert Pea, Tansy, Waratah, Wild Potato Bush, Wild Rose, Willow, Zinnia

nervous

Alpine Aster, Angelica, Angelsword, Aspen, Borage, Bottlebrush, Californian Valerian, Chamomile, Cherry Plum, Cosmos, Crowea, Elm, Garlic, Golden Yarrow, Hawthorn, Impatiens, Indian Pink, Kangaroo Paw, Larch, Lavender, Mallow, Mimulus, Monkshood, Morning Glory, Oregon Grape, Purple Monkeyflower, Red Chestnut, Red Clover, Red Penstemon, Rescue Remedy, Rock Rose, St John's Wort, Vervain, Violet, Waratah, YES formula

nostalgic

Bottlebrush, Chrysanthemum, Corn Lily, Fairy Lantern, Forget-Me-Not, Honeysuckle, Jasmine, Pretty Face, Walnut

obsessed

Angelsword, Billy Goat Plum, Californian Poppy, Californian Valerian, Canyon Dudleya, Cherry Plum, Crab Apple, Crowea, Dandelion, Filaree, Hawthorn, Heather, Hibbertia, Lilac, Manzanita, Nectarine, Opium Poppy, Pennyroyal, Petunia, Pretty Face, Purple Monkeyflower, Red Chestnut, Rock Water, Thyme, Vervain, White Chestnut

overwhelmed

Bottlebrush, Canyon Dudleya, Chamomile, Chaparral, Cherry Plum, Corn, Cosmos, Crowea, Dill, Elm, Filaree, Golden Yarrow, Harvest Brodiaea, Hornbeam, Indian Pink, Larkspur, Lavender, Nectarine, Paw Paw, Pink Yarrow, Rabbitbrush, Red Clover, Rue, Shasta Daisy, Walnut, YES formula

panicky *(see hysterical, overwhelmed, paranoid, terrified)*

Aspen, Bottlebrush, Californian Valerian, Chamomile, Cherry Plum, Cosmos, Crowea, Echinacea, Garlic, Glassy Hyacinth, Impatiens, Indian Pink, Lavender, Monkshood, Nectarine, Orange, Purple Monkeyflower, Red Clover, Rescue Remedy, Rock Rose, Rue, Star of Bethlehem, Sweet Chestnut, Waratah

paranoid *(see also fearful, hysterical, panicky)*

Angelsword, Aspen, Californian Valerian, Chamomile, Cherry Plum, Crowea, Fringed Violet, Glassy Hyacinth, Indian Pink, Lavender, Lilac, Monkshood, Nectarine, Oregon Grape, Purple Monkeyflower, Red Clover, Rock Rose, Rue, Star of Bethlehem, Sweet Chestnut, Waratah, YES formula

pessimistic

Baby Blue Eyes, Blazing Star, Bleeding Heart, Borage, Corn Lily, Explorer's Gentian, Gentian, Gorse, Green Cross Gentian, Honeysuckle, Hyssop, Lilac, Love-Lies-Bleeding, Nasturtium, Pansy, Petunia, Penstemon, Red Larkspur, Red Penstemon, Scotch Broom, Sturt Desert Pea, Sweet Chestnut, Tansy, Waratah, Wild Potato Bush, Wild Rose, Willow, Zinnia

possessive

Bleeding Heart, Bottlebrush, Chicory, Chrysanthemum, Holly, Quaking Grass, Star Thistle, Tiger Lily, Trillium, Walnut

pride (excessive)

Hibbertia, Lotus, Red Lily, Sunflower, Water Violet

rebellious

Almond, Goldenrod, Petunia, Saguaro, Sunflower, Tiger Lily, Water Violet

rejected *(see also abandoned, alone, unloved)*

Angelica, Baby Blue Eyes, Billy Goat Plum, Bleeding Heart, Buttercup, Cherry, Chicory, Crab Apple, Dogwood, Evening Primrose, Forget-Me-Not, Goldenrod, Hyssop, Kangaroo Paw, Lilac, Mallow, Milkweed, Mountain Forget-Me-Not, Mariposa Lily, Petunia, Pretty Face, Shooting Star, Sturt Desert Pea, Sweet Pea, Tall Yellow Top, Violet, Water Violet

repressed

Agrimony, Almond, Angelsword, Aster Lily, Black Eyed Susan, Blazing Star, Bottlebrush, Calla Lily, Centaury, Cherry Plum, Cosmos, Dogwood, Easter Lily, Fairy Lantern, Foxglove, Fuchsia, Golden Ears Drops, Icelandic Poppy, Lady's Slipper, Lilac, Nicotiana, Oak, Pink Monkeyflower, Purple Monkeyflower, Red Grevillea, Rock Water, Scarlet Monkeyflower, Snapdragon, Sticky Monkeyflower, Sturt Desert Pea, Tansy, Willow, Yerba Santa

THE **ESSENTIAL** FLOWER ESSENCE BOOK

resentment

Almond, Baby Blue Eyes, Bottlebrush, Chicory, Dogwood, Holly, Larkspur, Red Grevillea, Walnut, Willow

responsible (overly-) *(see also burdened)*

Boab, Borage, Bottlebrush, Centaury, Chicory, Crowea, Elm, Green Cross Gentian, Hornbeam, Hyssop, Joshua Tree, Larkspur, Love-Lies-Bleeding, Oak, Pine, Red Chestnut, Rock Water, Sturt Desert Pea, Walnut

restless

Almond, Bunchberry, Californian Poppy, Canyon Dudleya, Cerato, Corn, Crowea, Dill, Impatiens, Jacaranda, Lavender, Madia, Morning Glory, Onion, Rabbitbrush, Red Grevillea, Red Lily, Sagebrush, Scleranthus, Shasta Daisy, Shooting Star, Sweet Pea, Silver Princess, Tall Yellow Top, Walnut, Wedding Bush, White Chestnut, Wild Oat, YES formula

sad *(see also blue, gloomy and depressed)*

Baby Blue Eyes, Bleeding Heart, Borage, Corn Lily, Explorer's Gentian, Gentian, Glassy Hyacinth, Golden Ear Drops, Gorse, Green Cross Gentian, Harvest Brodiaea, Honeysuckle, Hound's Tongue, Hyssop, Iris, Lilac, Love-Lies-Bleeding, Mustard, Pansy, Petunia, Pine, Scotch Broom, Sturt Desert Pea, Sweet Chestnut, Waratah, Wild Rose, Willow, Yerba Santa

scattered *(see also concentration, distracted, erratic and focus)*

Blackberry, Bunchberry, Cerato, Chamomile, Clematis, Corn, Crowea, Dill, Echinacea, Filaree, Fringed Violet, Indian Pink, Jacaranda, Madia, Morning Glory, Rabbitbrush, Red Lily, Rescue Remedy, Rue, Scleranthus, Shasta Daisy, Silver Princess, Sundew, Sweet Pea, Wild Oat, YES formula

self-absorbed

Billy Goat Plum, Bottlebrush, Chicory, Clematis, Crab Apple, Crowea, Fawn Lily, Harvest Brodiaea, Heather, Hibbertia, Hound's Tongue, Kangaroo Paw, Lotus, Love-Lies-Bleeding, Red Lily, Sundew, Sunflower, Tall Yellow Top, Violet, Willow, Yellow Star Tulip, Zinnia

self-pity *(see also victim)*

Almond, Baby Blue Eyes, Boab, Cherry, Chicory, Dogwood, Evening Primrose, Hyssop, Iris, Joshua Tree, Love-Lies-Bleeding, Red Grevillea, Sage, Saguaro, Sturt Desert Pea, Willow

selfish

Bleeding Heart, Chicory, Heather, Hibbertia, Holly, Lilac, Lotus, Milkweed, Quaking Grass, Self-Heal, Star Thistle, Sunflower, Tall Yellow Top, Tiger Lily, Trillium, Water Violet, Wedding Bush

sensitive (over-) *(see also boundaries and protection)*

Angelica, Aspen, Beech, Calendula, Canyon Dudleya, Cherry, Chamomile, Fringed Violet, Garlic, Golden Yarrow, Indian Pink, Icelandic Poppy, Kangaroo Paw, Larch, Lavender, Lavender Yarrow, Mallow, Mimulus, Monkshood, Mountain Pennyroyal, Mugwort, Mullein, Nicotiana, Oregon Grape, Pennyroyal, Pink Monkeyflower, Pink Yarrow, Poison Oak, Purple Monkeyflower, Pretty Face, Prickly Pear Cactus, Queen Anne's Lace, Red Clover, Red Grevillea, Rue, St John's Wort, Self-Heal, Star Thistle, Sticky Monkeyflower, Stinging Nettle, Wallflower, Walnut, Yarrow, YES formula

serious (over-)

Borage, Californian Poppy, Canyon Dudleya, Corn Lily, Crab Apple, Dandelion, Explorer's Gentian, Flannel Flower, Green Cross Gentian, Harvest Brodiaea, Hawthorn, Hibbertia, Hornbeam, Hound's Tongue, Hyssop, Iris, Kangaroo Paw, Lemon, Nasturtium, Pansy, Petunia, Quince, Sage, Vervain, Wild Potato Bush, Zinnia

shame

Agrimony, Alpine Lily, Basil, Billy Goat Plum, Buttercup, Cherry, Chocolate Lily, Corn Lily, Crab Apple, Easter Lily, Flannel Flower, Green Cross Gentian, Hyssop, Manzanita, Mullein, Pine, Pink Monkeyflower, Pretty Face, Redbud, Sticky Monkeyflower, Sturt Desert Pea

shock *(see also trauma)*

Angelica, Angel's Trumpet, Arnica, Blazing Star, Cherry Plum, Clematis, Crowea, Echinacea, Fringed Violet, Glassy Hyacinth, Golden Ear Drops, Lavender, Monkshood, Nectarine, Rescue Remedy, Rock Rose, Rue, St John's Wort, Self-Heal, Star of Bethlehem, Sundew, Sweet Chestnut, Waratah, YES formula

shy *(see also timid)*

Billy Goat Plum, Blazing Star, Buttercup, Calla Lily, Cherry, Columbine, Fairy Lantern, Fawn Lily, Flannel Flower, Garlic, Kangaroo Paw, Larch, Mallow, Mimulus, Mountain Pride, Penstemon, Pretty Face, Trumpet Vine, Violet, Wallflower, Water Violet

sluggish

Blackberry, Cayenne, Fireweed, Hornbeam, Honeysuckle, Hound's Tongue, Indian Paintbrush, Iris, Macrocarpa, Madia, Morning Glory, Nasturtium, Red Grevillea, Silver Princess, Tansy, Waratah, Wild Potato Bush, Wild Rose

sorrow *(see grief, heart-broken, sad)*

Bleeding Heart, Borage, Bottle Brush, Evening Primrose, Forget-Me-Not, Glassy Hyacinth, Golden Ear Drops, Gorse, Honeysuckle, Hyssop, Jasmine, Lilac, Love-Lies-Bleeding, Mustard, Rescue Remedy, Star of Bethlehem, Sturt Desert Pea, Sweet Chestnut, Waratah, Wild Rose, Yerba Santa

stress *(see also overwhelm and tension)*

Aloe Vera, Bottlebrush, Bunchberry, Californian Valerian, Cassandra, Chamomile, Cherry Plum, Corn, Crab Apple, Crowea, Dandelion, Dill, Elm, Filaree, Hawthorn, Impatiens, Indian Paintbrush, Indian Pink, Jacaranda, Lavender, Nectarine, Opium Poppy, Orange, Paw Paw, Vervain, Rescue Remedy, Shasta Daisy, Walnut, Waratah, White Chestnut, YES formula, Zinnia

stuck

Almond, Angel's Trumpet, Blackberry, Boab, Bottlebrush, Cayenne, Cerato, Explorer's Gentian, Fairy Lantern, Forget-Me-Not, Indian Paintbrush, Iris, Joshua Tree, Morning Glory, Onion, Red Grevillea, Red Penstemon, Redwood, Sagebrush, Silver Princess, Tansy, Walnut, Watermelon, Wedding Bush, Wild Oat, Wild Potato Bush, Wild Rose

tension

Bottlebrush, Chamomile, Cherry Plum, Crab Apple, Crowea, Dandelion, Dogwood, Hawthorn, Impatiens, Indian Pink, Lavender, Orange, Passionflower, Rescue Remedy, Snapdragon, Vervain, Yerba Santa, Zinnia

terrified *(see also afraid, apprehensive and fearful)*

Aspen, Borage, Cherry Plum, Fringed Violet, Garlic, Glassy Hyacinth, Monkshood, Oregon Grape, Purple Monkeyflower, Red Clover, Rescue Remedy, Rock Rose, St John's Wort, Star of Bethlehem, Waratah

timid *(see also shy)*

Angelsword, Blazing Star, Buttercup, Calla Lily, Cherry, Columbine, Fairy Lantern, Fawn Lily, Fairy Lantern, Garlic, Icelandic Poppy, Kangaroo Paw, Larch, Mimulus, Mountain Pride, Penstemon, Pretty Face, Purple Monkeyflower, Red

Grevillea, Red Penstemon, Sunflower, Violet, Wallflower, Waratah, YES formula

tired *(see also exhausted and fatigued)*

Aloe Vera, Blackberry, Californian Peony, Cayenne, Coffee, Fireweed, Forget-Me-Not, Hornbeam, Lady's Slipper, Lemon, Macrocarpa, Madia, Morning Glory, Nasturtium, Olive, Peppermint, Red Larkspur, Silver Princess, Tansy, Wild Potato Bush, Wild Rose

trauma *(see also shock)*

Angelica, Angel's Trumpet, Arnica, Californian Valerian, Cherry Plum, Crowea, Echinacea, Fringed Violet, Glassy Hyacinth, Golden Ear Drops, Lavender, Lilac, Monkshood, Nectarine, Redwood, Rescue Remedy, Rock Rose, Rue, St John's Wort, Self-Heal, Star of Bethlehem, Sturt Desert Pea, Sweet Chestnut, Waratah, YES formula

unloved *(see also abandoned, alone and rejected)*

Angelica, Baby Blue Eyes, Billy Goat Plum, Bleeding Heart, Buttercup, Cherry, Chicory, Crab Apple, Evening Primrose, Forget-Me-Not, Goldenrod, Lilac, Mallow, Milkweed, Mountain Forget-Me-Not, Mariposa Lily, Pretty Face, Shooting Star, Sturt Desert Pea, Sweet Pea, Tall Yellow Top

vague *(see also day-dreamy)*

Angelsword, Blackberry, Bunchberry, Cayenne, Clematis, Corn, Cosmos, Deerbrush, Honeysuckle, Lotus, Madia, Morning Glory, Mugwort, Nicotiana, Peppermint, Rabbitbrush, Red Lily, Rosemary, Shasta Daisy, Shooting Star, Sundew, Wild Oat, Wild Rose

victim *(see also self-pity)*

Almond, Blazing Star, Boab, Borage, Bottlebrush, Cherry, Chicory, Dogwood, Evening Primrose, Heather, Hyssop, Iris, Joshua Tree, Love-Lies-Bleeding, Ocotillo, Pansy, Petunia, Red Grevillea, Sage, Saguaro, Self-Heal, Sturt Desert Pea, Willow

vulnerable *(see also insecure and protection)*

Alpine Aster , Angelica, Arnica, Aspen, Cotton, Daffodil, Echinacea, Forget-Me-Not, Fringed Violet, Garlic, Golden Yarrow, Icelandic Poppy, Indian Pink, Kangaroo Paw, Larch, Mallow, Mimulus, Monkshood, Mullein, Oregon Grape, Purple Monkeyflower, Red Clover, Redwood, Rock Rose, Rue, St John's Wort, Self-Heal, Star Thistle, Sticky Monkeyflower, Sunflower, Violet, Wallflower, Waratah, Yarrow, YES formula

weary *(see also exhausted, fatigued and tired)*

Aloe Vera, Blackberry, Californian Peony, Cayenne, Coffee, Explorer's Gentian, Fireweed, Forget-Me-Not, Hornbeam, Iris, Lady's Slipper, Lemon, Macrocarpa, Morning Glory, Nasturtium, Olive, Peppermint, Red Larkspur, Silver Princess, Wild Potato Bush, Wild Rose

worried *(see also anxious, nervous, tense)*

Agrimony, Cassandra, Chaparral, Chicory, Crab Apple, Crowea, Elm, Filaree, Harvest Brodiaea, Hound's Tongue, Lavender, Pansy, Paw Paw, Pear, Pennyroyal, Red Chestnut, Shasta Daisy, White Chestnut, Zinnia

worthless

Billy Goat Plum, Buttercup, Centaury, Crab Apple, Hyssop, Kangaroo Paw, Larch, Mallow, Pine, Pretty Face, Quince, Sage, Self-Heal, Silver Princess, Sunflower, Violet, Wallflower, Watermelon, Wild Rose, Wild Oat

Flower essences for your life situation, aspirations or stage of development

abundance

Blackberry, Bleeding Heart, Bottlebrush, Buttercup, Cherry Plum, Chrysanthemum, Chicory, Crowea, Foxglove, Milkweed, Nectarine, Oak, Opium Poppy, Quaking Grass, Rock Water, Silver Princess, Squash, Star Thistle, Sunflower, Tansy, Tiger Lily, Trillium, Vine, Wallflower, Watermelon, Wild Oat, Willow

adolescence

Almond, Alpine Lily, Baby Blue Eyes, Billy Goat Plum, Bottlebrush, Calla Lily, Cherry, Crab Apple, Fairy Lantern, Flannel Flower, Goldenrod, Kangaroo Paw, Larch, Manzanita, Pomegranate, Pretty Face, Red Grevillea, Saguaro, Sticky Monkeyflower, Sunflower, Turk's Cap, Walnut, Wild Oat, Wild Rose

addiction

Agrimony, Boab, Bottlebrush, Californian Poppy, Californian Valerian, Canyon Dudleya, Cayenne, Chestnut Bud, Coffee, Cotton, Golden Yarrow, Iris, Joshua Tree, Lavender, Milkweed, Morning Glory, Nicotiana, Opium Poppy, Pansy, Petunia, Red Grevillea, Sagebrush, Self-Heal, Walnut, YES

ageing

Angel's Trumpet, Angelica, Bottlebrush, Chrysanthemum, Corn Lily, Dogwood, Explorer's Gentian, Fairy Lantern, Forget-Me-Not, Gorse, Oak, Honeysuckle, Jasmine, Pretty Face, Redbud, Redwood, Rosemary, Sage, Star Tulip, Walnut

ambition

Almond, Aloe Vera, Angelsword, Californian Poppy, Chrysanthemum, Dandelion, Forget-Me-Not, Foxglove, Green Cross Gentian, Hawthorn, Indian Paintbrush, Larkspur, Lotus, Quaking Grass, Red Lily, Silver Princess, Sunflower, Tiger Lily, Trillium, Wedding Bush, Vine, Wild Oat, Zinnia

attachment

Angel's Trumpet, Bleeding Heart, Boab, Bottlebrush, Canyon Dudleya, Chestnut Bud, Chicory, Fairy Lantern, Fringed Violet, Honeysuckle, Jasmine, Joshua Tree, Lady's Slipper, Lavender, Milkweed, Morning Glory, Pansy, Petunia, Pink Yarrow, Red Chestnut, Red Grevillea, Sagebrush, Trillium, Walnut, YES

authority

Almond, Baby Blue Eyes, Centaury, Cerato, Chestnut Bud, Fairy Lantern, Forget-Me-Not, Mountain Forget-Me-Not, Goldenrod, Petunia, Purple Monkeyflower, Red Grevillea, Sage, Saguaro, Sunflower, Tall Mountain Larkspur, Tiger Lily, Turk's Cap, Vine

birth

Angel's Trumpet, Bottlebrush, Chrysanthemum, Manzanita, Rescue Remedy, Walnut, Watermelon

body image

Alpine Lily, Billy Goat Plum, Cherry, Chocolate Lily, Corn Lily, Crab Apple, Fairy Lantern, Lady's Mantle, Love-Lies-Bleeding, Manzanita, Pansy, Pomegranate, Pretty Face, Redwood, Self-Heal

boundaries (see also protection, sensitive (over), vulnerable)

Angelica, Aspen, Beech, Boab, Bottlebrush, Bunchberry, Calendula, Canyon Dudleya, Centaury, Cosmos, Flannel Flower, Fringed Violet, Garlic, Golden Yarrow, Indian Pink, Joshua Tree, Lavender, Lavender Yarrow, Mountain Pennyroyal, Mugwort, Mulla Mulla, Oregon Grape, Pennyroyal, Pink Monkeyflower, Pink Yarrow, Poison Oak, Opium Poppy, Prickly Pear Cactus, Queen Anne's Lace, Red Clover, Red

Grevillea, Rue, St John's Wort, Star Thistle, Sticky Monkeyflower, Stinging Nettle, Wallflower, Walnut, Yarrow, YES

challenge

Angelsword, Blackberry, Blazing Star, Borage, Cayenne, Elm, Gentian, Gorse, Larch, Mountain Pride, Penstemon, Red Penstemon, Scotch Broom, Waratah, Wild Rose

change *(see also transition)*

Angel's Trumpet, Aspen, Boab, Bottlebrush, Cherry Plum, Chrysanthemum, Cotton, Daffodil, Forget-Me-Not, Iris, Joshua Tree, Morning Glory, Nectarine, Sagebrush, Walnut

channelling

Alpine Aster, Angelica, Angel's Trumpet, Angelsword, Cassandra, Clematis, Deerbrush, Filaree, Forget-Me-Not, Garlic, Mountain Forget-Me-Not,, Lavender Yarrow, Monkshood, Mountain Pennyroyal, Mugwort, Pear, Pennyroyal, Peppermint, Purple Monkeyflower, Queen Anne's Lace, Rosemary, St John's Wort, Star Tulip, Sundew, Thyme

city living

Cherry Plum, Clematis, Corn, Dill, Echinacea, Impatiens, Indian Pink, Madia, Morning Glory, Nectarine, Nicotiana, Opium Poppy, Peppermint, Rabbitbrush, Red Clover, Red Lily, Rosemary, Shasta Daisy, Shooting Star, Silver Princess, Sundew, Sweet Pea, Thyme, all the Yarrows, Tall Yellow Top, YES formula, Wild Oat

cleansing

Agrimony, Almond, Billy Goat Plum, Bottlebrush, Chaparral, Cherry, Chocolate Lily, Crab Apple, Easter Lily, Fireweed, Morning Glory, Red Grevillea, Sagebrush, Self-Heal, Yerba Santa

co-dependency

Almond, Black Cohosh, Blazing Star, Bleeding Heart, Boab, Bottlebrush, Centaury, Cerato, Chestnut Bud, Chicory, Elm, Fairy Lantern, Joshua Tree, Milkweed, Pine, Pink Yarrow, Red Chestnut, Red Grevillea, Tansy, Walnut, YES formula

communication *(see also misunderstood)*

Almond, Angelica, Angelsword, Blazing Star, Buttercup, Calendula, Cerato, Columbine, Cosmos, Deerbrush, Fawn Lily, Forget-Me-Not, Goldenrod, Green Cross

Gentian, Larch, Lemon, Lotus, Mallow, Mountain Forget-Me-Not, Mullein, Pink Monkeyflower, Queen Anne's Lace, Red Lily, Shooting Star, Snapdragon, Trumpet Vine, Violet, Wallflower, Water Violet

confidence *(see also doubtful)*

Angelsword, Aspen, Blazing Star, Buttercup, Calla Lily, Cerato, Centaury, Cosmos, Crowea, Elm, Explorer's Gentian, Fairy Lantern, Fawn Lily, Garlic, Gentian, Gorse, Kangaroo Paw, Larch, Mimulus, Mountain Pride, Onion, Pansy, Penstemon, Pretty Face, Red Grevillea, Red Penstemon, St John's Wort, Scleranthus, Scotch Broom, Silver Princess, Sunflower, Self-Heal, Tansy, Trumpet Vine, Violet, Wallflower, Watermelon, Wild Oat

competitiveness

Almond, Angelsword, Blazing Star, Chicory, Dandelion, Hawthorn, Impatiens, Mountain Pride, Ocotillo, Penstemon, Poison Oak, Prickly Pear Cactus, Tiger Lily, Trillium, Turk's Cap, Vervain, Vine

concentration *(see also distracted and focus)*

Blackberry, Bunchberry, Californian Poppy, Canyon Dudleya, Cassandra, Cayenne, Clematis, Coffee, Corn, Forget-Me-Not, Honeysuckle, Jacaranda, Lemon, Madia, Morning Glory, Mugwort, Nicotiana, Peppermint, Rabbitbrush, Red Lily, Rosemary, Shasta Daisy, Shooting Star, Sundew, White Chestnut, Wild Oat, Wild Rose

conflict

Almond, Calendula, Chicory, Holly, Impatiens, Indian Pink, Mountain Pride, Ocotillo, Oregon Grape, Penstemon, Poison Oak, Pomegranate, Prickly Pear Cactus, Quaking Grass, Quince, Red Grevillea, Saguaro, Sunflower, Tiger Lily, Trillium, Turk's Cap, Vine, Walnut, Wedding Bush

cooperation

Almond, Bottle Brush, Calendula, Chicory, Corn, Filaree, Holly, Impatiens, Ocotillo, Pomegranate, Quaking Grass, Quince, Saguaro, Stinging Nettle, Sunflower, Sweet Pea, Tiger Lily, Trillium, Turk's Cap, Vine, Walnut, Water Violet, Wedding Bush

cravings

Apricot, Bleeding Heart, Boab, Bottlebrush, Californian Poppy, Cherry Plum, Coffee, Crowea, Joshua Tree, Love-Lies-Bleeding, Morning Glory, Nectarine, Nicotiana, Opium Poppy, Petunia, Walnut

creativity

Aloe Vera, Angelsword, Blackberry, Bleeding Heart, Cayenne, Cosmos, Fawn Lily, Fig, Fireweed, Forget-Me-not, Hibbertia, Kangaroo Paw, Indian Paintbrush, Iris, Larch, Mugwort, Nasturtium, Pansy, Passionflower, Pear, Pomegranate, Queen Anne's Lace, Red Penstemon, Shasta Daisy, Silver Princess, Trumpet Vine, Watermelon, Wild Oat

cynicism

Baby Blue Eyes, Chrysanthemum, Gentian, Explorer's Gentian, Forget-Me-Not, Green Cross Gentian, Hibbertia, Hibiscus, Mountain Forget-Me-Not, Pear, Sage, Saguaro, Self-Heal, Tall Yellow Top, Wild Rose, Willow

death and dying

Alpine Aster, Angelica, Angel's Trumpet, Bottlebrush, Cherry Plum, Chrysanthemum, Forget-Me-Not, Garlic, Glassy Hyacinth, Love-Lies-Bleeding, Monkshood, Mugwort, Nectarine, Red Clover, Rescue Remedy, St John's Wort, Star of Bethlehem, Thyme, Walnut, Waratah

denial

Agrimony, Almond, Black Cohosh, Black Eyed Susan, Bottlebrush, Californian Poppy, Chestnut Bud, Chocolate Lily, Deerbrush, Fairy Lantern, Fuchsia, Impatiens, Lady's Slipper, Lilac, Lotus, Milkweed, Monkshood, Mullein, Nicotiana, Orange, Pink Monkeyflower, Pretty Face, Purple Monkeyflower, Queen Anne's Lace, Red Grevillea, Self-Heal, Star Tulip, Thyme

dreams

Alpine Aster, Angelsword, Angelica, Aspen, Chaparral, Forget-Me-Not, Fringed Violet, Garlic, Lavender, Lavender Yarrow, Mugwort, Passionflower, St John's Wort, Star Tulip, YES formula

eating disorders

Apricot, Billy Goat Plum, Bottlebrush, Californian Pitcher Plant, Chestnut Bud, Coffee, Crab Apple, Fairy Lantern, Manzanita, Morning Glory, Nicotiana, Pretty Face, Rock Water, Tansy, Walnut, Wild Potato Bush

emergency

Angel's Trumpet, Angelica, Arnica, Cherry Plum, Crowea, Echinacea, Glassy Hyacinth, Indian Pink, Monkshood, Nectarine, Red Clover, Rescue Remedy, Rock Rose, Rue, St John's Wort, Star of Bethlehem, Sweet Chestnut, Waratah, Yarrow, YES formula

empathy

Baby Blue Eyes, Bleeding Heart, Calendula, Evening Primrose, Fawn Lily, Fringed Violet, Heather, Hibbertia, Hibiscus, Impatiens, Kangaroo Paw, Lotus, Love-Lies-Bleeding, Ocotillo, Pear, Petunia, Prickly Pear Cactus, Shooting Star, Star Tulip, Thyme, Violet, Water Violet, all the Yarrows, Yellow Star Tulip, YES formula

escapism *(see also denial)*

Agrimony, Black Cohosh, Black Eyed Susan, Bottlebrush, Californian Poppy, Canyon Dudleya, Chestnut Bud, Clematis Coffee, Fairy Lantern, Hibbertia, Honeysuckle, Impatiens, Lady's Slipper, Lilac, Lotus, Milkweed, Morning Glory, Nicotiana, Pretty Face, Queen Anne's Lace, Red Grevillea, Shooting Star, Star Tulip, Sundew, Sweet Pea, Tall Yellow Top, Thyme

faith *(see also trust)*

Angelica, Aspen, Baby Blue Eyes, Borage, Cherry Plum, Chrysanthemum, Explorer's Gentian, Forget-Me-Not, Garlic, Gentian, Glassy Hyacinth, Gorse, Green Cross Gentian, Hibiscus, Monkshood, Nectarine, Pink Monkeyflower, Sage, Scotch Broom, Self-Heal, Sweet Chestnut, Waratah

father and fathering

Agrimony, Baby Blue Eyes, Elm, Fairy Lantern, Flannel Flower, Kangaroo Paw, Pomegranate, Quince, Red Chestnut, Sage, Saguaro, Squash (Zucchini), Sunflower, Tiger Lily, Trillium, Vine, Zinnia

focus *(see also concentration and distracted)*

Blackberry, Bunchberry, Californian Poppy, Canyon Dudleya, Cassandra, Cayenne, Clematis, Coffee, Corn, Cotton, Forget-Me-Not, Honeysuckle, Jacaranda, Lemon, Madia, Morning Glory, Nicotiana, Peppermint, Rabbitbrush, Red Lily, Rosemary, Scleranthus, Shasta Daisy, Shooting Star, Sundew, White Chestnut, Wild Oat, Wild Rose

forgiveness

Almond, Baby Blue Eyes, Bottlebrush, Dogwood, Golden Ear Drops, Hibiscus, Holly, Hyssop, Pine, Stinging Nettle, Sturt Desert Pea, Walnut, Willow

groundedness

Blackberry, Bunchberry, Californian Poppy, Californian Pitcher Plant, Canyon Dudleya, Clematis, Corn, Crowea, Dill, Echinacea, Fawn Lily, Indian Pink, Lady's Slipper, Lilac, Lotus, Manzanita, Queen Anne's Lace, Red Lily, Rosemary,

Shooting Star, Sundew, Sweet Pea, Tall Yellow Top, Waratah, Water Lily, Wild Oat, Wild Rose, YES formula

higher Self

Alpine Aster, Angelica, Angel's Trumpet, Angelsword, Californian Poppy, Cerato, Chrysanthemum, Clematis, Crowea, Daffodil, Deerbrush, Fawn Lily, Filaree, Forget-Me-Not, Harvest Brodiaea, Hibbertia, Lilac, Lotus, Mountain Forget-Me-Not, Foxglove, Lavender Yarrow, Mugwort, Paw Paw, Peppermint, Purple Monkeyflower, Queen Anne's Lace, Red Lily, Rosemary, Silver Princess, Star of Bethlehem, Sundew, Thyme, Wild Oat

idealism

Beech, Blackberry, Crowea, Clematis, Dandelion, Fawn Lily, Hawthorn, Hibbertia, Larkspur, Lilac, Lotus, Manzanita, Pine, Red Lily, Rock Water, Sundew, Vervain

immunity (natural) *(see also boundaries and protection)*

Arnica, Aspen, Crab Apple, Cotton, Daffodil, Echinacea, Fringed Violet, Garlic, Golden Yarrow, Lavender, Lavender Yarrow, Morning Glory, Mountain Pennyroyal, Olive, Pansy, Pennyroyal, Pink Yarrow, Nasturtium, Red Clover, Rue, Self-Heal, Violet, Walnut, Yarrow, YES formula

inner child

Baby Blue Eyes, Centaury, Evening Primrose, Flannel Flower, Golden Ear Drops, Hibiscus, Lady's Mantle, Lilac, Mariposa Lily, Milkweed, Pink Yarrow, Sunflower, Tansy, Zinnia

inspiration *(see also creativity & higher self)*

Aloe Vera, Angelsword, Blackberry, Bleeding Heart, Californian Poppy, Cayenne, Cerato, Collumbine, Cosmos, Explorer's Gentian, Fig, Fireweed, Forget-Me-not, Foxglove, Hound's Tongue, Indian Paintbrush, Iris, Mountain Forget-Me-Not, Lemon, Madia, Mugwort, Nasturtium, Onion, Pansy, Paw Paw, Pear, Pomegranate, Queen Anne's Lace, Red Grevillea, Shasta Daisy, Silver Princess, Star Tulip, Wild Oat, Wild Potato Bush, Wild Rose

insight

Angelica, Angelsword, Apricot, Black Eyed Susan, Californian Poppy, Cerato, Chestnut Bud, Chrysanthemum, Fuchsia, Harvest Brodiaea, Hound's Tongue, Mugwort, Orange, Queen Anne's Lace, Sage, Scarlet Monkeyflower, Shasta Daisy, Star Tulip

passion

Aloe Vera, Buttercup, Californian Peony, Californian Poppy, Explorer's Gentian, Fawn Lily, Fig, Forget-Me-Not, Foxglove, Hornbeam, Green Cross Gentian, Indian Paintbrush, Iris, Lady's Slipper, Madia, Mountain Forget-Me-Not, Onion, Passionflower, Red Larkspur, Shasta Daisy, Silver Princess, Tansy, Watermelon, Wedding Bush, Wild Oat, Wild Rose, Zinnia

perfectionism

Crab Apple, Crowea, Dandelion, Hawthorn, Pine, Pretty Face, Rock Water, Vervain

pregnancy

Bottle Brush, Fairy Lantern, Filaree, Manzanita, Mariposa Lily, Pomegranate, Quince, Red Lily, St John's Wort, Self-Heal, She Oak, Walnut, Watermelon

procrastination

Boab, Cayenne, Blackberry, Bottlebrush, Hornbeam, Lady's Slipper, Madia, Morning Glory, Red Grevillea, Tansy, Walnut

protection (see also boundaries and immunity)

Angelica, Aspen, Cotton, Daffodil, Echinacea, Fringed Violet, Garlic, Golden Yarrow, Icelandic Poppy, Lavender Yarrow, Monkshood, Mountain Pennyroyal, Pansy, Pennyroyal, Purple Monkeyflower, Pink Yarrow, Red Clover, St John's Wort, Violet, Wallflower, Waratah, Yarrow, YES formula

purification *(see also cleansing)*

Agrimony, Almond, Angel's Trumpet, Basil, Billy Goat Plum, Bottlebrush, Chaparral, Cherry, Chocolate Lily, Crab Apple, Easter Lily, Fireweed, Holly, Mulla Mulla, Morning Glory, Pink Monkeyflower, Sagebrush, Self-Heal, Yerba Santa

purpose *(see also motivation)*

Angelsword, Buttercup, Californian Poppy, Cerato, Clematis, Cosmos, Explorer's Gentian, Fawn Lily, Forget-Me-Not, Foxglove, Green Cross Gentian, Iris, Lady's Slipper, Love-Lies-Bleeding, Mountain Forget-Me-Not, Onion, Red Lily, Sage, Scotch Broom, Shasta Daisy, Shooting Star, Silver Princess, Sundew, Sweet Pea, Tall Yellow Top, Wedding Bush, Wild Oat, Wild Rose

psychic protection

Angelica, Fringed Violet, Garlic, Lavender Yarrow, Monkshood, Mountain

THE **ESSENTIAL** FLOWER ESSENCE BOOK

Pennyroyal, Pennyroyal, Pink Yarrow, Purple Monkeyflower, Red Clover, St John's Wort, Self-Heal, Sunflower, Wallflower, Walnut, Waratah, Yarrow, YES formula

release *(see letting go)*

Angel's Trumpet, Bleeding Heart, Boab, Bottlebrush, Cherry Plum, Dandelion, Dogwood, Golden Ear Drops, Honeysuckle, Jasmine, Joshua Tree, Nectarine, Poison Oak, Red Grevillea, Sagebrush, Stinging Nettle, Tiger Lily, Vervain, Walnut, Willow

self-expression *(see also creativity)*

Almond, Aloe Vera, Angelsword, Bleeding Heart, Blazing Star, Boab, Columbine, Cosmos, Fawn Lily, Fig, Fireweed, Forget-Me-not, Joshua Tree, Kangaroo Paw, Indian Paintbrush, Iris, Lady's Slipper, Larch, Monkshood, Mountain Forget-Me-Not, Nasturtium, Pansy, Pear, Pomegranate, Queen Anne's Lace, Red Grevillea, Red Penstemon, Redwood, Sagebrush, Silver Princess, Squash, Sunflower, Trumpet Vine, Violet, Watermelon, Wild Oat

service

Centuary, Cosmos, Forget-Me-Not, Larkspur, Lotus, Quaking Grass, Red Larkspur, Red Lily, Wedding Bush, Wild Oat

sexuality

Alpine Lily, Basil, Billy Goat Plum, Californian Peony, Calla lily, Chocolate Lily, Crab Apple, Easter Lily, Flannel Flower, Hibiscus, Mallow, Manzanita, Orange, Passionflower, Queen Anne's Lace, Snapdragon, Squash, Sticky Monkeyflower, Trillium

speaking (public)

Angelsword, Blazing Star, Cherry Plum, Columbine, Cosmos, Garlic, Kangaroo Paw, Larch, Lemon, Mimulus, Mountain Pennyroyal, Mountain Pride, Penstemon, Red Grevillea, Red Penstemon, Redwood, Rescue Remedy, Rock Rose, Sunflower, Trumpet Vine, Violet, Wallflower, Waratah

spiritual awakening

Angelica, Angel's Trumpet, Angelsword, Alpine Aster, Bottlebrush, Chrysanthemum, Cotton, Daffodil, Fringed Violet, Forget-Me-Not, Garlic, Glassy Hyacinth, Icelandic Poppy, Lavender Yarrow, Lotus, Love-Lies-Bleeding, Monkshood, Mountain Forget-Me-Not, Mountain Pennyroyal, Nicotiana, Pear, Pennyroyal, Purple Monkeyflower, Red Clover, Red Lily, St John's Wort, Self-Heal, Sturt Desert

spontaneity

Agrimony, Angelica, Angelsword, Black Eyed Susan, Boab, Bottlebrush, Cherry Plum, Crowea, Dogwood, Flannel Flower, Fuchsia, Hibbertia, Hibiscus, Oak, Mimulus (and all the Monkeyflowers), Nasturtium, Nectarine, Red Grevillea, Red Penstemon, Rock Water, Sagebrush, Snapdragon, Sturt Desert Pea, Tansy, Willow, Zinnia

strength

Angelsword, Blazing Star, Borage, Cherry Plum, Elm, Mountain Pride, Penstemon, Red Penstemon, Redwood, Sunflower, Waratah

study

Bunchberry, Chestnut Bud, Clematis, Cosmos, Crowea, Forget-Me-Not, Elm, Iris, Lemon, Madia, Nasturtium, Paw Paw, Peppermint, Rabbitbrush, Rosemary, Shasta Daisy, Sundew, White Chestnut

surrender

Almond, Angelica, Angel's Trumpet, Bleeding Heart, Bottlebrush, Cherry Plum, Chrysanthemum, Dandelion, Flannel Flower, Hibiscus, Lotus, Love-Lies-Bleeding, Mallow, Nectarine, Quaking Grass, Sagebrush, Sunflower, Tiger Lily, Walnut, Wedding Bush, Willow

transformation

Almond, Angel's Trumpet, Boab, Angelsword, Bottlebrush, Chrysanthemum, Cotton, Daffodil, Easter Lily, Forget-Me-Not, Glassy Hyacinth, Joshua Tree, Love-Lies-Bleeding, Red Grevillea, Sagebrush, Self-Heal, Sweet Chestnut, Tansy, Walnut

transition *(see also change)*

Angel's Trumpet, Boab, Bottlebrush, Cherry Plum, Chrysanthemum, Cotton, Daffodil, Forget-Me-Not, Joshua Tree, Mountain Forget-Me-Not, Impatiens, Nectarine, Paw Paw, Sagebrush, Thyme, Walnut, Wild Oat

true to Self

Almond, Angelsword, Blazing Star, Boab, Buttercup, Columbine, Forget-Me-not, Goldenrod, Joshua Tree, Lady's Slipper, Larch, Mountain Forget-Me-Not, Mountain Pennyroyal, Mountain Pride, Mullein, Pansy, Pear, Pomegranate, Red Grevillea, Red Penstemon, Redwood, Sagebrush, Self-Heal, Silver Princess, Squash, Sunflower, Tansy, Violet, Walnut, Waratah, Wild Oat

trust

Alpine Aster, Angelica, Aspen, Baby Blue Eyes, Californian Valerian, Cherry Plum, Chrysanthemum, Crowea, Flannel Flower, Forget-Me-Not, Garlic, Glassy Hyacinth, Gorse, Hibiscus, Nectarine, Purple Monkeyflower, Self-Heal, Sticky Monkeyflower, Sweet Chestnut, Waratah, Wedding Bush

wisdom

Angelsword, Boab, Bottlebrush, Californian Poppy, Cerato, Chestnut Bud, Chrysanthemum, Hibbertia, Hound's Tongue, Icelandic Poppy, Joshua Tree, Lotus, Opium Poppy, Pear, Red Lily, Sage, Saguaro, Sagebrush, Shasta Daisy, Silver Princess, Star Tulip, Thyme, Walnut, Wild Oat

Bibliography

Alaskan Essences, *Healing Essences from the Heart of Nature* (alaskanessences.com), 2013.

Allardice, E, Bone, K., Hutchison, F., *Magic and Medicine of Plants*. Sydney: Reader's Digest Australia, 1994.

Bach, Dr E. *Collected Writings of Edward Bach*. Bach Educational Programme, 1987.

Bailey, Alice A., *Esoteric Healing (Vol.IV of A Treatise on the Seven Rays)*. London: Lucis Press, 1984.

Bailey, Alice A., *Glamour: A World Problem*. London: Lucis Press, 1984.

Barnard, J. and M. *The Healing Herbs of Edward Bach: An Illustrated Guide to the Flower Remedies*. Britain: Bach Educational Programme, 1988.

Barnard, J. *Bach Flower Remedies – The Essence Within*. California: Winter Press, 2010.

Blavatsky, H. P. *The Secret Doctrine: The Synthesis of Science, Religion & Philosophy*. California: Theosophical University Press, 1888.

Cram, J. R., (2001b) 'Flower Essence Therapy in the Treatment of Major Depression: Preliminary Findings'. *International Journal of Healing and Caring*.https://ijhc. org/2001/09/02/flower-essence-therapy-in-the-treatment-of-major-depression-preliminary-findings/

Culpeper, N. *Culpeper's Complete Herbal*. Omega Books, 1985.

Cunningham, D., Ramer, A. *The Spiritual Dimensions of Healing Addictions*. San Rafael: Cassandra Press, 1988.

Cunningham, D., Ramer, A. *Further Dimensions of Healing Addictions*. San Rafael: Cassandra Press, 1988.

Jacka, J. *Meditation: The Most Natural Therapy*. Melbourne: Lothian Books, 1995.

Kaminski, P., Katz, R. (Eds.). *Flower Essence Repertory – A comprehensive guide to North American and English flower essences for emotional and spiritual well-being.* Nevada City: The Flower Essence Society, 1994.

MacCulloch, D. *Thomas Cranmer: A life.* New Haven: Yale University Press, 1996.

McIntyre, A. *The Complete Floral Healer.* Sydney: Hodder Headline, 1996.

Moore, M. *Medicinal Plants of the Desert and Canyon West.* Santa Fe: Museum of New Mexico Press, 1990.

Souto, R. *Baby Blue Eyes: Healing the Father Archetype in the Soul.* Nevada City: The Flower Essence Society, 2009 https://www.flowersociety.org/baby_blue_eyes.htm

Steiner, R. *Agriculture Course: The Birth of the Biodynamic Method.* London: Rudolf Steiner Press, 2004.

Weeks, N. *The Medical Discoveries of Edward Bach, Physician.* Essex, England: C. W. Daniel Co, 1969.

Weeks, N., Butlen, V. *The Bach Flower Remedies, Illustrations and Preparations.* Essex, England: C. W. Daniel Co, 1973.

Wilber, K. *No Boundary – Eastern and Western approaches to personal growth.* Boston: Shambhala, 2001.

Wells, M. *The Bach Flowers Today.* Melbourne: Wells Naturopathic Centre, 1993.

Wells, M. *Twelve Dynamic Elements of Good Health – The Tissue Salts.* Melbourne: Wells Naturopathic Centre, 1995.

White, I. *Australian Bush Flower Healing.* Sydney: Bantam, 1999.

White Eagle. *Spiritual Unfoldment 2 – The Ministry of Angels and the Invisible World of Nature.* London: White Eagle Publishing Trust, 1998.

For further information on private consultations, books, courses (including by correspondence), seminars, workshops:

Mark Wells
PO Box 79
Kew East, 3102
Melbourne, Australia
Telephone 0409 985 970
hsphealth.com.au

Alaskan Flower Essences
Orders: 800-545-9309 (U.S. & Canada)
Customer Service: 406-642-3670
Fax: 406-642-3672
Alaskan Flower Essence Project
PO Box 1369
Homer, AK 99603
alaskanessences.com

Alaskan FE Australia Distributor:
"Rainbows and Bridges"
PO Box 123, Mansfield
Victoria 3724
(03) 5779 1778
wwwizardry.com.au/
rainbowsandbridges/

Bach Flowers
Australian Distributor:
Martin and Pleasance
7 Rocklea Drive, Port Melbourne
VIC 3207
(03) 9427 7422
martinandpleasance.com

Australian Bush Flower Essences
45 Booralie Road
Terrey Hills NSW 2084
Australia

Telephone: 61 2 9450 1388
Fax: 61 2 9450 2866
ausflowers.com.au

Flower Essence Services (FES)
P.O. Box 1769
Nevada City, CA 95959
(800) 548-0075
Fax (530) 265-6467
fesflowers.com

Australian Distributor (FES):
Oborne Health Supplies
5-9 Cleeland Road
Oakleigh South
VIC 3167
1300 887 188
oborne.com.au

Images and illustrations recognition and copyright conditions

Black and White images and illustrations throughout book

Borage *Borago officinalis* B/W image (page 12) provided by Flower Essence Society (FES) under copyright.

Mistletoe *Viscum album* sketch (page 15) by Louise Minahan.

Pomegranate *Punica granatum* sketch (page 16) by Louise Minahan.

Horsetail *Equisetum arvense* sketch (page 16) by Louise Minahan.

Bleeding Heart *Dicentra formosa* sketch (page 19) by Louise Minahan.

Aloe Vera sketch *Aloe vera* sketch (page 20) by Louise Minahan.

Star Thistle *Centaurea solstitialis* sketch (page 20) by Louise Minahan.

Violet *Viola odorata* sketch (page 21) by Louise Minahan.

Mariposa Lily *Calochortus leichtlinii* B/W image (page 22) provided by Flower Essence Society (FES) under copyright.

Chamomile *Matricaria recutita* sketch (page 22) by Louise Minahan.

Flannel Flower *Actinotus helianthi* B/W image (page 183) provided by Australian Bush Flower Essences under copyright.

Indian Pink *Silene californica* B/W image (page 218) provided by Flower Essence Society (FES) under copyright.

Madia *Madia elegans* B/W image (page 235) provided by Flower Essence Society (FES) under copyright.

Manzanita *Arctostaphylus viscida* B/W image (page 239) thank you Terry McFall.

Mariposa Lily *Calochortus leichtlinii* B/W image (page 241) provided by Flower Essence Society (FES) under copyright.

Shasta Daisy *Chrysanthemum maximum* B/W image (page 312) provided by Flower Essence Society (FES) under copyright.

Silver Princess *Eucalyptus caesia* B/W image (page 318) provided by Australian Bush Flower Essences under copyright.

Waratah *Telopea speciosissima* B/W image (page 357) provided by Australian Bush Flower Essences under copyright.

Yarrow *Achillea millefolium* B/W image (page 373) provided by Flower Essence Society (FES) under copyright.

Notes:

Notes:

Index/Glossary

Acupuncture Meridians, 33. Ethereal energy channels that carry and distribute life-force energy (chi) throughout the physical body.

Agrimony, 78

Alaskan Flower Essences, 71

Almond, 80

Aloe Vera, 83

Alpine Aster, 378

Alpine Lily, 379

Angelica, 85

Angel's Trumpet, 87

Angelsword, 89

Anima - In psychoanalyst Carl Jung's terms, the feminine side of a man or 'the woman in a man.'

Animus - Psychoanalyst Carl Jung described the Animus as the masculine side of a woman or 'the man in a woman.'

Apricot, 91

Archetype - An original and inherited mental aspect present in the unconscious, and so intrinsic in Nature. It is often reflected to us in the inner quality, form, dynamic and function of a plant.

Arnica, 93

Aspen, 95

Aura, 30. The energy that surrounds and interpenetrates the physical body, which is invisible to most people. It exists around all life forms, and is an amalgam of all the subtle bodies of each being.

Australian Bush Flower Essences, 72

Baby Blue Eyes, 97

Bach, Dr Edward, 1

Bach Flower Essences, 72

Basil, 100

Chakra, 38. An energy centre in our subtle anatomy. Humans have seven chakras, each one relating to particular elements, properties, hormones, emotions and spiritual states. The chakras both push out and pull in energy to the body.

Chi, 30. The ancient Chinese term for the subtle, life force energy in Nature. Chi circulates within the human being through the acupuncture meridians.

Clairaudience - A faculty of hearing in other dimensions beyond the usual sensory limits. (From the French, meaning 'clear hearing.')

Clairvoyance - A faculty of seeing subtle energy levels beyond the usual sensory range. (From the French, meaning 'clear seeing.')

Creative Visualisation - A meditative process in which we visualise within the mind images that are of benefit to us.

Gestalt Therapy - Based on the psychological theory that we are continually seeking to become 'whole' or form 'gestalts' at all levels of our experience. Gestalt therapists guide us to our fullest awareness of the present so that we can focus on how we construct our lives rather than why.

Hibiscus, 204

Higher self - The level at which our higher principles and experiences exist. It is the wise, all-knowing aspect of ourselves that accommodates the pure intentions of our soul.

Holistic (Vitalistic not Mechanistic), 30. A synergistic approach that integrates all human aspects – physical, mental, emotional and spiritual – in health and illness.

Holly, 206

Homeopathy, 31. A therapy that utilises minute doses of natural substances to treat people. It is based on the principle of 'like cures like' (law of similar) that informs the prescription of homoeopathic medicine for patients whose symptoms match the medicine's known symptoms.

Honeysuckle, 208

Hops, 388

Hornbeam, 210

Hound's Tongue, 212

Hyssop, 389

Icelandic Poppy, 389

Impatiens, 213

Indian Paintbrush, 215

Indian Pink, 217

Iris, 219

Jacaranda, 389

Jasmine, 390

Joshua Tree, 390

Jung, Dr Carl - A medical psychoanalyst who initially trained under Dr Sigmund Freud. Jungian psychology developed from his works and teachings in psychotherapy. There are many practising Jungian therapist in the world today.

Kangaroo Paw, 221

Karma - 'As ye sow, so shall ye reap' in Christian belief – or in contemporary terms, 'cause and effect.' It allows the soul to experience the full range of perspectives on life and continually provides opportunities for personal growth.

Lady's Mantle, 391

Lady's Slipper, 391

Larch, 223

Larkspur, 225

Lavender, 227

Lavender Yarrow, 391

Left-brain faculties - The faculties and senses governed by the left brain hemisphere. These faculties include the analytical, logical and linear modes of thought, or quantitative ways of perceiving.

Lemon, 229

Lilac, 392

Lotus, 231

Love-Lies-Bleeding, 392

Macrocarpa, 233

Madia, 235

Mallow, 237

Manzanita, 239

Mariposa Lily, 241

Meditation - A process or practice whereby deep mental relaxation and personal or transcendental insights can be achieved. Various mental techniques may be used to facilitate this process, such as mantra repetition, creative visualisation and progressive affirmations.

Mental Body, 37. The mental body houses our fundamental beliefs about ourselves – our concept of Self. The state of the mental body reflects the quality of our thought patterns and characteristic attitudes or personal mindset.

Milkweed, 393

Mimulus, 243

Mindfulness – 'Paying attention on purpose, in the moment, without judgment.' It is about being awake, aware and grounded in the present without dwelling on our worries and concerns.

Monkshood, 393

Potentisation, 31. This is the term used to describe the method for making homeopathic medicines. The original natural substance is diluted in water and/or alcohol base and then vigorously shaken manually or by machine. Repeated dilutions are made, each dilution undergoing the same process. The higher the dilution, the more potentised the remedy.

Psychoneuroimmunology - A medical term for a developing discipline that studies the mind-body interaction and its influence on the immune system and physical health.

Reincarnation - A philosophy (and belief in some religions) that the soul has multiple lives, through multiple incarnations on the physical plane. The soul continually evolves through experiencing different lives.

Relaxation techniques (*see* Bioenergetics, Meditation, Mindfulness) - Mental or physical processes or practices that allow the mind and body to reach deeper states of relaxation.

Right-brain faculties - The faculties and senses governed by the right brain hemisphere. These faculties include intuitive, artistic, symbolic, and lateral or non-linear thought – referred to as qualitative ways of perceiving.

Shadow - Dr Carl Jung's concept of the Shadow is made up of our ingrained habits, instinctive, automatic and compulsive drives, and the results of early childhood conditioning. The rapprochement with these shadow sides through conscious confrontation and acceptance can lead to possible transformation. Flower essences can act as catalysts here.

Spirit Guides - Sometimes referred to as our 'guardian angels'; individual or collective souls existing in other dimensions who assist us on the earthly plane. Our subtle nature is receptive to their assistance and guidance.

Subconscious - The part of our personality that dwells just below the surface of waking consciousness and controls automatic human functions. It subliminally records and absorbs through the senses all information from our environment. It develops and constructs an internal picture of how we really perceive ourselves in this world.

Subtle Body (*see* Aura), 31. A general term for the subtle energy bodies existing in and around the physical body at a higher vibrational frequency or octave than the physical realm.

Subtle Dimensions, 31

Subtle energy, 31. Energy that exists at a higher vibrational frequency and beyond the physical realm, so it cannot be seen.

Synchronicity, 23. Dr Carl Jung discussed parallel phenomena that are not related in a causal way. Spontaneous coincidences that defy statistical probability – where something other than chance is operating, highly abstract and not readily predictable.

Traditional Chinese Medicine (TCM), 31. A form of medicine and philosophy of healing with a tradition of use that goes back thousands of years. The concepts of chi, yin and yang and acupuncture meridians are integral parts of TCM philosophy and approach to life and health.

Vibrational energies, 28. The subtle energies in varying frequencies and amplitudes. Quantum physics has used this term when studying the energetic characteristics of matter at a subatomic level.

Vibrational medicine, 28. Any medicine or healing that is subtle in nature and can influence directly the subtle energies of a human being. It aims to treat the whole person – mind, body and spirit – by conveying measured amounts of frequency-specific energy to the human multidimensional system.

Wellbeing (Wellness) - A subjective quality that relates to how a person feels within. Our state of wellbeing is a consequence of our health, happiness and vitality.

Yin and yang - These terms represent complementary opposites (there is an element of the opposite in each) that are neither forces nor material entities, but philosophical concepts used to explain the continuous process of natural change. It is a system of thought within TCM in which all things are seen as part of an integrated whole and everything is relative. Yin and yang exist in everything in nature. For instance, moon (yin)/sun (yang), night/day, cold/hot, feminine/masculine, and so on.

www.ingramcontent.com/pod-product-compliance
Lightning Source LLC
Chambersburg PA
CBHW072040020426
42334CB00017B/1344